Clinical Biochemistry
Lecture Notes

Clinical Biochemistry
Lecture Notes

Peter Rae
BA, PhD, MBChB, FRCPE, FRCPath
Consultant Clinical Biochemist
Royal Infirmary of Edinburgh
Honorary Senior Lecturer in Clinical Biochemistry
University of Edinburgh

Mike Crane
BSc, PhD, MSc, FRCPath
Consultant Clinical Biochemist
Royal Hospital for Sick Children & Royal Infirmary of Edinburgh
Honorary Lecturer in Clinical Biochemistry
University of Edinburgh

Rebecca Pattenden
BSc, MSc, FRCPath
Consultant Clinical Biochemist
Western General Hospital, Edinburgh

Tenth Edition

WILEY Blackwell

This edition first published 2018 © 2018 by John Wiley & Sons Ltd

Edition History
John Wiley & Sons Ltd (9e, 2013)

Registered Office(s)
John Wiley & Sons, Inc., 111 River Street, Hoboken, NJ 07030, USA
John Wiley & Sons Ltd, The Atrium, Southern Gate, Chichester, West Sussex, PO19 8SQ, UK

Editorial Office
9600 Garsington Road, Oxford, OX4 2DQ, UK

For details of our global editorial offices, customer services, and more information about Wiley products visit us at www.wiley.com.

Wiley also publishes its books in a variety of electronic formats and by print-on-demand. Some content that appears in standard print versions of this book may not be available in other formats.

Library of Congress Cataloging-in-Publication Data

Names: Rae, Peter, 1953– author. | Crane, Mike, 1979– author. |
    Pattenden, Rebecca, 1974– author.
Title: Lecture notes. Clinical biochemistry/Peter Rae, Mike Crane, Rebecca Pattenden.
Other titles: Clinical biochemistry
Description: Tenth edition. | Hoboken, NJ : Wiley, 2018. | Preceded by Lecture notes.
    Clinical biochemistry. 9th ed./Geoffrey Beckett ... [et al.]. 2013. |
    Includes bibliographical references and index.
Identifiers: LCCN 2017013974 (print) | LCCN 2017014660 (ebook) | ISBN 9781119248699 (pdf) |
    ISBN 9781119248637 (epub) | ISBN 9781119248682
Subjects: | MESH: Biochemical Phenomena | Clinical Laboratory Techniques |
    Clinical Chemistry Tests | Pathology, Clinical–methods
Classification: LCC RB40 (ebook) | LCC RB40 (print) | NLM QU 34 | DDC 616.07/56–dc23
LC record available at https://lccn.loc.gov/2017013974

Cover design by Wiley
Cover image: © Miguel Malo/gettyimages

Set in 8.5/11pt Utopia by SPi Global, Pondicherry, India

10   9   8   7   6   5   4   3   2   1

Contents

Preface, vi

List of abbreviations, vii

About the companion website, x

1 Requesting and interpreting tests, 1
2 Disturbances of water, sodium and potassium balance, 12
3 Acid–base balance and oxygen transport, 30
4 Renal disease, 43
5 Disorders of calcium, phosphate and magnesium metabolism, 60
6 Diabetes mellitus and hypoglycaemia, 77
7 Disorders of the hypothalamus and pituitary, 91
8 Abnormalities of thyroid function, 105
9 Disorders of the adrenal cortex and medulla, 121
10 Investigation of gonadal function infertility, menstrual irregularities and hirsutism, 139
11 Pregnancy and antenatal screening, 158
12 Cardiovascular disorders, 167
13 Liver disease, 183
14 Gastrointestinal tract disease, 198
15 Nutrition, 208
16 Inflammation, immunity and paraproteinaemia, 224
17 Malignancy and tumour markers, 234
18 Disorders of iron and porphyrin metabolism, 241
19 Uric acid, gout and purine metabolism, 252
20 Central nervous system and cerebrospinal fluid, 259
21 Therapeutic drug monitoring and chemical toxicology, 263
22 Clinical biochemistry in paediatrics and the elderly, 276

Index, 295

Preface

This is the tenth edition of the book originally written by Professor Gordon Whitby, Dr Alistair Smith and Professor Iain Percy-Robb in 1975. It remains an Edinburgh-based book, but both the content and the authorship continue to evolve.

Ever since the first edition this book has been primarily aimed at medical students and junior doctors, but we also believe that it will be of value to specialist registrars, clinical scientists and biomedical scientists pursuing a career in clinical biochemistry and metabolic medicine, and studying for higher qualifications. It has continued to develop in line with changes that have both reshaped the undergraduate curriculum and taken place in medical practice.

Over the course of the book's existence changes in medical education have tended to reduce or abolish courses exclusively covering laboratory medicine disciplines, with their content being integrated into the relevant parts of a systems-based curriculum. This clearly places the laboratory disciplines at the heart of medical teaching in the diagnosis and management of patients, but risks losing the opportunity to take a closer view of the principles behind the use of diagnostic investigations. This book aims to focus on the choice and interpretation of investigations in the diagnosis and management of conditions where biochemical testing plays a key role, with a view to understanding not only their uses but also developing an appreciation of their limitations. This is underpinned by brief summaries of the relevant pathophysiology. There is an emphasis on commonly requested tests and commonly occurring pathology, but less common tests and disorders are also described.

We have reviewed and updated all chapters to ensure that they reflect current clinical practice, the availability of new tests, and where relevant the latest versions of national guidelines, with an emphasis on those published in the UK. Planning this new edition benefited from helpful feedback from a number of sources, including groups of both students and their teachers, commissioned by Wiley, and in response to this we have among other changes increased the numbers of diagrams and tables where these help to summarise useful information. We have also increased the numbers of clinical cases, as these remain a popular feature. Multiple choice questions with an explanation of the answers, and key learning points for each chapter are available as an on-line resource for revision.

Since the last edition, Geoff Beckett, Simon Walker and Peter Ashby have all retired. They were authors since the fourth, fifth and seventh editions, respectively, and have had an enormous effect on the development and success of this book. Their places have been ably taken by Mike Crane and Rebecca Pattenden, who have brought a fresh perspective to many of the topics covered. As ever, we are also indebted to a number of colleagues who read various chapters and provided valuable comment and advice, in particular Catriona Clarke and Jonathan Malo. We remain grateful for the continued interest and support provided by the staff at Wiley towards this title since its first appearance over forty years ago.

Peter Rae
Mike Crane
Rebecca Pattenden

List of abbreviations

α-MSH	α-melanocyte stimulating hormone	CKD	chronic kidney disease
AAT	α₁-antitrypsin	CNS	central nervous system
ABP	androgen-binding protein	CoA	coenzyme A
A&E	accident and emergency	COC	combined oral contraceptive
ACE	angiotensin-converting enzyme	COHb	carboxyhaemoglobin
ACTH	adrenocorticotrophic hormone	CRH	corticotrophin-releasing hormone
ADH	antidiuretic hormone	CRP	C-reactive protein
AFP	α-foetoprotein	CSF	cerebrospinal fl uid
AI	angiotensin I	CT	computed tomography
AII	angiotensin II	CV	coefficient of variation
AIII	angiotensin III	DDAVP	1-deamino,8-D-arginine vasopressin
AIP	acute intermittent porphyria		
AIS	androgen insensitivity syndrome	DHEA	dehydroepiandrosterone
ALA	aminolaevulinic acid	DHEAS	dehydroepiandrosterone sulphate
ALP	alkaline phosphatase	DHCC	dihydrocholecalciferol
ALT	alanine aminotransferase	DHT	dihydrotestosterone
AMA	anti-mitochondrial antibodies	DIT	di-iodotyrosine
AMH	anti-Mullerian hormone	DKA	diabetic ketoacidosis
AMP	adenosine 5-monophosphate	DPP	4 dipeptidyl peptidase-4
ANP	atrial natriuretic peptide	DSD	disorder of sexual differentiation
AST	aspartate aminotransferase	DVT	deep venous thrombosis
ATP	adenosine triphosphate	ECF	extracellular fluid
AT	Pase adenosine triphosphatase	ECG	electrocardiogram/electrocardiography
β-LPH	β-lipotrophin	ED	erectile dysfunction
BChE	butylcholinesterase	EDTA	ethylenediamine tetraacetic acid
BMI	body mass index	eGFR	estimated glomerular filtration rate
BMR	basal metabolic rate	EPH	electrophoresis
BNP	B-type natriuretic peptide	EPP	erythropoietic protoporphyria
CABG	coronary artery bypass grafting	ERCP	endoscopic retrograde cholangiopancreatography
CAH	congenital adrenal hyperplasia	ESR	erythrocyte sedimentation rate
cAMP	cyclic adenosine monophosphate	FAD	flavin adenine dinucleotide
CBG	cortisol-binding globulin	FAI	free androgen index
CCK	cholecystokinin	FBHH	familial benign hypocalciuric hypercalcaemia
CCK-PZ	cholecystokinin-pancreozymin		
CDT	carbohydrate-deficient transferrin	FIT	faecal immunochemical test
CEA	carcinoembryonic antigen	FMN	flavin mononucleotide
CFT	calculated free testosterone	FOB	faecal occult blood
ChE	cholinesterase	FPP	free protoporphyrin
CK	creatine kinase	FSH	follicle-stimulating hormone

FT3	free tri-iodothyronine		IFG	impaired fasting glucose
FT4	free thyroxine		Ig	immunoglobulin
GAD	glutamic acid decarboxylase		IGF	insulin-like growth factor
Gal-1-PUT	galactose-1-phosphate uridylyl-transferase		IGFBP	insulin-like growth factor-binding protein
GDM	gestational diabetes mellitus		IGT	impaired glucose tolerance
GFR	glomerular filtration rate		IM	intramuscular
GGT	γ-glutamyltransferase		INR	international normalised ratio
GH	growth hormone		IV	intravenous
GHD	growth hormone deficiency		LCAT	lecithin cholesterol acyltransferase
GHRH	growth hormone-releasing hormone		LDH	lactate dehydrogenase
GI	gastrointestinal		LDL	low-density lipoprotein
GIP	glucose-dependent insulinotrophic peptide/ gastric inhibitory polypeptide		LH	luteinising hormone
			Lp(a)	lipoprotein (a)
GLP-1	glucagon-like polypeptide-1		LSD	lysergic acid diethylamide
GnRH	gonadotrophin-releasing hormone		MCAD	medium chain acyl-CoA dehydrogenase
GP	general practitioner			
GSH	glucocorticoid-suppressible hyperaldosteronism		MCV	mean cell volume
			MDRD	Modification of Diet in Renal Disease
GTT	glucose tolerance test		MEGX	monoethylglycinexylidide
Hb	haemoglobin		MEN	multiple endocrine neoplasia
HC	hereditary coproporphyria		MGUS	monoclonal gammopathy of unknown significance
HCC	hydroxycholecalciferol			
hCG	human chorionic gonadotrophin		MI	myocardial infarction
HDL	high-density lipoprotein		MIT	mono-iodotyrosine
HGPRT	hypoxanthine-guanine phosphoribosyltransferase		MODY	maturity onset diabetes of the young
			MOM	multiples of the median
HHS	hyperosmolar hyperglycaemic state		MRCP	magnetic resonance cholangiopancreatography
5-HIAA	5-hydroxyindoleacetic acid			
HIV	human immunodeficiency virus		MRI	magnetic resonance imaging
HLA	human leucocyte antigen		MTC	medullary thyroid cancer
HMG-CoA	β-hydroxy-β-methylglutaryl-coenzyme A		MUST	Malnutrition Universal Screening Tool
HMMA	4-hydroxy-3-methoxymandelic acid		NABQI	N-acetyl-p-benzoquinoneimine
HNF	hepatic nuclear factor		NAC	N-acetylcysteine
HPA	hypothalamic–pituitary–adrenal		NAD	nicotinamide–adenine dinucleotide
HPLC	high-performance liquid chromatography		NADP	NAD phosphate
HRT	hormone replacement therapy		NAFLD	nonalcoholic fatty liver disase
hsCRP	highly sensitive C-reactive protein		NASH	nonalcoholic steatohepatitis
5-HT	5-hydroxytryptamine		NICE	National Institute for Health and Clinical Excellence
5-HTP	5-hydroxytryptophan			
IBS	irritable bowel syndrome		NIPT	noninvasive prenatal testing
ICF	intracellular fluid		NSAID	nonsteroidal anti-inflammatory agent
ICU	intensive care unit		NTD	neural tube defect
IDL	intermediate-density lipoprotein		NTI	nonthyroidal illness
IFCC	International Federation for Clinical Chemistry		OCP	oral contraceptive pill
			OGTT	oral glucose tolerance test

PAPP-A	pregnancy-associated plasma protein A	SGLT	sodium-glucose cotransporter
PBG	porphobilinogen	SUR	sulphonylurea receptor
PCI	percutaneous coronary intervention	T3	tri-iodothyronine
PCOS	polycystic ovarian syndrome	T4	thyroxine
PCSK9	proprotein convertase subtilisin/kexin type 9	TBG	thyroxine-binding globulin
		TDM	therapeutic drug monitoring
PCT	porphyria cutanea tarda	TDP	thiamin diphosphate
PE	pulmonary embolism	TGN	6-thioguanine nucleotide
PEG	percutaneous endoscopic gastrostomy	THR	thyroid hormone resistance
PEM	protein-energy malnutrition	TIBC	total iron-binding capacity
PIIINP	pro-collagen type III	TNF	tumour necrosis factor
PKU	phenylketonuria	TPMT	thiopurine S-methyltransferase
PLP	pyridoxal 5′-phosphate	TPN	total parenteral nutrition
POCT	point of care testing	TPOAb	thyroid peroxidase antibody
POP	progestogen-only pill	TPP	thiamin pyrophosphate
PRPP	5-phosphoribosyl-1-pyrophosphate	TRAb	thyrotrophin receptor antibody
PSA	prostate-specific antigen	TRH	thyrotrophin-releasing hormone
PT	prothrombin time	TSH	thyroid-stimulating hormone
PTH	parathyroid hormone	TSI	thyroid-stimulating immunoglobulin
PTHrP	PTH-related protein	tTG	tissue transglutaminase
RBP	retinol-binding protein	U&Es	urea and electrolytes
RDA	recommended dietary allowance	UFC	urinary free cortisol
RF	rheumatoid factor	UV	ultraviolet
RMI	risk of malignancy index	VIP	vasoactive intestinal peptide
ROC	receiver operating characteristic	VLDL	very low density lipoprotein
SAAG	serum-ascites albumin gradient	VMA	vanillylmandelic acid
SAH	subarachnoid haemorrhage	VP	variegate porphyria
SD	standard deviation	WHO	World Health Organization
SHBG	sex hormone-binding globulin	XO	xanthine oxidase
SIADH	inappropriate secretion of ADH	ZPP	zinc protoporphyrin

About the companion website

This book is accompanied by a companion website:

 www.lecturenoteseries.com/clinicalbiochemistry

The website includes:
- Interactive multiple-choice questions
- Key revision points for each chapter

Requesting and interpreting tests

Learning objectives

To understand:

✔ how sample handling, analytical and biological factors can affect test results in health and disease and how these relate to the concept of a test reference range;

✔ the concepts of accuracy, precision, test sensitivity, test specificity in the quantitative assessment of test performance.

Introduction

Biochemical tests are crucial to modern medicine. Most biochemical tests are carried out on blood using plasma or serum, but urine, cerebrospinal fluid (CSF), faeces, kidney stones, pleural fluid, etc. are sometimes required. Plasma is obtained by collecting blood into an anticoagulant and separating the fluid, plasma phase from the blood cells by centrifugation. Serum is the corresponding fluid phase when blood is allowed to clot. For many (but not all) biochemical tests on blood, it makes little difference whether plasma or serum is used.

There are many hundreds of tests available in clinical biochemistry but a core of common tests makes up the majority of tests requested. These core tests are typically available from most clinical laboratories throughout the 24-h period. Tests are sometimes brought together in profiles, especially when a group of tests provides better understanding of a problem than a single test (e.g. the liver function test profile). More specialist tests may be restricted to larger laboratories or specialist centres offering a national or regional service.

In dealing with the large number of routine test requests, the modern clinical biochemistry laboratory depends heavily on automated instrumentation linked to a laboratory computing system. Test results are assigned to electronic patient files that allow maintenance of a cumulative patient record. Increasingly, test requests can be electronically booked at the ward, clinic or in General Practice via a terminal linked to the main laboratory computer. Equally, the test results can be displayed on computer screens at distant locations, removing the need to issue printed reports.

In this first chapter, we set out some of the principles of requesting tests and of the interpretation of results. The effects of analytical errors and of physiological factors, as well as of disease, on test results are stressed. Biochemical testing in differential diagnosis and in screening is discussed.

Collection of specimens

Test requests require unambiguous identification of the patient (patient's name, sex, date of birth and, increasingly, a unique patient identification number), together with the location, the name of the

---

Clinical Biochemistry Lecture Notes, Tenth Edition. Peter Rae, Mike Crane and Rebecca Pattenden.
© 2018 John Wiley & Sons Ltd. Published 2018 by John Wiley & Sons Ltd.
Companion website: www.lecturenoteseries.com/clinicalbiochemistry

requesting doctor and the date and time of sampling. Each test request must specify the analyses requested and provide details of the nature of the specimen itself and relevant clinical diagnostic information. This may be through a traditional request form and labelled specimen or be provided electronically in which case only the sample itself need be sent to the laboratory with its own unique identifier (typically a bar code which links it to the electronic request).

Clinical laboratories have multiple procedures at every step of sample processing to avoid errors. Regrettably, errors do occur and these arise at different stages between the sample being taken and the result being received:

- Pre-analytical. These arise prior to the actual test measurement and can happen at the clinical or laboratory end. Most errors fall into this category (see Table 1.1).
- Analytical. Laboratory based analytical errors are rare but may occur, e.g. reagent contamination, pipetting errors related to small sample volumes, computing errors.
- Post-analytical. These are increasingly rare because of electronic download of results from the analyser but include, for example, transcription errors when entering results from another laboratory into the computer manually; results misheard when these are telephoned to the clinician.

Despite the scale of requesting of biochemical tests, errors are fortunately very rare. However, occasional blunders do arise and, if very unexpected results are obtained, it is important that the requesting doctor contacts the laboratory immediately to check whether the results are indeed correct or whether some problem may have arisen. Occasionally this reveals that more than one problem has occurred, for example two samples were labelled with each other's details on the ward, so querying the results can have wider benefits.

The use of clinical biochemistry tests

Biochemical tests are most often *discretionary*, meaning that the test is requested for defined diagnostic purposes. The justification for discretionary testing is well summarised by Asher (1954):

1. Why do I request this test?
2. What will I look for in the result?
3. If I find what I am looking for, will it affect my diagnosis?

Table 1.1 **Some more common causes of pre-analytical errors arising from use of the laboratory.**

Error	Consequence
Crossover of addressograph labels between patients	This can lead to two patients each with the other's set of results. Where the patient is assigned a completely wrong set of results, it is important to investigate the problem in case there is a second patient with a corresponding wrong set of results.
Timing error	There are many examples where timing is important but not considered. Sending in a blood sample too early after the administration of a drug can lead to misleadingly high values in therapeutic monitoring. Interpretation of some tests (e.g. cortisol) is critically dependent on the time of day when the blood was sampled.
Sample collection tube error	For some tests the nature of the collection tube is critical, which is why the Biochemistry Laboratory specifies this detail. For example, using a plasma tube with lithium–heparin as the anti-coagulant is not appropriate for measurement of a therapeutic lithium level. Electrophoresis requires a serum sample rather than plasma so that fibrinogen does not interfere with the detection of any monoclonal bands. Topping up a biochemistry tube with a haematology (potassium ethylenediamine tetraacetic acid [EDTA]) sample will lead to high potassium and low calcium values in the biochemistry sample.
Sample taken from close to the site of an intravenous (IV) infusion	The blood sample will be diluted so that all the tests will be correspondingly low with the exception of those tests that might reflect the composition of the infusion fluid itself. For example, using normal saline as the infusing fluid would lead to a lowering of all test results, but with sodium and chloride results that are likely to be raised.

4 How will this investigation affect my management of the patient?

5 Will this investigation ultimately benefit the patient?

The main reasons for this type of testing are summarised in Table 1.2. Tests may also be used to help evaluate the future risk of disease (e.g. total cholesterol and HDL-cholesterol levels contribute to assessment of an individual's risk of cardiovascular disease), or in disease prognosis (e.g. biochemical tests to assess prognosis in acute pancreatitis or liver failure), or to screen for a disease, without there being any specific indication of its presence in the individual (e.g. maternal screening for foetal neural tube defects).

Screening may take several forms:

• In well-population screening a spectrum of tests is carried out on individuals from an apparently healthy population in an attempt to detect pre-symptomatic or early disease. It is easy to miss significant abnormalities in the large amount of data provided by the laboratory, even when the abnormalities are highlighted in some way. For these and other reasons, the value of well-population screening has been called into question and certainly should only be initiated under certain specific circumstances (Table 1.3).

Table 1.3 **Requirements for well-population screening.**

• The disease is common or life-threatening
• The tests are sensitive and specific
• The tests are readily applied and acceptable to the population to be screened
• Clinical, laboratory and other facilities are available for follow-up
• Economics of screening have been clarified and the implications accepted

Table 1.4 **Examples of tests used in case-finding programmes.**

Programmes to detect diseases in	Chemical investigations
Neonates	
Phenylketonuria (PKU)	Serum phenylalanine
Hypothyroidism	Serum TSH
Adolescents and young adults	
Substance abuse	Drug screen
Pregnancy	
Diabetes mellitus in the mother	Plasma glucose
Open neural tube defect (NTD) in the foetus	Maternal serum α-foetoprotein
Industry	
Industrial exposure to lead	Blood lead
Industrial exposure to pesticides	Serum cholinesterase activity
Elderly	
Malnutrition	Serum vitamin D levels
Thyroid dysfunction	Serum TSH and thyroxine

Table 1.2 **Test selection for the purposes of discretionary testing.**

Category	Example
To confirm a diagnosis	Serum free T4 and thyroid-stimulating hormone (TSH) in suspected hyperthyroidism
To aid differential diagnosis	To distinguish between different forms of jaundice
To refine a diagnosis	Use of adrenocorticotrophic hormone (ACTH) to localise Cushing's syndrome
To assess the severity of disease	Serum creatinine or urea in renal disease
To monitor progress	Plasma glucose and serum K^+ to follow treatment of patients with diabetic ketoacidosis (DKA)
To detect complications or side effects	Alanine aminotransferase (ALT) measurements in patients treated with hepatotoxic drugs
To monitor therapy	Serum drug concentrations in patients treated with anti-epileptic drugs

• In case-finding screening programmes appropriate tests are carried out on a population sample known to be at high risk of a particular disease. These are inherently more selective and yield a higher proportion of useful results (Table 1.4).

Point of care testing (POCT)

These are tests conducted close to the patient, for example in the emergency department, an out-patient clinic, or a general practitioner's surgery.

Table 1.5 Examples of POCT that are in common use.

Common POCT in blood	Common POCT in urine
Blood gases	Glucose
Glucose	Ketones
Urea and creatinine	Red cells/haemoglobin
Na, K and Ca	Bilirubin
Bilirubin	Protein
Alcohol	hCG

Table 1.6 Advantages and disadvantages of point-of-care testing (POCT).

Advantages	Disadvantages
Rapid results on acutely ill patients	More expensive than centralised tests
Allows more frequent monitoring	Wide staff training may be needed
Immediate patient feedback	Nontrained users may have access, with potential for errors
Available 24 h if required	Calibration and quality control may be less robust
	Health and Safety may be less well monitored
	Results less often integrated into patient electronic record

The instrumentation used is typically small and fits on a desk or may even be handheld. This approach can be helpful where there is a need to obtain a result quickly (e.g. blood gas results in the emergency department in a breathless patient), or where a result can be used to make a real-time clinical management decision (e.g. whether to adjust someone's statin dose on the basis of a cholesterol result). A further attraction is the immediate feedback of clinical information to the patient. POCT can be used to monitor illness by the individual patient and help identify if a change in treatment is needed (e.g. blood glucose monitoring in a diabetic patient). There is also an increasing number of urine test sticks that are sold for home use (e.g. pregnancy and ovulation testing by measuring human chorionic gonadotrophin (hCG) and luteinising hormone (LH), respectively). Table 1.5 shows examples of POCT tests in common use.

The introduction of POCT methodology requires attention to cost, ease of use, staff training, quality, health and safety as well as need. The advantages and disadvantages of POCT are summarised in Table 1.6.

Interpretation of clinical biochemistry tests

Most reports issued by clinical biochemistry laboratories contain numerical measures of concentration or activity, expressed in the appropriate units. Typically, the result is interpreted in relation to a reference range (see Chapter 1: Reference ranges) for the analyte in question. Results within and outside the reference range may be subject to variation caused by a number of factors. These include analytical variation, normal biological variation, and the influence of pathological processes.

Sources of variation in test results

Analytical sources of variation

Analytical results are subject to error, no matter how good the laboratory and no matter how skilled the analyst. The words "accuracy" and "precision" have carefully defined meanings in this context.

An *accurate* method will, on average, yield results close to the true value of what is being measured. It has no systematic bias. Lack of accuracy means that results will always tend to be either high or low.

A *precise* method yields results that are close to one another (but not necessarily close to the true value) on repeated analysis. If multiple measurements are made on one specimen, the spread of results will be small for a precise method and large for an imprecise one. Lack of precision means that results may be scattered, and unpredictably high or low.

A 'dartboard' analogy is often used to illustrate the different meanings of the terms accuracy and precision, and this is illustrated in Figure 1.1.

The standard deviation (SD) is the usual measure of scatter around a mean value. If the spread of results is wide, the SD is large, whereas if the spread is narrow, the SD is small. For data that have a Gaussian distribution, as is nearly always the case for analytical errors, the shape of the curve (Figure 1.2) is completely defined by the mean and the SD, and these characteristics are such that:

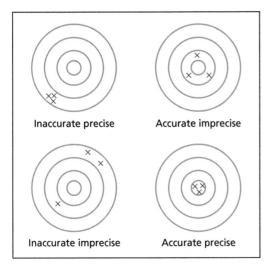

Figure 1.1 The 'dartboard' analogy can be used to illustrate accuracy and precision.

Inaccurate precise

Accurate imprecise

Inaccurate imprecise

Accurate precise

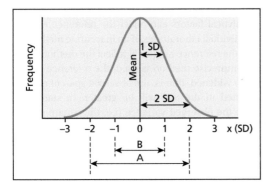

Figure 1.2 Diagram of a Gaussian (normal or symmetrical) distribution curve. The span (A) of the curve, the distance between the mean ± 2 SD, includes about 95% of the 'population'. The narrower span (B), the distance between the mean ± 1 SD, includes about 67% of the 'population'.

- About 67% of results lie in the range mean ± 1 SD.
- About 95% of results lie in the range mean ± 2 SD.
- Over 99% of results lie in the range mean ± 3 SD.

Blunders are grossly inaccurate results that bear no constant or predictable relationship to the true value. They arise, for instance, from mislabelling of specimens at the time of collection, or transcription errors when preparing or issuing reports (see Table 1.1).

If different results for the same test are obtained on two or more occasions on the same patient, then an important question that arises is whether that difference is due to analytical imprecision or to a true change in the patient's clinical condition. Statistically, if the results differ by more than 2.8 times the analytical SD then there is a chance of over 95% that a genuine change in concentration of the substance has occurred.

Biological causes of variation

Test results also show biological variation in both health and disease. The concentrations of all analytes in blood vary with time due to diverse physiological factors *within* the individual. There are also differences *between* individuals.

The following may be important causes of within-individual variation:

1 *Diet:* Variations in diet can affect the results of many tests, including serum triglyceride, the response to glucose tolerance tests and urinary calcium excretion.
2 *Time of day:* Several plasma constituents show diurnal variation (variation with the time of day), or a sleep/wake cycle. Examples include iron, adrenocorticotrophic hormone (ACTH) and cortisol concentrations.
3 *Posture:* Proteins and all protein-bound constituents of plasma show modest differences in concentration between blood collected from upright individuals and blood from recumbent individuals. Examples include serum calcium, cholesterol, cortisol and total thyroxine concentrations.
4 *Muscular exercise:* Recent exercise, especially if vigorous or unaccustomed, may increase serum creatine kinase (CK) activity and blood lactate, and lower blood pyruvate.
5 *Menstrual cycle:* Several substances show variation with the phase of the cycle. Examples include serum iron, and the serum concentrations of the pituitary gonadotrophins, ovarian steroids and their metabolites, as well as the amounts of these hormones and their metabolites excreted in the urine.
6 *Drugs:* These can have marked effects on chemical results. Attention should be drawn particularly to the many effects of oestrogen-containing oral contraceptives on serum constituents (Chapter 10: Steroid contraceptives).

Even after allowing for known physiological factors that may affect plasma constituents and for analytical imprecision, there is still considerable residual individual

CASE 1.1

A 52-year-old man taking a statin drug to reduce his cholesterol level attended for a routine follow-up appointment. He was well, and had recently started training for a half-marathon as part of his determination to get fitter and reduce his risk of future cardiovascular problems. Statins sometimes cause muscle side effects, so among his other blood tests a creatine kinase (CK) was checked and it was very high. Should his statin be stopped?

Comments: Muscular exertion, especially if unaccustomed or severe, can give rise to high CK results. He was asked to refrain from training for a few days, and on repeat a CK level was normal.

variation (Table 1.7). The magnitude of this variation depends on the analyte, but it may be large and must be taken into account when interpreting successive values from a patient.

Differences between individuals can affect the concentrations of analytes in the blood. The following are the main examples:

1 *Age:* Examples include serum phosphate and alkaline phosphatase (ALP) activity, and serum and urinary concentrations of the gonadotrophins and sex hormones.
2 *Sex:* Examples include serum creatinine, iron and urate concentrations, and serum and urinary concentrations of the sex hormones.
3 *Race:* Racial differences have been described for serum cholesterol and protein. It may be difficult to distinguish racial from environmental factors, such as diet.

Reference ranges

When looking at results, we need to compare each result with a set of results from a particular defined (or reference) population. This reference range is determined, in practice, by measuring a set of reference values from a sample of that population, usually of healthy individuals. The nature of the reference population should be given whenever reference ranges are quoted, although a healthy population is usually assumed. Even age-matched and sex-matched reference ranges are often difficult to obtain, since fairly large numbers of individuals are needed.

When results of analyses for a reference population are analysed, they are invariably found to cluster around a central value, with a distribution that may be symmetrical (often Gaussian, Figure 1.3a) or asymmetrical (often log-Gaussian, Figure 1.3b). However, reference ranges can be calculated from these data without making any assumptions about the distribution of the data, using nonparametric methods.

Because of geographical, racial and other biological sources of variation between individuals, as well as differences in analytical methods, each laboratory should ideally define and publish its own reference ranges. By convention, these encompass the central 95% of the results obtained for each analysis from the reference population.

Analytical factors can affect the reference ranges for individual laboratories. If an inaccurate method is used, the reference range will reflect the method bias. If an imprecise method is used, the reference range will be widened, that is, the observed span of results (reflected in the SD) will be greater. In statistical terms, the observed variance (i.e. the square of the SD) of the population results will equal the sum of the true or biological variance of the population plus the analytical variance of the method.

How do results vary in disease?

Biochemical test results do not exist in isolation, and when laboratory tests are requested, the clinician will often have made a list of differential diagnoses based on the patient's history, symptoms and signs, and may have a provisional diagnosis that is the likeliest possibility from this list

Table 1.7 Residual individual variation of some serum constituents (expressed as the approximated day-to-day, within-individual coefficient of variation). CV = coefficient of variation.

Serum constituent	CV (%)	Serum constituent	CV (%)
Sodium	1	ALT activity	25
Calcium	1–2	AST activity	25
Potassium	5	Iron	25
Urea	10		

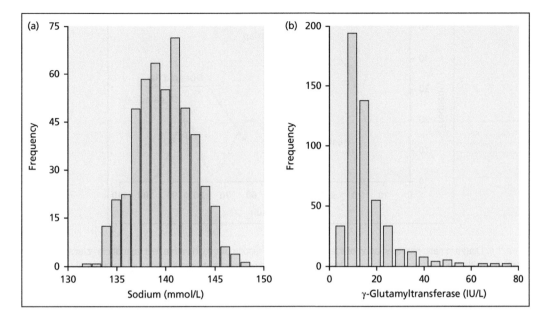

Figure 1.3 Histograms showing the relative frequency with which results with the values indicated were obtained when serum Na⁺ and γ-glutamyltransferase (GGT) activities were measured in a reference population of healthy adult women. (a) The sodium data are symmetrically distributed about the mean whereas (b) the GGT data show a log-Gaussian distribution.

For example, in a patient with severe abdominal pain, tenderness and rigidity, there may be several diagnoses to consider including acute pancreatitis, perforated peptic ulcer and acute cholecystitis. In all three conditions, the serum amylase activity may be raised above the upper reference value for healthy adults. We need to know how the serum amylase activity might vary in the clinically likely diagnoses. It would be useful to know, for instance, that very high serum amylase activities are more likely to be associated with one of these diagnostic possibilities (pancreatitis), than with the other two.

To summarise, to interpret results on patients adequately, we need to know:

- the reference range for healthy individuals of the appropriate age range and sex;
- the values to be expected for patients with the disease, or diseases, under consideration;
- the prevalence of the disease, or diseases, in the population to which the patient belongs.

The assessment of diagnostic tests – sensitivity and specificity

In evaluating and interpreting a test, it is necessary to know how it behaves in health and disease. Central to this understanding are the terms "sensitivity" and "specificity." These define how well a test performs in the diagnosis of a disease, but in order to calculate them it is necessary to know whether the disease is present or not by some method (this could be some other definitive test, or may be a diagnosis made later once the clinical course has made this more obvious).

- Test sensitivity refers to how effective the test is in detecting individuals who have the disease in question. It is expressed as the percentage of true positives in all the individuals who have disease (all the individuals with disease will encompass the true positives (TP) and false negatives (FN)). So:

$$\text{Sensitivity} = \text{TP} / (\text{TP} + \text{FN}) \times 100\%$$

- Test specificity is a measure of how good the test is at providing a negative result in the absence of disease. It is expressed as the percentage of true negatives in all those without the disease (all the individuals without disease will encompass the true negatives (TN) and the false positives (FP)). So:

$$\text{Specificity} = \text{TN} / (\text{TN} + \text{FP}) \times 100\%$$

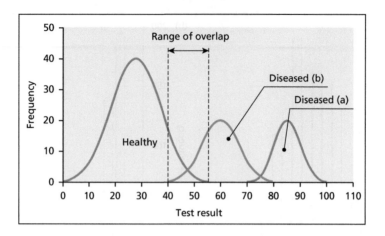

Figure 1.4 Diagrammatic representation of the distributions of results obtained with a test (a) that completely separates healthy people from people with a disease without any overlap between the distribution curves (i.e. an ideal test with 100% sensitivity and 100% specificity), and a test (b) that is less sensitive and less specific, in which there is an area of overlap between the distribution curves for healthy people and people with disease.

The ideal test is 100% sensitive (positive in all patients with the disease) and 100% specific (negative in all patients without the disease). We can illustrate this by means of the following hypothetical example shown diagrammatically in Figure 1.4a. This ideal is rarely achieved; there is usually overlap between the healthy and diseased populations (Figure 1.4b). In practice, we have to decide where to draw dividing lines that most effectively separate 'healthy' from 'diseased' groups, or disease A from disease B.

In evaluating tests for decision making, it is important to decide on the relative importance of sensitivity versus specificity in the context for which a test is used, and to compare the performance of different tests. In defining the presence or absence of a disease, a cut-off may be assigned to a test. Consider the situation where a high value for a particular test equates with the presence of a particular disease. A value above the cut-off would then define the presence of the disease and a value below the cut-off, the absence of disease. A cut-off set at a higher level will increase the test specificity at the expense of test sensitivity (more false negatives), while a cut-off set at a lower value will increase test sensitivity at the expense of test specificity (more false positives).

One way of comparing different tests and of visualising the balance between sensitivity and specificity at different test cut-offs is to plot the test sensitivity against specificity in a so-called 'receiver operating characteristic' (ROC) curve.

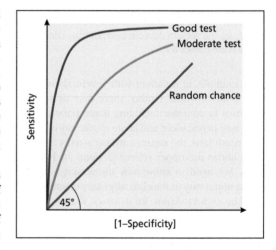

Figure 1.5 Schematic representation of a receiver operating characteristic (ROC) plot. A random test produces a straight line set at 45° to the axes. A discriminatory, good test produces a graph with a steep slope from the origin, displaying high sensitivity at high specificity. Less discriminatory tests produce curves at intermediate positions, as shown. (Adapted from: Roulston, J.E. and Leonard, R.F.C. (1993). Serological Tumour Markers: An Introduction. Reproduced with permission from Elsevier.)

These curves will highlight which test is best suited to which requirement and will also help to define which cut-off to select in order to balance specificity versus sensitivity. This is illustrated in Figure 1.5.

The assessment of diagnostic tests – positive and negative predictive values

The effectiveness of a test can also be defined in terms of the predictive value of a positive result and the predictive value of a negative result. These reflect the reality of clinical practice more than sensitivity and specificity do, in that the presence of a positive or negative test provides information about how likely a disease is to be present or not.

The positive predictive value is the proportion of the positive results that are true positives:

$$TP/(TP+FP)\times100\%.$$

A test with a high positive predictive value will, by definition, have few false positives. This would be important in a situation where a high number of false positives would otherwise lead to extensive and costly further investigation.

The negative predictive value is the proportion of the negative results that are true negatives:

$$TN/(TN+FN)\times100\%.$$

A test with a high negative predictive value would, by definition, have few false negatives. This would be particularly important, for example, in a test that was used for a screening programme where it is essential not to miss a case of the disease in question.

What is not immediately intuitive is that the predictive values depend not just on the sensitivity and specificity of a test but on the prevalence of the condition being tested for in the population of patients being tested.

To illustrate this, first consider screening neonates for an inherited metabolic disorder with an incidence of 1:5000; this is similar to that of some of the more common, treatable, inherited metabolic diseases such as phenylketonuria (PKU) or congenital hypothyroidism. Assume that we have a test with excellent performance, defined by sensitivity and specificity each of 99.5%, and that 1 000 000 neonates are tested (Table 1.8). The known incidence of the condition means that there will be 200 affected babies: 199 of these 200 babies will have a positive result (this is the sensitivity of 99.5%); 999 800 of the babies screened will not have the condition, and of these 994 801 will have a negative result (this is the specificity of 99.5%). However, there will be 4999 babies without the condition who receive a positive result, despite the apparently excellent specificity of the test, because the test

Table 1.8 **A hypothetical set of results of a screening test for a relatively common inherited metabolic disorder in neonates.**

Diagnostic category	Positive results	Negative results	Total
Disease present	199	1	200
Disease absent	4999	994801	999800
Total	5198	994802	1000000
Predictive value	3.8%	100%	

Assumptions: sensitivity of the test 99.5%; specificity 99.5%; prevalence of the disorder 1:5000; 1 000 000 neonates screened. Note that the prevalence of PKU and of hypothyroidism in the UK is about 1:5000 live births, and that about 800 000 neonates in the UK are screened annually.

Table 1.9 **A hypothetical set of results of a test for a myocardial infarction.**

Diagnostic category	Positive results	Negative results	Total
Disease present	225	25	250
Disease absent	75	675	750
Total	300	700	1000
Predictive value	75%	96%	

Assumptions: sensitivity of the test 90%, specificity 90%, prevalence of the disorder 1:4; 1000 patients tested.

has been performed on so many babies. This means that the predictive value of a positive result is as low as 3.8%, while the predictive value of a negative result is virtually 100%. For every neonate affected by the disorder who has a positive test result, there will be about 25 (4999/199) neonates who also have a positive test but who do not have the disease.

Next consider a new test for myocardial infarction (MI) that has been shown to have slightly lower (but still acceptable) sensitivity and specificity of 95%. This is used to test patients presenting at an emergency department with severe central chest pain and it has previously been established in this department that 25% of such patients have suffered an MI (Table 1.9). The known incidence of MI in this population means that there will be 250 affected patients: 225 of these 250 patients will have a positive result (this is the sensitivity of 95%); 750 of the patients tested will not have had an MI and will be suffering from some other cause of chest pain, and of these 675 will have a negative result (this is the specificity of 95%). There will be 75 patients without an MI who receive a positive result, meaning that the predictive value of a positive result is 75% (225 out of 300 patients), while the predictive value of a negative result is 96% (675 out of 700 patients). A negative result has virtually excluded the possibility of an MI, while a positive result has made an MI more than likely.

The second of these examples has shown a much higher positive predictive value (75%) than the first (3.8%) despite the lower sensitivity of the test used. This is because the condition being tested for was much more likely to be present. This provides an important lesson about how laboratory investigations can be used to make diagnoses, showing that tests perform better when a diagnosis is at least a likely possibility, and less well when a test is performed speculatively looking for an unlikely diagnosis.

Two important points regarding screening tests (those used to look for a condition in a basically healthy population) follow on from this. First, tests with very high sensitivity and with very low false-positive rates are required. Secondly, a heavy investigative load will result from the screening programme, since all the false positives will have to be followed up to determine whether or not they indicate the presence of disease. The traditional 95% reference range is not relevant to screening for rare conditions, since the rate of false positives would be far too high. The cut-off value has to be altered to decrease the false-positive rate, at the probable expense of missing some patients who have the condition for which screening is being carried out.

Comment: This is best examined by constructing a table as follows:

	Positive results	Negative results	Totals
Heart failure present	190 TP	10 FN	200
Heart failure absent	240 FP	560 TN	800
Total	430	570	1000

Because the test has a relatively high sensitivity, the table shows that it identifies the majority of patients with heart failure which is what is required in a test to rule out heart failure. Because the test lacks specificity, it can also be seen from the table that it identifies a considerable number of patients with positive results who do not have heart failure. In fact, the test is positive on more occasions in patients who do not have heart failure than in those with heart failure. Because other tests are available to the clinician, the false-positive patients can be separated from the true-positive patients on the basis of these further investigations. The 560 patients where the result is a true negative would then not need to go through more expensive further investigations. In this example, the test has been valuable in ruling out patients who would not require further investigation but ruling in those who would benefit. Clearly, it is not a perfect test but it would potentially prevent costly further investigations in a significant number of patients and, provided that the test itself is not too expensive, ultimately be worthy of consideration in terms of health economics.

CASE 1.2

A new test is marketed which claims to diagnose heart failure. The test has a specificity of 70% and a sensitivity of 95% at the manufacturer's recommended cut-off for diagnosis. The Admissions Unit decides to use the test as part of an admission profile on breathless patients over the age of 65 years admitted for further assessment in order to exclude heart failure. Assuming a prevalence of 20% for heart failure in this population, calculate how many false negatives would be recorded after the first 1000 patients meeting the testing criteria had passed through the unit. Given that other tests can be used to establish a diagnosis of heart failure, do you think that the cut-off selected is sensible? (Prevalence figures are for illustrative purposes only.)

Clinical audit in laboratory medicine

Clinical audit is a process that monitors the procedures involved in patient care to improve the delivery of the service. The principles are applicable to all clinical and investigational specialties (e.g. radiology), as well as laboratory-based specialties such as clinical biochemistry. For example, the monitoring of laboratory performance may identify a delay in analysing samples from the emergency department. This would precipitate a review of the way tests are requested, how samples are delivered to the department, the possible need for these samples to be prioritised in some way, and the way results are communicated back to the clinicians. Any necessary changes would

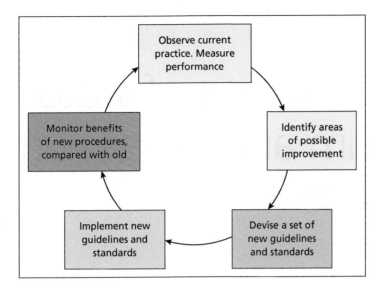

Figure 1.6 The audit cycle.

be instituted, and the process re-monitored to ensure that the original problem had been overcome.

The audit cycle

There is an essential sequence to auditing activities (Figure 1.6):

1 Identify an area of concern or interest, particularly if it is felt that there is room for improvement in the service, or if the same quality of service can be provided more economically.
2 Review and analyse the present procedures.
3 Identify specific aspects that might be capable of improvement.
4 Identify alternative procedures or standards that might lead to improvement.
5 Take the practical steps necessary to implement any changes proposed.
6 Compare the performance after the changes with that before them.

It must be emphasised that the final stage of analysis of the effects of any change is an integral part of the audit process; it is essential to know whether the measures taken have improved the service or made it more cost-effective. Sometimes, changes have no effect, or even have adverse effects.

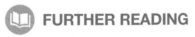 **FURTHER READING**

Asher, R. (1954) Straight and crooked thinking in medicine. *British Medical Journal* **2**, 460–2.

2

Disturbances of water, sodium and potassium balance

Learning objectives

To understand:

✔ the distribution of water, Na⁺ and K⁺ in the different fluid compartments of the body, and their control by hormonal and other factors;

✔ the clinical effects and management of different types of loss, retention or redistribution of fluid;

✔ the causes of hypernatraemia, hyponatraemia, hyperkalaemia and hypokalaemia, and what further investigations might be useful.

Introduction

Fluid loss, retention or redistribution are common clinical problems in many areas of clinical practice. The management of these conditions is often urgent, and requires a rapid assessment of the history and examination, and of biochemical and other investigations. Both internal and external balance of these analytes must be considered. The internal balance is the distribution between different body compartments, while the external balance matches input with output.

Water and sodium balance

The continuous movements of Na⁺ and water between plasma and glomerular filtrate, or between plasma and gastrointestinal (GI) secretions, provide the potential for large losses, with consequent serious and rapid alterations in internal balance. For example, about 25 000 mmol of Na⁺ are filtered at the glomerulus over 24 h, normally with subsequent reabsorption of more than 99%. Likewise, 1000 mmol of Na⁺ enter the GI tract in various secretions each day, but less than 0.5% (5 mmol) is normally lost in the faeces.

Internal distribution of water and sodium

In a 70 kg adult, total body water is about 42 L comprising about 28 L of intracellular fluid (ICF) and 14 L of extracellular fluid (ECF) water. ECF water is distributed as 3 L of plasma water and 11 L of interstitial water. Total body Na⁺ is about 4200 mmol and is mainly extracellular – about 50% is in the ECF, 40% in bone and 10% in the ICF.

Clinical Biochemistry Lecture Notes, Tenth Edition. Peter Rae, Mike Crane and Rebecca Pattenden.
© 2018 John Wiley & Sons Ltd. Published 2018 by John Wiley & Sons Ltd.
Companion website: www.lecturenoteseries.com/clinicalbiochemistry

Two important factors influence the distribution of fluid between the ICF and the intravascular and extravascular compartments of the ECF:

- *Osmolality:* This affects the movement of water across cell membranes.
- *Colloid osmotic pressure:* Together with hydrodynamic factors, this affects the movement of water and low molecular mass solutes (predominantly NaCl) between the intravascular and extravascular compartments.

Osmolality and tonicity

The *osmolality* is the number of solute particles per unit weight of water, irrespective of the size or nature of the particles. Therefore, a given weight of low molecular weight solutes contributes much more to the osmolality than the same weight of high molecular weight solutes. The units are mmol/kg of water. This determines the osmotic pressure exerted by a solution across a membrane. Most laboratories can measure plasma osmolality, but it is also possible to calculate the approximate osmolality of plasma using a number of formulae of varying complexity. The following formula has the benefit of being easy to calculate and performs approximately as well as more complex versions (all concentrations must be in mmol/L):

Calculated osmolality

$$= 2\left[Na^+\right] + 2\left[K^+\right] + \left[glucose\right] + \left[urea\right]$$

This formula includes all the low molecular weight solutes that contribute to plasma osmolality. Values for Na^+ and K^+ are doubled in order to make allowance for their associated anions, such as chloride. The formula is approximate and is not a complete substitute for direct measurement. Calculated osmolality is usually close to measured osmolality, but they may differ considerably for two different types of reason:

- There may be a large amount of unmeasured low molecular mass solute (e.g. ethanol) present in plasma. This will contribute to the measured osmolality, but will obviously not be taken into account in the osmolality calculated from this formula. This will cause an 'osmole gap', with measured osmolality being greater than calculated osmolality.
- Alternatively, there may be a gross increase in plasma protein or lipid concentration, both of which decrease the plasma water per unit volume. This affects some methods of measurement of Na^+, giving an artefactually low result ('pseudohyponatraemia', see Chapter 2: Other causes of

hyponatraemia). This will result in an erroneously low calculated osmolality.

The osmolality of urine is usually measured directly, but is also linearly related to its specific gravity (which can be measured using urine dipsticks), unless there are significant amounts of glucose, protein or X-ray contrast media present.

Tonicity is a term often confused with osmolality. It relates to the osmotic pressure due to those solutes (e.g. Na^+) that exert their effects across cell membranes, thereby causing movement of water into or out of the cells. Substances that can readily diffuse into cells down their concentration gradients (e.g. urea, alcohol) contribute to plasma osmolality but not to plasma tonicity, since after equilibration their concentration will be equal on both sides of the cell membrane. Tonicity is not readily measurable.

The tonicity of ICF and ECF equilibrate with one another by movement of water across cell membranes. An increase in ECF tonicity causes a reduction in ICF volume as water moves from the ICF to the ECF to equalise the tonicity of the two compartments, whereas a decrease in ECF tonicity causes an increase in ICF volume as water moves from the ECF to the ICF.

 CASE 2.1

A 45-year-old man was brought into the A&E department late at night in a comatose state. It was impossible to obtain a history from him, and clinical examination was difficult, but it was noted that he smelt strongly of alcohol. The following analyses were requested urgently.

Why is his measured osmolality so high?

Serum	Result	Reference ranges (adult male)
Urea	4.7	2.5–6.6 mmol/L
Na^+	137	135–145 mmol/L
K^+	4.3	3.6–5.0 mmol/L
Total CO_2	20	22–30 mmol/L
Glucose	4.2	mmol/L
Osmolality	465	280–296 mmol/kg

Comments: The osmolality can be calculated as 291.5, using the formula in Chapter 2: Osmolality and tonicity. The difference between this figure and the value for the directly measured osmolality (465 mmol/L) could be explained by the presence of another low molecular mass solute in plasma.

From the patient's history, it seemed that ethanol might be contributing significantly to the plasma osmolality, and plasma ethanol was measured the following day, on the residue of the specimen collected at the time of emergency admission. The result was 170 mmol/L, very close to the difference between the measured and calculated osmolalities.

Colloid osmotic pressure (oncotic pressure)

The osmotic pressure exerted by plasma proteins across cell membranes is negligible compared with the osmotic pressure of a solution containing NaCl and other small molecules, since they are present in much lower molar concentrations. In contrast, small molecules diffuse freely across the capillary wall, and so are not osmotically active at this site, but plasma proteins do not readily do so. This means that plasma protein concentration and hydrodynamic factors together determine the distribution of water and solutes across the capillary wall, and hence between the intravascular and interstitial compartments (Figure 2.1).

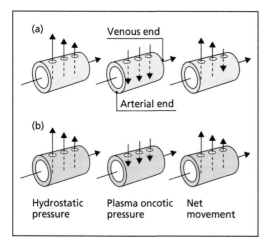

(a) Venous end / Arterial end

(b) Hydrostatic pressure / Plasma oncotic pressure / Net movement

Figure 2.1 Movements of water and low molecular mass solutes across the capillary wall when the plasma protein concentration is (a) normal and (b) low. The effects shown are: hydrostatic pressure, which drives water and low molecular mass solutes *outwards* and decreases along the length of the capillary; and plasma oncotic pressure, which attracts water and low molecular mass solutes *inwards* and is constant along the length of the capillary. The net movement of water and low molecular mass solutes across the capillary wall is governed by the net effect of hydrostatic and plasma oncotic pressures.

Regulation of external water balance

Typical daily intakes and outputs of water are given in Table 2.1. Water intake is largely a consequence of social habit and is very variable, but is also controlled by the sensation of thirst. Its output is controlled by the action of vasopressin, also known as antidiuretic hormone (ADH). In states of pure water deficiency, plasma tonicity increases, causing a sensation of thirst and stimulating vasopressin secretion, both mediated by hypothalamic osmoreceptors. Vasopressin then promotes water reabsorption in the distal nephron, with consequent production of small volumes of concentrated urine. Conversely, a large intake of water causes a fall in tonicity, suppresses thirst and reduces vasopressin secretion, leading to a diuresis, producing large volumes of dilute urine.

Table 2.1 Average daily water intake and output of a normal adult in the UK.

Intake of water	mL	Output of water	mL
Water drunk	1500	Urine volume	1500
Water in food	750	Water content of faeces	50
Water from metabolism of food	250	Losses in expired air and insensible perspiration	950
Total	2500	Total	2500

Secretion of vasopressin is normally sensitively controlled by small changes in ECF tonicity, but it is also under tonic inhibitory control from baroreceptors in the left atrium and in the great vessels on the left side of the heart. When haemodynamic factors (e.g. excessive blood loss, heart failure) reduce the stretch on these receptors, often without an accompanying change in ECF tonicity, a reduction in tonic inhibitory control stimulates vasopressin secretion. The resulting water retention causes hyponatraemia, and is relatively ineffective in expanding the intravascular compartment, since water diffuses freely throughout all compartments (Figure 2.2).

Regulation of external sodium balance

Dietary intakes of Na⁺ (and Cl⁻) are very variable worldwide. A typical 'Western' diet provides 100–200 mmol

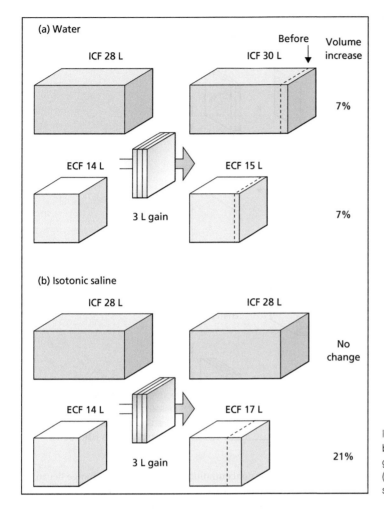

(a) Water

Before | Volume increase

ICF 28 L | ICF 30 L

7%

ECF 14 L | ECF 15 L

3 L gain | 7%

(b) Isotonic saline

ICF 28 L | ICF 28 L

No change

ECF 14 L | ECF 17 L

3 L gain | 21%

Figure 2.2 Different effects on the body's fluid compartments of fluid gains of 3 L of (a) water and (b) isotonic saline. The volumes shown relate to a 70 kg adult.

of both Na^+ and Cl^- daily, but a normal total body Na^+ can be maintained even if intake is less than 5 mmol or greater than 750 mmol daily. Urinary losses of Na^+ normally closely match intake. There is normally little loss of these ions through the skin or in the faeces, but in disease the GI tract can become a major source of Na^+ loss.

The amount of Na^+ excreted in the urine controls the ECF volume since, when osmoregulation is normal, the amount of extracellular water is controlled to maintain a constant concentration of extracellular Na^+. A number of mechanisms are important regulators of Na^+ excretion:

- *The renin–angiotensin–aldosterone system:* Renin is secreted in response to a fall in renal afferent arteriolar pressure or to a reduction in supply of Na^+ to the distal tubule. It converts angiotensinogen in plasma to angiotensin I (AI), which in turn is

converted to angiotensin II (AII) by angiotensin-converting enzyme (ACE). Both AII and its metabolic product angiotensin III (AIII) are physiologically active, and stimulate the release of aldosterone from the adrenal cortex. Aldosterone acts on the distal tubule to promote Na^+ reabsorption in exchange for urinary loss of H^+ or K^+. Since Na^+ cannot enter cells freely, its retention (with iso-osmotically associated water) contributes solely to ECF volume expansion, unlike pure water retention (Figures 2.2 and 2.3). Although the renin–angiotensin–aldosterone system causes relatively slow responses to Na^+ deprivation or Na^+ loading, evidence suggests that this is the main regulatory mechanism for Na^+ excretion.

- *The glomerular filtration rate (GFR):* The rate of Na^+ excretion is often related to the GFR. When the GFR falls acutely, less Na^+ is filtered and excreted, and

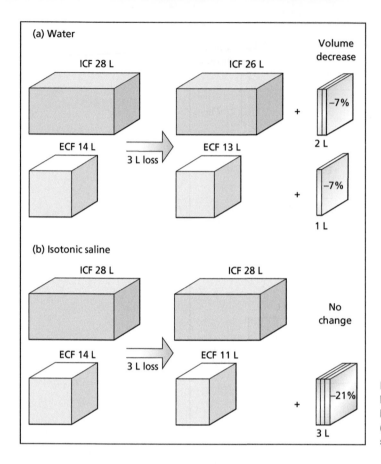

Figure 2.3 Different effects on the body's fluid compartments of fluid losses of 3 L of (a) water and (b) isotonic saline. The volumes shown relate to a 70 kg adult.

vice versa. However, this only becomes a limiting factor in Na⁺ excretion at very low levels of GFR.

- *Atrial natriuretic peptide (ANP):* This peptide secreted by cardiocytes of the right atrium of the heart promotes Na⁺ excretion by the kidney, apparently by causing a marked increase in GFR. The importance of the ANP regulatory mechanism is not yet clear, but it probably only plays a minor role. Other structurally similar peptides have been identified, including brain or B-type natriuretic peptide (BNP), secreted by the cardiac ventricles and with similar properties to ANP. BNP is increasingly being used in the assessment of patients suspected of having cardiac failure (see Chapter 12: The diagnosis of heart failure).

Disorders of water and sodium homeostasis

It is important to remember that the concentration of any substance is a consequence of the amount both of the solute (here Na⁺) and of the solvent (here water).

The concentration of the solute may change because of changes in either the amount of solute, the amount of solvent, or both. Although the physiological control mechanisms for water and for Na⁺ are distinct, they need to be considered together when seeking an understanding of a patient's Na⁺ and water balance, and of the plasma Na⁺ concentration.

Whereas losses or gains of pure water are distributed across all fluid compartments, losses or gains of Na⁺ and water, as isotonic fluid, are borne by the much smaller ECF compartment (Figures 2.2 and 2.3). Thus, it is usually more urgent to replace losses of isotonic fluid than losses of water. For the same reason, circulatory overload is more likely with excessive administration of isotonic Na⁺-containing solutions than with isotonic dextrose (effectively water administration, since the dextrose is metabolised, leaving water).

Plasma Na⁺ concentration cannot be used as a simple measure of body Na⁺ status since it is very often abnormal as a result of losses or gains of water rather than of Na⁺. The plasma Na⁺ concentration must be interpreted in relation to the patient's history and the

Table 2.2 **Causes of depletion of and excess water.**

Categories	Examples
Depletion of water	
• Inadequate intake	Infants, patients in coma or who are very sick, or have symptoms such as nausea or dysphagia
• Abnormal losses via	
Lungs	Inadequate humidification in mechanical ventilation
Skin	Fevers and in hot climates
Renal tract	Diabetes insipidus, lithium therapy
Excess water	
• Excessive intake	
Oral	Psychogenic polydipsia
Parenteral	Hypotonic infusions after operations
• Renal retention	Excess vasopressin (SIADH, Table 2.6), hypoadrenalism, hypothyroidism

Table 2.3 **Causes of depletion of and excess sodium.**

Categories	Examples
Depletion of sodium	
• Inadequate oral intake	Rare, by itself
• Abnormal losses via	
Skin	Excessive sweating, dermatitis, burns
GI tract	Vomiting, aspiration, diarrhoea, fistula, paralytic ileus, blood loss
Renal tract	Diuretic therapy, osmotic diuresis, renal tubular disease, mineralocorticoid deficiency
Excess of sodium	
• Excessive intake	
Oral	Sea water (drowning), salt tablets, hypertonic NaCl administration (this is rare)
Parenteral	Post-operatively, infusion of hypertonic NaCl
• Renal retention	Acute and chronic renal failure, primary and secondary hyperaldosteronism, Cushing's syndrome

findings on clinical examination, and if necessary backed up by other investigations.

The main causes of depletion and excess of water are summarised in Table 2.2, and of Na$^+$ in Table 2.3. Although some of these conditions may be associated with abnormal plasma Na$^+$ levels, it must be emphasised that this is not necessarily always the case. For example, patients with acute losses of isotonic fluid (e.g. plasma, ECF, blood) may be severely and dangerously hypovolaemic and Na$^+$ depleted, and very possibly in shock, but their plasma Na$^+$ concentration may nevertheless be normal or even raised.

Hyponatraemia

Hyponatraemia is the most common clinical biochemical abnormality, occurring in up to 30% of hospitalised patients, with a wide spectrum of clinical symptoms from mild to life-threatening. It is usually primarily a disorder of water balance, with a relative excess of total body water. Most patients with hyponatraemia also have a low plasma osmolality. Unless an unusual cause of hyponatraemia is suspected (see Chapter 2: Other causes of hyponatraemia), measurement of plasma osmolality contributes little or no extra information.

Patients with hyponatraemia can be divided into three categories, on the basis of the ECF volume being low, normal or increased. These categories in turn reflect a total body Na$^+$ that is low, normal or increased, respectively. The value of this classification is two-fold. First, the clinical history and examination often indicate the ECF volume and therefore the total body Na$^+$ status. Secondly, treatment often depends on the total body Na$^+$ status rather than the Na$^+$ concentration. One possible way of narrowing the differential diagnosis of a patient with hyponatraemia, based on this subdivision, is shown in Figure 2.4.

It is also helpful to assess the rate at which the hyponatraemia is likely to have developed, and the severity of any symptoms, since these are important factors in determining treatment. Acute hyponatraemia develops over a period of less than 48h, with chronic hyponatraemia developing over a longer period. Neurological symptoms of hyponatraemia are due to the development of cerebral oedema (Table 2.4).

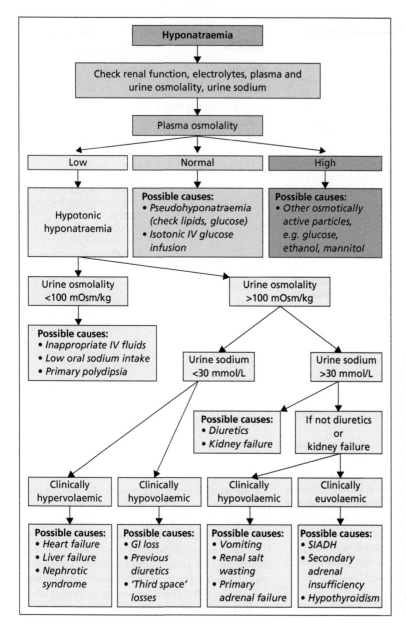

Figure 2.4 Schematic diagram to assist in the diagnosis of some of the more common causes of hyponatraemia. In practice more than one cause may be present, and the findings may be influenced by the recent clinical history and oral or IV fluid intake. (GI, gastrointestinal; SIADH, syndrome of inappropriate secretion of antidiuretic hormone; 'third space' losses, leakage of fluid from intravascular to extravascular space, seen in bowel obstruction, pancreatitis, sepsis, etc.)

Table 2.4 Neurological symptoms of hyponatraemia.

Severity	Symptoms
Moderately severe	Nausea without vomiting, headache, confusion
Severe	Vomiting, cardio-respiratory distress, drowsiness, seizures, coma

Cerebral oedema is less likely to have developed in acute hyponatraemia, so treatment is aimed at preventing this from developing. In chronic hyponatraemia, rapid correction of a low sodium can result in osmotic demyelination syndrome, with consequences including dysarthria, dysphagia, spastic quadriparesis, seizures and death. Correction of hyponatraemia should therefore be performed at a controlled rate, in a setting where biochemical monitoring can be performed. It

Table 2.5 **Causes of hyponatraemia.**

ECF volume	Categories	Examples
Decreased total body Na$^+$ (loss of Na$^+$ > H$_2$O)		
• Extrarenal losses of Na$^+$ (urine Na$^+$ < 20 mmol/L)	GI tract	Vomiting, diarrhoea
	Skin	Burns, severe dermatitis
	'Internal'	Paralytic ileus, peritoneal fluid
• Renal losses of Na$^+$ (urine Na$^+$ > 20 mmol/L)	Diuretics	
	Kidneys	Diuretic phase of renal tubular necrosis
	Adrenals	Mineralocorticoid deficiency
Normal or near-normal total body Na$^+$	Acute conditions	Parenteral administration of water, after surgery or trauma, or during or after delivery
	Chronic conditions	
	Anti-diuretic drugs	Opiates, chlorpropamide
	Kidneys	Chronic renal failure
	Adrenals	Glucocorticoid deficiency
	Vasopressin excess	SIADH (Table 2.6)
	Osmoregulator	Low setting in carcinomatosis
Increased total body Na$^+$	Acute conditions	Acute renal failure
	Chronic conditions	Oedematous states (see Chapter 2: Hyponatraemia with increased ECF volume)

should be directed at the underlying cause where possible. Possible treatments include infusion of hypertonic saline, fluid restriction and stopping contributory drugs. The use of drugs such as demeclocycline or vasopressin antagonists is not usually recommended.

Hyponatraemia with low ECF volume

The patient has lost Na$^+$ and water in one or more body fluids (e.g. GI tract secretions, urine, inflammatory exudate) or may have been treated with a diuretic (Table 2.5). The low ECF volume leads to tachycardia, orthostatic hypotension, reduced skin turgor and oliguria. The hypovolaemia causes secondary aldosteronism with a low urinary Na$^+$ concentration (usually <20 mmol/L), unless diuretic treatment is the cause, when urinary Na$^+$ remains high. The hypovolaemia also provides a 'volume stimulus' to vasopressin secretion, resulting in oliguria and a concentrated urine. The consequent water retention can further contribute to the hyponatraemia. Treatment is usually straightforward here and requires administration of isotonic saline.

Hyponatraemia with normal ECF volume

The hyponatraemia results from excessive water retention, due to inability to excrete a water load. This may develop acutely, or it may be chronic (Table 2.5).

- *Acute water retention:* Plasma vasopressin is acutely increased after trauma or major surgery, as part of the metabolic response to trauma, and during delivery and post-partum. Administration of excessive amounts of water (e.g. as 5% dextrose) in these circumstances may exacerbate the hyponatraemia and cause acute water intoxication.
- *Chronic water retention:* Perhaps the most widely known chronic 'cause' of this form of hyponatraemia is dilutional hyponatraemia, often known as the syndrome of inappropriate secretion of ADH (SIADH) (Table 2.6). Whether this concept is of value in understanding its aetiology, or valid in terms of altered physiology, is uncertain. As the name implies, ADH (or rather vasopressin) is being secreted in the absence of an 'appropriate' physiological stimulus, of either fluid depletion or hypernatraemia. As water is

Table 2.6 SIADH.

Characteristics of the syndrome	Causes (and examples)
Low plasma Na$^+$ and osmolality	Malignant disease of the bronchus, prostate, pancreas, etc.
Inappropriately high urine osmolality	Chest diseases, e.g. pneumonia, bronchitis, tuberculosis
Excessive renal excretion of Na$^+$	Central nervous system (CNS) diseases, including brain trauma, tumours, meningitis
No evidence of volume depletion	
No evidence of oedema	Drug treatment, e.g. carbamazepine, chlorpropamide, opiates
Normal renal and adrenal function	Miscellaneous conditions, including porphyria, psychosis, post-operative states

What is the most likely cause of this man's low plasma Na$^+$ concentration?

Serum	Result	Reference ranges (adult male)
Urea	4.3	2.5–6.6 mmol/L
Na$^+$	128	135–145 mmol/L
K$^+$	4.3	3.6–5.0 mmol/L
Total CO$_2$	25	22–30 mmol/L

Comments: Hyponatraemia is often seen in post-operative patients receiving IV fluids. At this time the ability to excrete water is reduced as part of the metabolic response to trauma. If excessive amounts of hypotonic fluids (usually 5% dextrose) are given, hyponatraemia will result. It may also be at least partly due to the 'sick cell syndrome'. There are usually no clinical features of water intoxication, and all that is required is review of the patient's fluid balance, and adjustment of the prescription for IV fluids. This man had received a total of 4.5L of fluid since his operation, and his fluid balance chart showed that he had a positive balance of 2L.

retained, the potential for expansion of the ECF volume is limited by a reduction in renin and an increase in sodium excretion. A new steady state is achieved, with essentially normal, or only mildly increased, ECF volume. If the causative disorder (Table 2.6) is transient, plasma Na$^+$ returns to normal when the primary disorder (e.g. pneumonia) is treated. However, in patients with cancer, the hyponatraemia is presumably due to production of vasopressin or a related substance by the tumour, and is usually persistent. If symptoms are mild, they may be treated by fluid restriction. Increased solute intake with urea or a combination of oral sodium chloride and a low dose loop diuretic can also be used in more profound hyponatraemia. Other causes of chronic retention of water include:

     CASE 2.2

A 76-year-old man was making reasonable post-operative progress following major abdominal surgery for a carcinoma of the colon. Two days after the operation he appeared well, and there were no signs of dehydration or oedema. The following results were obtained:

     CASE 2.3

A 63-year-old coal miner had had a persistent chest infection, with cough and sputum, for the previous 2 months. He was a smoker. Clinical examination revealed finger clubbing, crackles and wheezes throughout the chest, and a small pleural effusion. There were no signs of dehydration or oedema.

Examination of blood and of a simultaneous urine specimen yielded the following results:

Serum	Result	Reference ranges (adult male)
Urea	2.3	2.5–6.6 mmol/L
Na$^+$	118	135–145 mmol/L
K$^+$	4.3	3.6–5.0 mmol/L
Total CO$_2$	26	22–30 mmol/L
Osmolality	260	280–296 mmol/L
Urine	Result	
Na$^+$	74	mmol/L
Osmolality	625	mmol/kg

What is the most likely cause of this man's low plasma Na$^+$ and osmolality?

Comments: This patient is not diluting his urine in response to low plasma osmolality and hyponatraemia: this suggests inappropriate ADH secretion. There tends to be a continuing natriuresis despite the hyponatraemia in these patients, as the retention of water leads to mild expansion of the ECF, and hence reduced aldosterone secretion. The presence of a dilutional hyponatraemia is also supported by the low plasma urea concentration. Before diagnosing the syndrome of inappropriate ADH secretion (SIADH – see Chapter 2: Hyponatraemia with normal ECF volume and Table 2.6), it is important to exclude adrenal, pituitary and renal disease. In this patient, possible explanations include the recurrent chest infections, and/or an underlying bronchogenic carcinoma, with ectopic secretion of ADH.

- *Chronic renal disease:* Damaged kidneys may be unable to concentrate or to dilute urine normally, tending to produce a urin e of osmolality about that of plasma. Thus, the ability to excrete a water load is severely impaired, and excess water intake (oral or IV) readily produces a dilutional hyponatraemia. These patients may also be overloaded with Na⁺.
- *Glucocorticoid deficiency:* Whether due to anterior pituitary disease or abrupt withdrawal of long-term glucocorticoid therapy, this may lead to inability to excrete a water load, and to hyponatraemia.
- *Resetting of the osmostat:* Some patients with malnutrition, carcinomatosis or tuberculosis seem to have their osmostat reset at a low level, with plasma Na⁺ of 125–130 mmol/L. The cause is uncertain.

Hyponatraemia with increased ECF volume

Significant increases in total body Na⁺ give rise to clinically detectable oedema (Table 2.5). Generalised oedema is usually associated with secondary aldosteronism, caused by a reduction in renal blood flow, which stimulates renin production. Patients fall into at least three categories:

- *Renal failure:* Excess water intake in a poorly controlled patient with acute or chronic renal disease can lead to hyponatraemia with oedema.
- *Congestive cardiac failure:* In cardiac failure there is reduced renal perfusion and an 'apparent' volume deficit, and also increased venous pressure, with altered fluid distribution between the intravascular and interstitial compartments (Figure 2.1). These

lead to secondary aldosteronism and increased vasopressin secretion, causing Na⁺ overload and hyponatraemia.

- *Hypoproteinaemic states:* Low plasma protein, especially low albumin, leads to excessive losses of water and low molecular mass solutes from the intravascular to the interstitial compartments (Figure 2.1). Hence interstitial oedema is accompanied by reduced intravascular volume, with consequent secondary aldosteronism and stimulation of vasopressin release.

'Sick cell syndrome'

Some ill patients may have a hyponatraemia that is very resistant to treatment, and has no immediately obvious cause. The effective arterial plasma volume may be contracted, with a consequent secondary hyperaldosteronism and Na⁺ retention. The total ECF volume may in contrast be increased, possibly because of stress-induced vasopressin secretion, or other causes of SIADH. These, however, may not be the whole explanation for the observed pathophysiology, since plasma aldosterone and vasopressin concentrations are not always raised. The hyponatraemia may be due, at least in part, to the 'sick cell syndrome', in which there is an inability to maintain a Na⁺ gradient across the cell membrane, because of an increase in permeability, with or without impaired Na⁺ pump activity.

Other causes of hyponatraemia

In all the examples of hyponatraemia discussed above, the low plasma Na⁺ occurs in association with reduced plasma osmolality. Where this is not the case, the following possibilities should be considered:

- *Artefact:* 'Hyponatraemia' is often caused by collection of a blood specimen from a vein close to a site at which fluid (typically 5% dextrose) is being administered intravenously.
- *Pseudohyponatraemia:* This is an artefactual result due to a reduction in plasma water caused by marked hyperlipidaemia or hyperproteinaemia (e.g. multiple myeloma). Normally, lipids and proteins make up a relatively small proportion, by volume, of plasma. Na⁺ and other electrolytes are dissolved in the plasma water, and do not enter the lipid or protein fraction of the plasma. This means that methods which measure Na⁺ concentration in the plasma water give similar results to those that measure Na⁺ concentration in total plasma. Most commonly used methods for measuring Na⁺ measure the amount of Na⁺ in a given volume of plasma. These methods include

flame photometry, and ion-selective electrode methods in which the plasma is diluted before measurement. If the lipid or protein fraction is markedly increased, even if the Na$^+$ concentration in plasma water is normal, the amount of Na$^+$ in a given volume of plasma will be lower than normal, since there will be less water present than normal. The diagnosis can be confirmed by measuring plasma Na$^+$ in undiluted plasma using a direct ion-selective electrode, which measures the Na$^+$ in the plasma water (strictly speaking, the Na$^+$ activity), or by measuring plasma osmolality. In the absence of another cause of true hyponatraemia, the results of these measurements will be normal.

- *Hyperosmolar hyponatraemia:* This may be due to hyperglycaemia, administration of mannitol or occasionally other causes. The hyponatraemia mainly reflects the shift of water out of the cells into the ECF in response to osmotic effects, other than those due to Na$^+$, across cell membranes. Treatment should be directed to the cause of the hyperosmolality rather than to the hyponatraemia.

Hypernatraemia

This is the most common cause of increased tonicity of body fluids. It is nearly always due to water deficit rather than Na$^+$ excess. The ICF volume is decreased due to movement of water out of cells.

Hypernatraemia with decreased body sodium

This is the most common group (Table 2.7). It is usually due to extrarenal loss of hypotonic fluid. The nature and effects of the disturbance of fluid balance can be thought of as comprising the consequences of the combination of two components:

- Loss of isotonic fluid, which causes reduction in ECF volume, with hypotension, shock and oliguria. The physiological response is high urine osmolality and low urine Na$^+$ of less than 20 mmol/L.
- Loss of water, which causes volume reduction of both ICF and ECF and consequent hypernatraemia.

Urinary loss of hypotonic fluid sometimes occurs due to renal disease or to osmotic diuresis; in these patients, urine Na$^+$ is likely to be greater than 20 mmol/L. The most common cause of hypernatraemia associated with an osmotic diuresis is hyperglycaemia.

Treatment should initially aim to replace the deficit of isotonic fluid by infusing isotonic saline or, if the deficit is large, hypotonic saline.

Hypernatraemia with normal body sodium

These patients (Table 2.7) have a pure water deficit, as may occur when insensible water losses are very high and insufficient water is drunk as replacement (e.g. in hot climates, in unconscious patients or in patients with a high fever). The urine has a high osmolality, and its Na$^+$ content depends on Na$^+$ intake.

Hypernatraemia with normal body Na$^+$ also occurs in diabetes insipidus (see Chapter 4: Interpretation of tests of renal concentrating ability) due to excessive renal water loss. This loss is normally replaced by drinking. However, dehydration may develop if the patient is unable to drink, as may occur in very young children or in unconscious patients. The urine has a low osmolality and its Na$^+$ content depends on Na$^+$ intake.

Treatment should aim to rehydrate these patients fairly slowly, to avoid causing acute shifts

---

Table 2.7 **Causes of hypernatraemia.**

Body sodium	Categories	Examples
Decreased body Na$^+$ (loss of H_2O > Na$^+$)	Extrarenal	Sweating, diarrhoea
	Renal	Osmotic diuresis (e.g. diabetes mellitus)
Normal body Na$^+$ (loss of H_2O only)	Extrarenal	Fever, high-temperature climates
	Via kidneys	Diabetes insipidus, prolonged unconsciousness
Increased body Na$^+$ (retention of Na$^+$ > H_2O)	Steroid excess	Steroid treatment, Cushing's syndrome, Conn's syndrome
	Intake of Na$^+$	Self-induced or iatrogenic, oral or parenteral

of water into cells, especially those of the brain, which may have accommodated to the hyperosmolality by increasing its intracellular solute concentration. Water, administered orally, is the simplest treatment. IV therapy may be necessary, with 5% glucose or glucose–saline.

Hypernatraemia with increased body sodium

This is relatively uncommon (Table 2.7). Mild hypernatraemia may be caused by an excess of mineralocorticoids or glucocorticoids. More often, it occurs if excess Na^+ is administered therapeutically (e.g. $NaHCO_3$ during resuscitation). Treatment may be with diuretics or, rarely, by renal dialysis.

Other chemical investigations in fluid balance disorders

Several other chemical investigations, in addition to plasma Na^+, may help when the history or clinical examination suggests that there is a disorder of fluid balance.

Blood specimens

Plasma urea and plasma creatinine: Hypovolaemia is usually associated with a reduced GFR, and so with raised plasma urea and creatinine. Plasma urea may increase before plasma creatinine in the early stages of water and Na^+ depletion (see Chapter 4: High plasma urea concentration).

Plasma chloride: Alterations in plasma Cl^- parallel those in plasma Na^+, except in the presence of some acid–base disturbances (see Chapter 3: Plasma chloride). Chloride measurements are rarely of value in assessing disturbances of fluid balance.

Plasma albumin: This may help to assess acute changes in intravascular volume, and may be useful in following changes in patients with fluid balance disorders over time. Plasma albumin should be measured in patients with oedema, to find out whether hypoalbuminaemia is present as a contributory cause, and to determine its severity.

Plasma osmolality: Plasma osmolality usually parallels plasma Na^+ concentration and can be estimated by calculation (see Chapter 2: Osmolality and tonicity), but may be of value when a defect in vasopressin action is suspected to be responsible for a fluid-electrolyte disorder. Plasma osmolality measurements are also of interest when it seems likely that the calculated osmolality and measured osmolality might differ significantly. This occurs when:

 CASE 2.4

A neighbour found a 78-year-old woman to be drowsy and unwell. She had had an upper respiratory tract infection several weeks previously, and had been very slow to recover from this. She had been increasingly thirsty over this period. The only past history was of diabetes mellitus, diagnosed about 5 years previously and controlled by diet. On examination, she was very dehydrated, but her breath did not smell of ketones. The following results were obtained:

Why is her sodium so high?

Serum	Result	Reference ranges (adult female)
Urea	28.2	2.5–6.6 mmol/L
Na^+	156	135–145 mmol/L
K^+	4.4	3.6–5.0 mmol/L
Total CO_2	26	22–30 mmol/L
Glucose	38.2	mmol/L

Comments: She has hyperosmolar hyperglycaemic decompensation of her diabetes. The onset of this is usually slower than that of ketoacidosis and, possibly because vomiting is less likely, patients do not become acutely ill so rapidly. The prolonged osmotic diuresis due to the severe hyperglycaemia results in large losses of water, often in excess of the sodium loss, resulting in hypernatraemia. GFR is reduced, causing raised plasma urea. Treatment requires the replacement of the fluid and electrolyte losses, and the use of insulin to restore the glucose concentration to normal and prevent the continuing osmotic diuresis. (See also Chapter 12.)

- there is marked hyperproteinaemia or hypertriglyceridaemia, causing a low plasma water concentration;
- significant amounts of exogenous low molecular mass materials (e.g. ethanol, ethylene glycol, glycine) which will not contribute to calculated osmolality are present in plasma;
- in both these examples, the finding of a marked discrepancy between the measured osmolality and the calculated osmolality may be of diagnostic value.

Urine specimens

Urine osmolality: Measurements of urine osmolality are of value in the investigation of:

- *Polyuria:* A relatively concentrated urine suggests that polyuria is due to an osmotic diuretic (e.g. glucose), whereas a dilute urine suggests that there is primary polydipsia or diabetes insipidus (see Chapter 4: Urine osmolality and renal concentration tests). Patients with chronic renal failure may also have polyuria, with a urine osmolality that is usually within 50 mmol/kg of the plasma value.

- *Oliguria:* Where acute renal failure is suspected (see Chapter 4: Acute kidney injury).
- *SIADH:* In patients with SIADH (see Chapter 2: Hyponatraemia with normal ECF volume and Table 2.5) the urine osmolality is not maximally dilute, despite a dilutional hyponatraemia.

Urine sodium: This normally varies with Na^+ intake. Measurements of 24 h output, taken with the clinical findings, may be useful in the diagnosis of disturbances in Na^+ and water handling, and in planning fluid replacement.

- *Patients with low urine Na^+ concentration:* This is an appropriate response in patients who are volume depleted, with oliguria and normally functioning kidneys; urine Na^+ is usually less than 10 mmol/L, and urine flow increases after volume repletion. Na^+ retention and low urine Na^+ occur in the secondary hyperaldosteronism associated with congestive cardiac failure, liver disease and hypoproteinaemic states, and in Cushing's syndrome and Conn's syndrome.
- *Patients with natriuresis:* In hyponatraemic patients with evidence of ECF volume depletion, continuing natriuresis (i.e. urine Na^+ >20 mmol/L) suggests either:
  - Volume depletion that is so severe as to have led to acute renal failure. The patient will be oliguric, with rising plasma urea and creatinine concentrations; diuresis fails to occur after volume repletion.
  - In the absence of acute renal failure, this occurs with overzealous diuretic use, with salt-losing nephritis and with defects in the hypothalamic–pituitary–adrenal (HPA) axis, including Addison's disease.

Natriuresis may also occur in hyponatraemic states associated with SIADH or acute water intoxication and where ECF volume is normal or even increased.

Potassium balance

Potassium is the main intracellular cation. About 98% of total body K^+ is in cells, the balance (~50 mmol) being in the ECF. There is a large concentration gradient across cell membranes, the ICF K^+ being about 150 mmol/L compared with about 4 mmol/L in ECF.

Internal distribution

This is determined by movements across the cell membrane. Factors causing K^+ to move out of cells include hypertonicity, acidosis, insulin lack and severe cell damage or cell death. Potassium moves into cells if there is alkalosis, or when insulin is given.

External balance

This is mainly determined, in the absence of GI disease, by intake of K^+ and by its renal excretion. A typical 'Western' diet contains 20–100 mmol of K^+ daily; this intake is normally closely matched by urinary excretion. The control of renal K^+ excretion is not fully understood, but the following points have been established:

- Nearly all the K^+ filtered at the glomerulus is reabsorbed in the proximal tubule. Less than 10% reaches the distal tubule, where the main regulation of K^+ excretion occurs. Secretion of K^+ in response to alterations in dietary intake occurs in the distal tubule, the cortical collecting tubule and the collecting duct.
- The distal tubule is an important site of Na^+ reabsorption. When Na^+ is reabsorbed, the tubular lumen becomes electronegative in relation to the adjacent cell, and cations in the cell (e.g. K^+, H^+) move into the lumen to balance the charge. The rate of movement of K^+ into the lumen depends on there being sufficient delivery of Na^+ to the distal tubule, as well as on the rate of urine flow and on the concentration of K^+ in the tubular cell.
- The concentration of K^+ in the tubular cell depends largely on adenosine triphosphatase-dependent (ATPase-dependent) Na^+/K^+ exchange with peritubular fluid (i.e. the ECF). This is affected by mineralocorticoids, by acid–base changes and by ECF K^+ concentration. The tubular cell K^+ tends to be increased by hyperkalaemia, by mineralocorticoid excess and by alkalosis, all of which tend to cause an increase in K^+ excretion.

Abnormalities of plasma potassium concentration

The reference range for plasma K^+ is 3.6–5.0 mmol/L in adults. The important, and often life-threatening, clinical manifestations of abnormalities of plasma K^+

concentration are those relating to disturbances of neuromuscular excitability and of cardiac conduction. Any patient with an abnormal plasma K^+ concentration, who also shows signs of muscle weakness or of a cardiac arrhythmia, should have cardiac monitoring with electrocardiography (ECG). The abnormal plasma K^+ level should be corrected, with appropriate monitoring during treatment.

Hypokalaemia (Table 2.8) must not be equated with K^+ depletion, and hyperkalaemia (Table 2.9) must not be equated with K^+ excess. Although most patients with K^+ depletion have hypokalaemia, and most patients with K^+ excess may have hyperkalaemia, acute changes in the distribution of K^+ in the body can offset any effects of depletion or excess. To generalise, acute changes in plasma K^+ are usually caused by redistribution of K^+ across cell membranes, whereas chronic changes in plasma K^+ are usually due to abnormal external K^+ balance.

Hypokalaemia

Altered internal distribution: shift of K^+ into cells

- *Acute shifts* of K^+ into the cell may occur in alkalosis, but the hypokalaemia may be more closely related to the increased renal excretion of K^+. Patients with respiratory alkalosis caused by voluntary hyperventilation rarely show hypokalaemia, but patients on prolonged assisted ventilation may have low plasma K^+ if the alveolar P_{CO_2} is low for a relatively long period.
- *Insulin* in high dosage, given intravenously, promotes the uptake of K^+ by liver and muscle. Acute shifts of K^+ into cells may occur in diabetic ketoacidosis (DKA) shortly after starting treatment.

- *Adrenaline* and other β-adrenergic agonists stimulate the uptake of K^+ into cells. This may contribute to the hypokalaemia appearing in patients after myocardial infarction, since catecholamine levels are likely to be increased in these patients. Hypokalaemic effects of salbutamol (a synthetic β-adrenergic agonist) have also been described.
- *Cellular incorporation of K^+* may cause hypokalaemia in states where cell mass rapidly increases. Examples include the treatment of severe megaloblastic anaemia with vitamin B_{12} or folate, and the parenteral re-feeding of wasted patients (especially if insulin is also administered). It also occurs when there are rapidly proliferating leukaemic cells.

Altered external balance: deficient intake of K^+

Prolonged deficient intake of K^+ can lead to a decrease in total body K^+, eventually manifested as hypokalaemia. This may occur in chronic and severe malnutrition in the developing world, in the elderly on deficient diets, and in anorexia nervosa.

Altered external balance: excessive losses of K^+

- *Hyperaldosteronism*, both primary and secondary, and Cushing's syndrome (including that due to steroid administration) cause excessive renal K^+ loss due to increased K^+ transfer into the distal tubule in response to increased reabsorption of Na^+ from the tubular lumen. Mineralocorticoid excess also favours transfer of K^+ into the tubular cell from the interstitial fluid in exchange for Na^+. Urinary K^+ loss in hyperaldosteronism returns to normal if

Table 2.8 **Causes of hypokalaemia.**

Cause	Categories	Examples
Artefact		Specimen collected from an infusion site or near to one
Redistribution of K^+ between ECF and ICF		Alkalosis, familial periodic paralysis (hypokalaemic form), treatment of hyperglycaemia with insulin
Abnormal external balance	Inadequate intake	Anorexia nervosa, alcoholism (both rare)
	Abnormal losses from the GI tract	Vomiting, nasogastric aspiration, diarrhoea, fistula, laxative abuse, villous adenoma of the colon
	Abnormal losses from the renal tract	Diuretics, osmotic diuresis, renal tubular acidosis, aldosteronism, Cushing's syndrome, Bartter's syndrome

Table 2.9 Causes of hyperkalaemia.

Cause	Categories	Examples
Artefact		Trauma during blood collection, delay in separating plasma/serum, freezing blood
Redistribution of K⁺ between ECF and ICF		Acidosis, hypertonicity, tissue and tumour necrosis (e.g. burns, leukaemia), haemolytic disorders, hyperkalaemic familial periodic paralysis, insulin deficiency
Abnormal external balance	Increased intake Decreased renal output*	Excessive oral intake of K⁺ (rare by itself)
	Renal causes	1 Renal failure, oliguric (acute and chronic); inappropriate oral intake in chronic failure
		2 Failure of renal tubular response, due to systemic lupus erythematosus, K⁺-sparing diuretics, chronic interstitial nephritis
	Adrenal causes	Addison's disease, selective hypoaldosteronism

*With or without inappropriate intake.

there is dietary Na⁺ restriction, which limits distal tubular delivery of Na⁺.

- *Diuretic therapy* increases renal K⁺ excretion by causing increased delivery of Na⁺ to the distal tubule and increased urine flow rate. Diuretics may also cause hypovolaemia, with consequent secondary hyperaldosteronism.
- *Acidosis and alkalosis* both affect renal K⁺ excretion in ways that are not fully understood. Acute acidosis causes K⁺ retention, and acute alkalosis causes increased K⁺ excretion. However, chronic acidosis and chronic alkalosis both cause increased K⁺ excretion.
- *GI fluid losses* often cause K⁺ depletion. However, if gastric fluid is lost in large quantity, renal K⁺ loss (due to the combined effects of the resultant secondary hyperaldosteronism and the metabolic alkalosis) is the main cause of the K⁺ depletion, rather than the direct loss of K⁺ in gastric juice. In diarrhoea or laxative abuse, the increased losses of K⁺ in faeces may cause K⁺ depletion.
- *Renal disease* does not usually cause excessive K⁺ loss. However, a few tubular abnormalities are associated with K⁺ depletion, in the absence of diuretic therapy:
  - *Renal tubular acidosis* The K⁺ loss is caused both by the chronic acidosis and, in patients with proximal renal tubular acidosis (Chapter 4, Renal tubular acidosis), by increased delivery of Na⁺ to the distal tubule. In distal renal tubular acidosis, the inability to excrete H⁺ may cause a compensatory transfer of K⁺ to the tubular fluid.

- *Bartter's syndrome* The syndrome consists of persistent hypokalaemia with secondary hyperaldosteronism in association with a metabolic alkalosis; patients are normotensive. There is increased delivery of Na⁺ to the distal tubule, caused by an abnormality of chloride reabsorption in the loop of Henle.
- *Excessive sweating* Sweat K⁺ is higher than ECF concentrations, so excessive sweat losses can result in potassium depletion and hypokalaemia.

Other causes of hypokalaemia

Artefact: Collection of a blood sample from a vein near to a site of an IV infusion, where the fluid has a low K⁺.

Hyperkalaemia

Plasma K⁺ over 6.5 mmol/L requires urgent treatment, especially if it has developed rapidly. IV calcium gluconate has a rapid but short-lived effect in countering the neuromuscular effects of hyperkalaemia. Treatment with glucose and insulin lowers plasma K⁺ by causing K⁺ to pass into the ICF. Treatment with cation-exchange resins promotes K⁺ loss from the body, and any drugs that might cause K⁺ retention should be stopped. Renal dialysis offers definitive treatment by removing K⁺, and may be needed.

Altered internal distribution of K⁺

- *Acidosis:* The effects of acidosis on internal K⁺ balance are complicated. As a general rule, acidotic states are often accompanied by hyperkalaemia, as K⁺ moves from the ICF into the ECF. Although this is the case for acute respiratory acidosis, and for both acute and chronic metabolic acidosis, it is more unusual to find hyperkalaemia in chronic respiratory acidosis. It is important to note that a high plasma K⁺ concentration may be accompanied by a reduced total body K⁺ as a result of excessive urinary K⁺ losses in both chronic respiratory acidosis and metabolic acidosis.
- *Hypertonic states:* In these, K⁺ moves out of cells, possibly because of the increased intracellular K⁺ caused by the reduction in ICF volume.
- *Uncontrolled diabetes mellitus:* The lack of insulin prevents K⁺ from entering cells. This results in hyperkalaemia, despite the K⁺ loss caused by the osmotic diuresis.
- *Cellular necrosis:* This may lead to excessive release of K⁺ and may result in hyperkalaemia. Extensive cell damage may be a feature of rhabdomyolysis (e.g. crush injury), haemolysis, burns or tumour necrosis (e.g. in the treatment of leukaemias).
- *Digoxin poisoning:* Causes hyperkalaemia by inhibiting the Na⁺/K⁺ ATPase pump. Therapeutic doses do not have this effect.

Altered external balance: increased intake of K⁺

Increased K⁺ intake only rarely causes accumulation of K⁺ in the body, since the normal kidney can excrete a large K⁺ load. However, if there is renal impairment, K⁺ may accumulate if salt substitutes are administered, or excessive amounts of some fruit drinks are drunk or if excessive potassium replacement therapy accompanies diuretic administration.

Altered external balance: decreased excretion of K⁺

- *Intrinsic renal disease:* This is an important cause of hyperkalaemia. It may occur in acute renal failure and in the later stages of chronic renal failure. In patients with renal disease that largely affects the renal medulla, hyperkalaemia may occur earlier. This may be because increased K⁺ secretion from the collecting duct, an important adaptive response in the damaged kidney, is lost earlier in patients with medullary disease.
- *Mineralocorticoid deficiency:* This may occur in Addison's disease and in secondary adrenocortical hypofunction. In both, K⁺ retention may occur. This is not an invariable feature, presumably because other mechanisms can facilitate K⁺ excretion. Selective hypoaldosteronism, accompanied by normal glucocorticoid production, may occur in patients with diabetes mellitus in whom juxtaglomerular sclerosis probably interferes with renin production. ACE inhibitors, by reducing AII (and therefore aldosterone) levels, may lead to increased plasma K⁺, but severe problems are only likely to occur in the presence of renal failure.
- Patients treated with *K⁺-sparing diuretics* (e.g. spironolactone, amiloride) may fail to respond to aldosterone. If the K⁺ intake is high in these patients, or if they have renal insufficiency or selective hypoaldosteronism, this can lead to dangerous hyperkalaemia.

Other causes of hyperkalaemia

- *Artefact* This is the most common cause of hyperkalaemia. When red cells, or occasionally white cells or platelets, are left in contact with plasma or serum for too long, K⁺ leaks from the cells. In any blood specimen that does not have its plasma or serum separated from the cells within about 3 h, K⁺ concentration is likely to be spuriously high. Blood specimens collected into potassium EDTA, an anti-coagulant widely used for haematological specimens, have greatly increased plasma K⁺. Sometimes, doctors decant part of a blood specimen initially collected by mistake into potassium EDTA into another container, and send this for biochemical analysis. A clue to the source of this artefact, which may increase plasma K⁺ to 'lethal' levels (e.g. >8 mmol/L), is an accompanying very low plasma calcium, due to chelation of Ca^{2+} with EDTA.
- *Pseudohyperkalaemia:* Pseudohyperkalaemia can occur in acute and chronic myeloproliferative disorders, chronic lymphocytic leukaemia and severe thrombocytosis as a result of cell lysis during venepuncture, or if there is any delay in the separation of plasma following specimen collection, since there are large numbers of abnormally fragile white cells present.

CASE 2.5

A young man was trapped underneath a car in a road traffic accident, and suffered multiple fractures. Despite adequate fluid intake over the next 36 h, he was noted to be oliguric. The following results were obtained:

Serum	Result	Reference ranges (adult male)
Urea	22.1	2.5–6.6 mmol/L
Creatinine	214	64–111 μmol/L
Na$^+$	133	135–145 mmol/L
K$^+$	6.1	3.6–5.0 mmol/L

Why is the potassium high?

Comments: The crush injuries, with associated rhabdomyolysis, may have caused hyperkalaemia for at least two reasons: (1) release of K$^+$ from the damaged muscle, and (2) acute renal failure caused by release of myoglobin, which is filtered at the glomerulus but precipitates in the distal nephron. This impairs the ability of the kidney to excrete K$^+$.

 CASE 2.6

A 64-year-old man was admitted on a Sunday for an elective operation on his nasal sinuses; his previous hospital notes were not available. He appeared to be fit for operation on clinical examination, and his preoperative ECG was normal, but the following results were obtained on a blood specimen analysed as part of the routine pre-operative assessment:

How would you interpret the hyperkalaemia in relation to the findings on clinical examination and the normal ECG recording? Would your comments be influenced by the information that became available later that day, when the patient's medical records were received, that he had chronic lymphocytic leukaemia?

Serum	Result	Reference ranges (adult male)
Creatinine	93	64–111 μmol/L
Na$^+$	135	135–145 mmol/L
K$^+$	8.8	3.6–5.0 mmol/L
Total CO$_2$	28	22–30 mmol/L

Comments: The ECG changes that are associated with hyperkalaemia are not correlated closely with the level of plasma K$^+$, but it would be most unlikely for the ECG to be normal in a patient whose plasma K$^+$ was 8.8 mmol/L. It is much more likely that the hyperkalaemia was an artefact caused by release of K$^+$ from blood cells (in this case from lymphocytes).

Other investigations in disordered K$^+$ metabolism

- *Urine* K$^+$ measurements may be of help in determining the source of K$^+$ depletion in patients with unexplained hypokalaemia, but are otherwise of little value. A 24-h urine collection should be made. If the patient is Na$^+$ depleted, this will induce aldosterone secretion, making the results difficult or impossible to interpret, so urine Na$^+$ should also be checked to ensure this is adequate.
- *Plasma total CO$_2$* (see Chapter 3: Total CO$_2$) may prove helpful in the investigation of disorders of K$^+$ balance, since metabolic acidosis and metabolic alkalosis are commonly associated with abnormalities of K$^+$ homeostasis. It is rarely necessary to assess acid–base status fully when investigating disturbances of K$^+$ metabolism; plasma total CO$_2$ often suffices.
- Other investigations may be indicated by the history of the patient's illness and the findings on clinical examination. Hypomagnesaemia may be associated with hypokalaemia, so Mg^{2+} concentration should be checked in cases of prolonged or unexplained hypokalaemia.

Fluid and electrolyte balance in surgical patients

Accidental and operative trauma produce several metabolic effects. These include breakdown of protein, release of K$^+$ from cells and a consequent K$^+$ deficit due to urinary loss, temporary retention of water, use of glycogen reserves, gluconeogenesis, mobilisation of fat reserves and a tendency to ketosis that sometimes progresses to a metabolic acidosis. Hormonal responses include increased secretion of adrenal corticosteroids, with temporary abolition of negative feedback control and increased secretion of aldosterone and vasopressin.

These metabolic responses to trauma are physiological and appropriate. They are the reason why post-operative states are such frequent causes of temporary disturbances in electrolyte metabolism. Most

Table 2.10 Composition of intravenous fluids.

	Na⁺ (mmol/L)	K⁺ (mmol/L)	Cl⁻ (mmol/L)	Osmolality (mosm/L)
Plasma	135–145	3.6–5.0	95–107	280–296
0.9% ('normal') saline	154	0	154	308
5% dextrose	0	0	0	278
Dextrose 4%, saline 0.18%	30	0	30	283
Ringer's lactate	130	4	109	273
Hartmann's	131	5	111	275

patients after major surgery have a temporarily impaired ability to excrete a water load or a Na⁺ load; they also have a plasma urea that is often raised due to tissue catabolism. Injudicious fluid therapy, especially in the first 48 h after operation, may 'correct' the chemical abnormalities, for example by lowering the plasma urea, but only by causing retention of fluid and the possibility of acute water intoxication.

Patients who present for emergency surgery with disturbances of water and electrolyte metabolism already developed should have the severity of the disturbances assessed and corrective measures instituted pre-operatively. This usually involves clinical assessment and the measurement of plasma urea, creatinine, Na⁺ and K⁺ as an emergency. Ideally, fluid and electrolyte disturbances should be corrected before surgery.

Patients admitted for major elective surgery, who may be liable to develop disturbances of water and electrolyte balance post-operatively, require pre-operative determination of baseline values for plasma urea, creatinine, Na⁺ and K⁺.

Post-operatively, any tendency for patients to develop disturbances of water and electrolyte balance can be minimised by regular clinical assessment. In addition to plasma 'electrolytes', fluid balance charts and measurement of 24-h urinary losses of Na⁺ and K⁺, or losses from a fistula, can provide information of value in calculating the approximate volume and composition of fluid needed to replace continuing losses.

Intravenous fluid administration

Fluid administration, whether oral or intravenous, may be required for normal daily maintenance, the replacement of abnormal losses, or for resuscitation. Food and fluids should be provided orally or enterally when possible, and any intravenous infusion should not be continued longer than necessary. Decisions regarding prescription of fluids should take the stress responses

described in the previous section into account as well as an assessment of any current excesses or deficits, normal maintenance requirements, and the volumes and compositions of any abnormal (e.g. intestinal) losses.

The most reliable assessment of patients' fluid status uses invasive cardiac monitoring, but this is unlikely to be practical except in the setting of intensive care. Under most circumstances fluid requirements are assessed and monitored by the usual clinical approaches of history, examination and laboratory measurements. Items of note in the history and examination are any abnormal losses or excesses, changes in weight, fluid balance charts, urine output, blood pressure, capillary refill, autonomic responses, skin turgor and dry mouth. Laboratory measurements include serum Na⁺, K⁺, HCO₃⁻ and Cl⁻ (the latter two on point of care blood gas machines) and urine Na⁺ (and possibly urine K⁺ and urea).

Normal daily maintenance requirements for an adult are 50–100 mmol of sodium, 40–80 mmol of potassium and 1.5–2.5 L of water. Historically these requirements have been met using a combination of 0.9% saline and 5% dextrose with added potassium as required (see Table 2.10). Current guidelines encourage the use of balanced salt solutions such as Hartmann's solutions or Ringer's lactate/acetate (see Further Reading), especially for the purposes of crystalloid fluid resuscitation or replacement of abnormal losses.

 ## FURTHER READING

National Institute of Health and Care Excellence (2013) Intravenous fluid therapy in adults in hospital. Clinical guideline [CG174]. NICE, London.

National Institute of Health and Care Excellence (2015) Clinical Knowledge Summary: Hyponatraemia. NICE, London.

Spasovski, G., Vanholder, R., Allolio, B. et al. (2014) Clinical practice guideline on diagnosis and treatment of hyponatraemia. *European Journal of Endocrinology* **170**, G1–G47.

3

Acid–base balance and oxygen transport

Learning objectives

To understand:

✔ acid-base homeostasis, its disorders and how they might be further investigated;

✔ oxygen transport and respiratory insufficiency.

Introduction

The hydrogen ion concentration of ECF is normally maintained within very close limits. To achieve this, each day the body must dispose of:

1 about 20000 mmol of CO_2 generated by tissue metabolism; CO_2 itself is not an acid, but combines with water to form the weak acid, carbonic acid;
2 about 40–80 mmol of nonvolatile acids, mainly sulphur-containing organic acids, which are excreted by the kidneys.

This chapter deals with the clinical disturbances that may arise in respiratory disorders, when gaseous exchange in the lung of O_2 or CO_2 or both is impaired, and in metabolic disorders when there is either an excessive production, or loss, of nonvolatile acid or an abnormality of excretion.

Transport of carbon dioxide

The CO_2 produced in tissue cells diffuses freely down a concentration gradient across the cell membrane into the ECF and red cells. This gradient is maintained because red blood cell metabolism is anaerobic, so that no CO_2 is produced there, and the concentration remains low. The following reactions then occur:

$$CO_2 + H_2O \leftrightarrow H_2CO_3 \qquad (3.1)$$

$$H_2CO_3 \leftrightarrow H^+ + HCO_3^- \qquad (3.2)$$

Reaction 3.1, the hydration of CO_2 to form carbonic acid (H_2CO_3), is slow, except in the presence of the catalyst carbonate dehydratase (also known as carbonic anhydrase). This limits its site in the blood mainly to erythrocytes, where carbonate dehydratase is located. Reaction 3.2, the ionisation of carbonic acid, then occurs rapidly and spontaneously. The H^+ ions are mainly buffered inside the red cell by haemoglobin (Hb). Hb is a more effective buffer when deoxygenated, so its buffering capacity increases as it passes through the capillary beds and gives up oxygen to the tissues. Bicarbonate ions, meanwhile, pass from the erythrocytes down their concentration gradient into plasma, in exchange for chloride ions to maintain electrical neutrality.

In the lungs, the P_{CO_2} in the alveoli is maintained at a low level by ventilation. The P_{CO_2} in the blood of the pulmonary capillaries is therefore higher than the P_{CO_2} in the alveoli, so the P_{CO_2} gradient is reversed. CO_2 diffuses into the alveoli down its concentration

---

Clinical Biochemistry Lecture Notes, Tenth Edition. Peter Rae, Mike Crane and Rebecca Pattenden.
© 2018 John Wiley & Sons Ltd. Published 2018 by John Wiley & Sons Ltd.
Companion website: www.lecturenoteseries.com/clinicalbiochemistry

gradient, and is excreted by the lungs. The above reaction sequence shifts to the left, carbonate dehydratase again catalysing Reaction 3.1, but this time in the reverse direction.

Renal mechanisms for HCO_3^- reabsorption and H^+ excretion

Glomerular filtrate contains the same concentration of HCO_3^- as plasma. At normal HCO_3^-, renal tubular mechanisms are responsible for reabsorbing virtually all this HCO_3^-. If this failed to occur, large amounts of HCO_3^- would be lost in the urine, resulting in an acidosis and reduction in the body's buffering capacity. In addition, the renal tubules are responsible for excreting 40–80 mmol of acid per day under normal circumstances. This will increase when there is an acidosis.

The mechanism of reabsorption of HCO_3^- is shown in Figure 3.1. HCO_3^- is not able to cross the luminal membrane of the renal tubular cells. H^+ is pumped from the tubular cell into the lumen, in exchange for Na^+. The H^+ combines with HCO_3^- to form H_2CO_3 in the lumen. This dissociates to give water and CO_2, which readily diffuses into the cell. In the cell, CO_2 recombines with water under the influence of carbonate dehydratase to give H_2CO_3. This dissociates to H^+ and HCO_3^-. The HCO_3^- then passes across the basal membrane of the cell into the interstitial fluid. This mechanism results in the reabsorption of filtered HCO_3^-, but no net excretion of H^+.

The net excretion of H^+ relies on the same renal tubular cell reactions as HCO_3^- reabsorption, but occurs after luminal HCO_3^- has been reabsorbed, and depends on the presence of other suitable buffers in the urine (Figure 3.2). The main urinary buffer is phosphate, most of which is present as HPO_4^{2-}, which can combine with H^+ to form $H_2PO_4^-$.

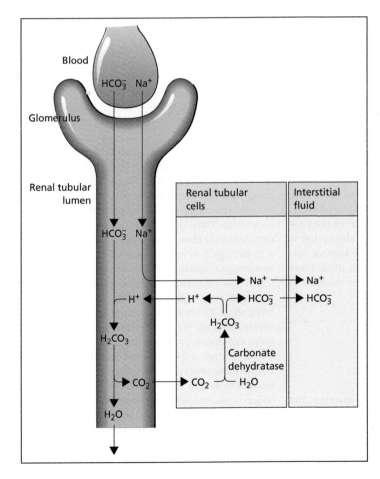

Figure 3.1 Reabsorption of bicarbonate in the renal tubule.

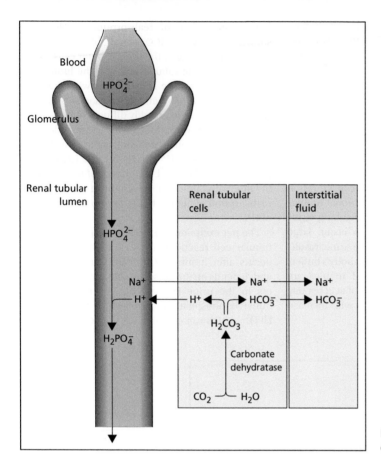

Figure 3.2 Renal hydrogen ion excretion.

Ammonia can also act as a urinary buffer, and is formed by the deamination of glutamine in renal tubular cells under the influence of the enzyme glutaminase. Ammonia readily diffuses across the cell membrane into the tubular lumen, where it combines with H^+ to form NH_4^+. This does not pass across cell membranes, so passive reabsorption is prevented. Glutaminase is induced in chronic acidoses, stimulating increased ammonia production and therefore increased H^+ excretion in the form of NH_4^+ ions.

Buffering of hydrogen ions

The lungs and the kidneys together maintain the overall acid–base balance. However, the ECF needs to be protected against rapid changes in H^+ concentration. This is achieved by various buffer systems. A buffer system consists of a weak (incompletely dissociated) acid in equilibrium with its conjugate base and H^+. The capacity of a buffer for H^+ is related to its concentration and the position of its equilibrium, being most effective at the H^+ concentration at which the acid and conjugate base are present in equal concentrations. Thus, Hb and plasma proteins act as efficient buffers in blood, since they are abundant, and at a physiological H^+ of approximately 40 nmol/L have side groups that exist in an appropriate equilibrium. At this H^+, the bicarbonate buffer system has an equilibrium that is far removed from the ideal, with HCO_3^- being about 20 times greater than H_2CO_3. However, the effectiveness of the bicarbonate system is greatly enhanced *in vivo* by the fact that H_2CO_3 is readily produced or disposed of by interconversion with CO_2. Furthermore, physiological control mechanisms act on this buffer system to maintain both P_{CO_2} and HCO_3^- within limits, and hence to control H^+.

Any physiological buffer system could be used to investigate and define acid–base status, but the H_2CO_3 / HCO_3^- buffer system is the most appropriate for this purpose, due to its physiological importance.

The Henderson equation simply applies the law of mass action to this buffer system, to give

$$[H^+] = K \times [H_2CO_3]/[HCO_3^-]. \qquad (3.3)$$

The H_2CO_3 term can be replaced by SP_{CO_2}, where S is the solubility coefficient of CO_2, since H_2CO_3 is in equilibrium with dissolved CO_2. Substituting numerical values, at $37\,°C$, this equation becomes

$$[H^+] = 180 \times [P_{CO_2}]/[HCO_3^-] \qquad (3.4)$$

(where H^+ is measured in nmol/L, P_{CO_2} in kilopascals (kPa) and HCO_3^- in mmol/L).

The changes discussed above are caused by changes in the equilibria of chemical reactions, and must be distinguished from the acid–base changes that occur as a result of respiratory or renal physiological mechanisms operating to return plasma H^+ towards normal. For example, if there is a rise in P_{CO_2}, this will be reflected immediately by a rise in both plasma H^+ and HCO_3^- due to a shift to the right in Reactions 3.1 and 3.2 above. The concentrations of H^+ and HCO_3^- are very different, H^+ being measured in nanomoles per litre while HCO_3^- is measured in millimoles per litre. The same rise in each may therefore result in a substantial relative increase in the concentration of H^+, but a relatively imperceptible increase in that of HCO_3^-. Only after several hours would the effect of physiological renal compensatory changes become evident.

Investigating acid–base balance

The acid–base status of a patient can be fully characterised by measuring H^+ concentration and P_{CO_2} in arterial or arterialised capillary blood specimens; HCO_3^- is then obtained by calculation (Equation 3.4). Although standard bicarbonate, and base excess or deficit are still sometimes reported, these derived values are not necessary for the understanding of acid–base disturbances.

Collection and transport of specimens

Arterial blood specimens are the most appropriate for assessing acid–base status. However, unless an arterial cannula is *in situ*, these specimens may be difficult to obtain for repeated assessment of patients whose clinical condition is changing rapidly. Arterialised capillary blood specimens are also widely used, especially in infants and children. It is essential for the capillary blood to flow freely, and collection of satisfactory samples may be impossible if there is peripheral vasoconstriction or the blood flow is sluggish.

Patients must be relaxed, and their breathing pattern should have settled after any temporary disturbance (e.g. due to insertion of an arterial cannula) before specimens are collected. Some patients may hyperventilate temporarily because they are apprehensive.

Blood is collected in syringes or capillary tubes that contain sufficient heparin to act as an anti-coagulant; excess heparin, which is acidic, must be avoided. If ionised Ca^{2+} is to be measured on the same specimen, as is possible with some instruments, calcium-balanced heparin must be used. Specimens must be free of air bubbles, since these will equilibrate with the sample causing a rise in P_{O_2} and a fall in P_{CO_2}.

Acid–base measurements should be performed immediately after the sample has been obtained, or the specimen should be chilled until analysis. Otherwise, glycolysis (with the production of lactic acid) occurs, and the acid–base composition of the blood alters rapidly. Specimens chilled in iced water can have their analysis delayed for as long as 4 h. However, the clinical reasons that gave rise to the need for acid–base measurements usually demand more rapid answers.

Temperature effects

Acid–base measurements are nearly always made at $37\,°C$, but some patients may have body temperatures that are higher or lower than $37\,°C$. Equations are available to relate H^+ concentration, P_{CO_2} and P_{O_2} determined at $37\,°C$, to 'equivalent' values that correspond to the patient's body temperature. However, reference ranges for acid–base data have only been established by most laboratories for measurements made at $37\,°C$. Analytical results adjusted to values that would have been obtained at the patient's temperature, according to these equations, may therefore be difficult to interpret. If treatment aimed at reducing an acid–base disturbance (e.g. bicarbonate administration) is given to a severely hypothermic patient, the effects of the treatment should be monitored frequently by repeating the acid–base measurements (at $37\,°C$).

Disturbances of acid–base status

Acid–base disorders fall into two main categories:

- *Respiratory disorders:* A primary defect in ventilation affects the P_{CO_2}
- *Metabolic disorders:* The primary defect may be the production of nonvolatile acids, or ingestion of

Table 3.1 Illustrative data for patients with simple disturbances of acid–base balance.

	H⁺ (nmol/L)	P_{CO_2} (kPa)	Plasma HCO₃ (mmol/L)	Plasma total CO₂ (mmol/L)
Reference ranges (adult males)	37–45	4.67–6.40	21–29	22–30
Respiratory acidosis	58	9.3	31	33
Respiratory alkalosis	29	3.2	19	20
Metabolic acidosis	72	3.2	8	11
Metabolic alkalosis	28	6.0	39	43

substances that give rise to them, in excess of the kidney's ability to excrete these substances. Alternatively, the primary defect may be the loss of H⁺ from the body, or it may be the loss or retention of HCO₃⁻.

Acid–base status can be understood and described on the basis of the relationships represented by Reactions 3.1 and 3.2, and consideration of the Henderson equation. The following discussion is restricted mainly to consideration of simple acid–base disturbances, in which there is a single primary disturbance, normally accompanied by compensatory physiological changes that usually tend to correct plasma H⁺ towards normal. We shall not consider mixed disturbances, where two or more primary simple disturbances are present, in any detail. Sets of illustrative acid–base results for patients with the four categories of simple disorders of acid–base status are given in Table 3.1.

Respiratory acidosis

This is caused by CO_2 retention due to hypoventilation (Table 3.2). It may accompany intrinsic lung

disease, or defects in the control of ventilation, or diseases affecting the nerve supply or muscles of the chest wall or diaphragm, or disorders affecting the ribcage.

In acute respiratory acidosis, a rise in P_{CO_2} causes the equilibria in Reactions 3.1 and 3.2 to shift to the right, as a result of which plasma H⁺ and HCO₃⁻ concentrations both increase (although, as explained above, because of the large difference in their basal concentrations, the immediate change in HCO₃⁻ will be small or imperceptible). Equilibration of H⁺ with body buffer systems limits the potential rise in H⁺, and a new steady state is achieved within a few minutes.

Unless the cause of the acute episode of acidosis is resolved, or is treated quickly and successfully, renal compensation causes HCO₃⁻ retention and H⁺ excretion, thereby returning plasma H⁺ towards normal while HCO₃⁻ increases. These compensatory changes can occur over a period of hours to days, by which time a new steady state is achieved and the daily renal H⁺ excretion and HCO₃⁻ retention return to normal. The patient then has the acid–base results of chronic respiratory acidosis.

Table 3.2 Respiratory acidosis.

Mechanism	Examples of causes
Alveolar P_{CO_2} increased due to defect in respiratory function	Pulmonary disease – chronic bronchitis, severe asthma, pulmonary oedema, fibrosis Mechanical disorders – thoracic trauma, pneumothorax, myopathies
Alveolar P_{CO_2} increased due to defect in respiratory control mechanisms	CNS disease – stroke, trauma CNS depression – anaesthetics, opiates, severe hypoxia Neurological disease – motor neuron disease, spinal cord lesions, poliomyelitis

CASE 3.1

A 75-year-old widow, a known heavy smoker and chronic bronchitic, and a patient in a long-stay hospital, became very breathless and wheezy. The senior nurse called the doctor who was on duty, but he was unable to come at once because he was treating another emergency. He asked the nurse to start the patient on 24% oxygen. One hour later, when the doctor arrived, he examined the patient and took an arterial specimen to determine her blood gases. The results were as follows:

Blood gas analysis	Result	Reference ranges (adult female)
H^+	97	37–45 nmol/L
P_{CO_2}	21.8	4.27–6.00 kPa
HCO_3^-	42	21–29 mmol/L
P_{O_2}	22.5	11.1–14.4 kPa

How would you describe the patient's acid–base status? Do you think that she was breathing 24% oxygen?

Comments: This patient had a respiratory acidosis. Although she gave a long history of chest complaints, the history of her recent illness was short, and it was most unlikely that renal compensation could have accounted in that short time for the very high arterial plasma HCO_3^-. From the arterial P_{O_2} result, it was apparent that the patient was breathing a much higher concentration of O_2 than 24%. Atmospheric pressure is approximately 100 kPa, so the P_{O_2} of inspired air (in kilopascals) is numerically equal, approximately, to the percentage of O_2 inspired. Further, it is approximately true that:

Inspired P_{O_2} = alveolar P_{O_2} + alveolar P_{CO_2}

Since alveolar P_{CO_2} equals arterial P_{CO_2}, this equation can be rewritten as:

Inspired P_{O_2} = alveolar P_{O_2} + arterial P_{CO_2}

Alveolar P_{O_2} *must* be greater than arterial P_{O_2}, so it was possible to conclude that the patient must have been breathing O_2 at a concentration of at least 40%. On checking, it was found that the wrong mask had been fitted, and that O_2 was being delivered at 60%.

It was concluded that the patient had an underlying chronic (compensated) respiratory acidosis with CO_2 retention (type II respiratory failure), and that the administration of oxygen at high concentration had removed the hypoxic drive to ventilation, thereby superimposing an acute respiratory acidosis on the underlying chronic acid–base disturbance.

Respiratory alkalosis

This is due to hyperventilation (Table 3.3). The reduced P_{CO_2} that results causes the equilibrium positions of Reactions 3.1 and 3.2 to move to the left. As a result, plasma H^+ and HCO_3^- both fall, although the relative change in HCO_3^- is small.

If conditions giving rise to a low P_{CO_2} persist for more than a few hours, the kidneys increase HCO_3^- excretion and reduce H^+ excretion. Plasma H^+ returns

Table 3.3 Respiratory alkalosis.

Mechanism	Examples of causes
Alveolar P_{CO_2} lowered due to hyperventilation	Voluntary hyperventilation, mechanical ventilation Reflex hyperventilation – chest wall disease, decreased pulmonary compliance Stimulation of respiratory centre – pain, fever, salicylate overdose, hepatic encephalopathy, hypoxia

towards normal, whereas plasma HCO_3^- falls further. A new steady state will be achieved in hours to days if the respiratory disorder persists. It is unusual for chronic respiratory alkalosis to be severe, and plasma HCO_3^- rarely falls below 12 mmol/L.

Metabolic acidosis

Increased production or decreased excretion of H^+ leads to accumulation of H^+ within the ECF (Table 3.4). The extra H^+ ions combine with HCO_3^- to form H_2CO_3, disturbing the equilibrium in Reaction 3.2, with a shift to the left. However, since there is no ventilatory abnormality, any increase in plasma H_2CO_3 concentration is only transient, as the related slight increase in dissolved CO_2 is immediately excreted by the lungs. The net effect is that a new equilibrium rapidly establishes itself in which the product, $[H^+]\times[HCO_3^-]$,

Table 3.4 Metabolic acidosis.

Mechanism	Examples of causes
Increased H^+ production in excess of body's excretory capacity	Ketoacidosis – diabetic, alcoholic Lactic acidosis – hypoxic, shock, drugs, inherited metabolic disease Poisoning – methanol, salicylate
Failure to excrete H^+ at the normal rate	Acute and chronic renal failure Distal renal tubular acidosis
Loss of HCO_3^-	Loss from the GI tract – severe diarrhoea, pancreatic fistula Loss in the urine – ureteroenterostomy, proximal renal tubular acidosis, carbonate dehydratase inhibitors (acetazolamide)

remains unchanged, since H_2CO_3 concentration is unchanged. In consequence, the rise in plasma H^+ is limited, but at the expense of a fall in HCO_3^-, which has been consumed in this process and may be very low. Its availability for further buffering becomes progressively more limited. Less often, metabolic acidosis arises from loss of HCO_3^- from the renal system or GI tract. Typically in these conditions, HCO_3^- does not fall to such a great extent, rarely being less than 15 mmol/L.

The rise in ECF H^+ stimulates the respiratory centre, causing compensatory hyperventilation. As a result, due to the fall in P_{CO_2}, plasma H^+ returns towards normal, while plasma HCO_3^- falls even further. It is quite common for patients with metabolic acidosis to have very low plasma HCO_3^-, often below 10 mmol/L. Plasma H^+ levels will not, however, become completely normal through this mechanism, since it is the low H^+ that drives the compensatory hyperventilation – as the H^+ falls, the hyperventilation becomes correspondingly reduced. In addition, if renal function is normal, H^+ will be excreted by the kidney.

 CASE 3.2

A young woman was admitted in a confused and restless condition. History taking was not easy, but it seemed that she had been becoming progressively unwell over the preceding week or two. Acid–base analysis was performed and results were as follows:

Blood gas analysis	Result	Reference ranges (adult female)
H^+	78	37–45 nmol/L
P_{CO_2}	3.2	4.27–6.00 kPa
HCO_3^-	6	21–29 mmol/L
P_{O_2}	11.8	11.1–14.4 kPa

What is her acid–base disorder? What are the most likely causes, and what investigations could narrow this down?

Comments: She has a metabolic acidosis. Despite the long list of possible causes of metabolic acidosis, the most common causes are relatively few, and are DKA, renal failure, salicylate overdose and lactic acidosis. Usually these can be differentiated on the basis of the history; by measuring urea and electrolytes (U&Es) and glucose (and salicylate if indicated); and performing urinalysis (using a dipstick, and looking especially for ketones). Lactate can also be measured if required, but is often not necessary. This woman was a newly presenting type 1 diabetic.

Table 3.5 Metabolic alkalosis.

Mechanism	Examples of causes
Saline-responsive	H^+ loss from GI tract – vomiting, nasogastric drainage
	H^+ loss in urine – thiazide diuretics (especially in cardiac failure), nephrotic syndrome
	Alkali administration – sodium bicarbonate
Saline-unresponsive	Associated with hypertension – primary and secondary aldosteronism, Cushing's syndrome
	Not associated with hypertension – severe K^+ depletion, Bartter's syndrome

Metabolic alkalosis

This is most often due to prolonged vomiting, but may be due to other causes (Table 3.5). The loss of H^+ upsets the equilibrium in Reaction 3.2, causing it to shift to the right as H_2CO_3 dissociates to form H^+ (which is being lost) and HCO_3^-. However, because there is no primary disturbance of ventilation, plasma HCO_3^- remains constant, with the net effect that plasma H^+ falls and HCO_3^- rises. Respiratory compensation (i.e. hypoventilation) for the alkalosis is usually minimal, since any resulting rise in P_{CO_2} or fall in P_{O_2} will be a potent stimulator of ventilation. HCO_3^- is freely filtered at the glomerulus, and is therefore available for excretion in the urine, which would rapidly tend to restore the acid–base status towards normal. The continuing presence of an alkalosis means there is inappropriate reabsorption of filtered HCO_3^- from the distal nephron. This can be due to ECF volume depletion, potassium deficiency or mineralocorticoid excess.

 CASE 3.3

A 70-year-old man was admitted to a hospital as an emergency. He gave a history of dyspepsia and epigastric pain extending over many years. He had never sought medical attention for this. One week prior to admission, he had started to vomit, and had since vomited frequently, being unable to keep down any food. He was clinically dehydrated, and had marked epigastric tenderness, but no sign of abdominal rigidity. Analysis of venous and arterial blood specimens gave the following results:

Serum	Result	Reference ranges (adult male)
Urea	17.3	2.5–6.6 mmol/L
Na$^+$	131	135–145 mmol/L
K$^+$	2.2	3.6–5.0 mmol/L
Creatinine	250	64–111 µmol/L

Blood gas analysis	Result	Reference ranges (adult male)
H$^+$	26	37–45 nmol/L
P_{CO_2}	6.2	4.67–6.40 kPa
HCO$_3^-$	44	21–29 mmol/L
P_{O_2}	9.5	11.1–14.4 kPa

How would you describe this patient's acid–base status? What might have caused the various abnormalities revealed by these results? Why is the plasma K$^+$ so low?

Comments: The patient had a metabolic alkalosis. This was caused by his persistent vomiting, the vomit being likely to consist almost entirely of gastric contents. In this age group, the cause could be carcinoma of the stomach or chronic peptic ulceration with associated scarring and fibrosis, leading to obstruction of gastric outflow.

Gastric juice K$^+$ is about 10 mmol/L. Also, in the presence of an alkalosis, K$^+$ shifts from the ECF into cells. Furthermore, dehydration causes secondary hyperaldosteronism in order to maintain ECF volume, and Na$^+$ is avidly retained by the kidneys in exchange for H$^+$ and K$^+$. Patients such as this man, despite having an alkalosis and despite being hypokalaemic, often excrete an acid urine containing large amounts of K$^+$.

Interpretation of results of acid–base assessment

Results of acid–base measurements must be considered in the light of clinical findings, and the results of other chemical tests (e.g. plasma creatinine, urea, Na$^+$ and K$^+$); other types of investigation (e.g. radiological) may also be important.

Interpretation of acid–base results is based on the equilibria represented by Reactions 3.1 and 3.2 and the related Henderson equation. After reviewing the

clinical findings, acid–base results can be considered in the following order:

- Plasma H$^+$. Reference range 37–45 nmol/L.
- Plasma P_{CO_2}. Reference ranges 4.67–6.40 kPa (adult male), 4.27–6.00 kPa (adult female).
- Plasma HCO$_3^-$. Reference range 21–29 mmol/L.

This procedure immediately identifies those patients in whom there is an uncompensated acidosis or alkalosis, and is the starting point for their further classification, as considered below.

Alternatively, the results can be plotted on a diagram of H$^+$ concentration against P_{CO_2} (Figure 3.3). In this diagram, simple acid–base disturbances fall within bands of results, as shown. Results falling between the bands due to metabolic acidosis and respiratory alkalosis, or between those due to respiratory acidosis and metabolic alkalosis need careful consideration. These may represent either a combination of two acid–base disorders, or compensation for a single disorder.

Plasma H$^+$ is increased

The patient has an acidosis. The P_{CO_2} result is considered next, as follows:

- P_{CO_2} is decreased. The patient has a *metabolic acidosis*. The reduced P_{CO_2} is due to hyperventilation, the physiological compensatory response (e.g. overbreathing in patients with DKA). Plasma HCO$_3^-$ is reduced in these patients, sometimes to below 10 mmol/L.
- P_{CO_2} is normal. The patient has an *uncompensated metabolic acidosis*. Plasma HCO$_3^-$ will be decreased. However, the normal compensatory response should lower the P_{CO_2} in patients with a simple metabolic acidosis (see above), so there is a co-existing respiratory pathology causing CO$_2$ retention – in other words, there is a simultaneous respiratory acidosis. This combination of results is seen, for example, in patients with combined respiratory and circulatory failure, such as occurs during a cardiac arrest.
- P_{CO_2} is increased. The patient has a *respiratory acidosis*. The pattern of results will depend on whether the respiratory acidosis is acute or chronic:
  - *Acute* The patient will have a high plasma H$^+$ and a high P_{CO_2}, with a slightly raised plasma HCO$_3^-$, since the renal response has not yet had time to develop.
  - *Chronic* The patient will have a normal or slightly raised plasma H$^+$, a high P_{CO_2} and a markedly raised plasma HCO$_3^-$ concentration, due to renal retention of HCO$_3^-$.

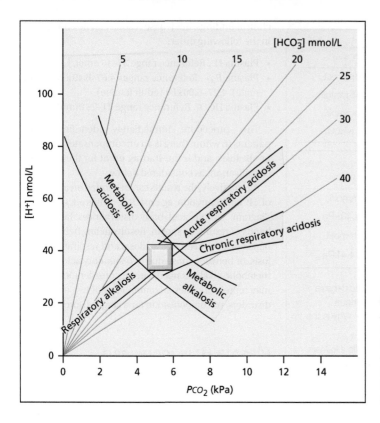

Figure 3.3 On this plot of H⁺ against P_{CO_2}, lines of equal HCO_3^- radiate from the origin, increasing in value towards the bottom right corner. The bands of values marked show the expected results in patients with simple acid–base disorders.

Plasma H⁺ is decreased

The patient has an alkalosis. The P_{CO_2} result should be assessed next:

- P_{CO_2} is decreased. The patient has a *respiratory alkalosis*. If this is a simple disturbance, plasma HCO_3^- will be somewhat decreased (not below ~12 mmol/L).
- P_{CO_2} is normal. The patient has an *uncompensated metabolic alkalosis*, and the plasma HCO_3^- will be increased.
- P_{CO_2} is increased. The patient may have a metabolic alkalosis with some respiratory compensation. However, it is unlikely that this patient has a simple acid–base disturbance since significant hypoventilation is not often a marked feature of the compensatory response to a metabolic alkalosis. A more common explanation for a low plasma H⁺ and an increased P_{CO_2} is that the patient has a mixed acid–base disturbance, consisting of a metabolic alkalosis and a respiratory acidosis. Plasma HCO_3^- will also be increased.

Plasma H⁺ is normal

The patient either has no acid–base disturbance, or no net acid–base disturbance, as a result of one of the mechanisms described below. Considering the P_{CO_2} result next:

- P_{CO_2} is decreased. The patient most probably has a mixed acid–base disturbance consisting of a respiratory alkalosis and a metabolic acidosis. Both these types of acid–base disturbance cause a decreased plasma HCO_3^-, and the distinction can usually be made on clinical grounds. A fully compensated respiratory alkalosis is another possibility.
- P_{CO_2} is normal. There is no significant acid–base disturbance. Since both plasma H⁺ and P_{CO_2} are normal, plasma HCO_3^- must be normal; see 3.4.
- P_{CO_2} is increased. The patient either has a fully compensated respiratory acidosis, or there is a mixed acid–base disturbance consisting of a respiratory acidosis and a metabolic alkalosis. Both these possibilities give rise to increased plasma HCO_3^-, to over 30 mmol/L. They can usually be distinguished on clinical grounds.

Mixed acid–base disturbances

It may not always be possible to differentiate some mixed acid–base disturbances from simple ones by the scheme described above. For instance, some

CASE 3.4

An elderly man was brought into the A&E department after collapsing in the street. He was deeply comatose and cyanosed, with unrecordable blood pressure. The results of acid–base analysis were as follows:

Blood gas analysis	Result	Reference ranges (adult male)
H^+	124	37–45 nmol/L
P_{CO_2}	10.4	4.67–6.40 kPa
HCO_3^-	15.4	21–29 mmol/L
P_{O_2}	4.8	11.1–14.4 kPa

What is his acid–base status? What are the possible causes?

Comments: He has a combined metabolic and respiratory acidosis. The combination of the elevated H^+ and P_{CO_2} may initially suggest that he has respiratory acidosis, but the bicarbonate would not be reduced in a simple respiratory acidosis. This means that there is an additional component of metabolic acidosis present. The same conclusion can be reached by plotting these results on Figure 3.3. Results of this sort are seen in patients with markedly impaired circulatory and respiratory function, such as that which occurs after a cardiac arrest. This man had a large abdominal aortic aneurysm that had ruptured.

patients with chronic renal failure (which causes a primary metabolic acidosis) may also have chronic obstructive airways disease (which causes a primary respiratory acidosis). Plasma H^+ will be increased in these patients, but the results for plasma P_{CO_2} and HCO_3^- cannot be predicted. The history and clinical findings must be taken into account.

Plotting the results on a diagram of H^+ against P_{CO_2} (Figure 3.3) may help. Results falling between the bands of respiratory and metabolic acidoses are due to a combination of these two conditions. Similarly, results between the bands due to respiratory and metabolic alkaloses are due to a combination of these.

Other investigations in acid–base assessment

The full characterisation of acid–base status requires arterial or arterialised capillary blood samples, since venous blood P_{CO_2} (even if 'arterialised') bears no constant relationship to alveolar P_{CO_2}. However, other investigations can provide some useful information.

Total CO_2

This test, performed on venous plasma or serum, includes contributions from HCO_3^-, H_2CO_3, dissolved CO_2 and carbamino compounds. However, about 95% of 'total CO_2' is contributed by HCO_3^-. Total CO_2 measurements have the advantages of ease of sample collection and suitability for measurement in large numbers, but they cannot define a patient's acid–base status, since plasma H^+ and P_{CO_2} are both unknown. For example, an increased plasma total CO_2 concentration may be due to either a respiratory acidosis or a metabolic alkalosis. However, when interpreted in the light of clinical findings, plasma total CO_2 can often give an adequate assessment of whether an acid–base disturbance is present and, if one is present, provide an indication of its severity. This is particularly true when there is a metabolic disturbance.

 CASE 3.5

A 60-year-old man with type 1 diabetes experienced severe central chest pain, associated with nausea. He refused to let his wife call the doctor, but went to bed and, since he felt too ill to eat, he stopped taking his insulin. Two days later, he had another episode of chest pain and became breathless. His wife called an ambulance, and he was admitted. He was shocked, with central cyanosis, pulse 120/min, blood pressure 66/34, respiratory rate 30/min. An ECG demonstrated a large anterior myocardial infarct. The results of acid–base analyses were as follows:

Blood gas analysis	Result	Reference ranges (adult male)
H^+	39	37–45 nmol/L
P_{CO_2}	2	4.67–6.40 kPa
HCO_3^-	9.4	21–29 mmol/L
P_{O_2}	7	11.1–14.4 kPa

What is his acid–base status, and what may have caused it?

Comments: The 'normal' H+ concentration in someone so obviously very ill may initially appear surprising, but the P_{CO_2} is very low. He has a combination of metabolic acidosis (causing elevated H+ and low P_{CO_2}) and respiratory alkalosis (causing low H+ and low P_{CO_2}). The combination explains the normal H+ with very low P_{CO_2}. The metabolic acidosis could be due to DKA (caused by inappropriately stopping insulin in the face of his severe illness) and/or to lactic acidosis (caused by impaired tissue perfusion because of his circulatory failure). The respiratory alkalosis is due to hyperventilation caused by pulmonary oedema and/or hypoxia and/or anxiety.

Anion gap

The anion gap is obtained from plasma electrolyte results, as follows:

$$AG = \left([Na^+]+[K^+]\right)-\left([Cl^-]+[total\ CO_2]\right)$$

The difference between the cations and the anions represents the unmeasured anions, or anion gap, and includes proteins, phosphate, sulphate and lactate ions. The anion gap may be increased because of an increase in unmeasured anions. This may be of help in narrowing the differential diagnosis in a patient with metabolic acidosis (Table 3.6). In the presence of metabolic acidosis, a raised anion gap points to the cause being excessive production of hydrogen ions or failure to excrete them. As the acid accumulates in the ECF (e.g. in DKA), the HCO_3^- is titrated and replaced with unmeasured anions (e.g. acetoacetate) and the anion gap increases. In contrast, if the cause is a loss of HCO_3^- (e.g. renal tubular acidosis), there is a compensatory increase in Cl^- and the anion gap remains unchanged (Table 3.4, and see Chapter 3: Plasma chloride).

Plasma chloride

The causes of metabolic acidosis are sometimes divided into those with an increased anion gap (Table 3.6) and those with a normal anion gap. In the latter group, the fall in plasma total CO_2 that accompanies the metabolic acidosis is associated with an approximately equal rise in plasma Cl^-. Patients with metabolic acidosis and a normal anion gap are sometimes described as having hyperchloraemic acidosis.

Increased plasma Cl^-, out of proportion to any accompanying increase in plasma Na^+, may occur in patients with chronic renal failure, ureteric transplants into the colon or renal tubular acidosis, or in patients treated with carbonic anhydrase inhibitors. Increased plasma Cl^- may also occur in patients who develop respiratory alkalosis as a result of prolonged assisted ventilation. An iatrogenic cause of increased plasma Cl^- is the IV administration of excessive amounts of isotonic or 'physiological' saline, which contains 155 mmol/L NaCl.

Patients who lose large volumes of gastric secretion (e.g. due to pyloric stenosis) often show a disproportionately marked fall in plasma Cl^- concentration compared with any hyponatraemia that may develop. They develop metabolic alkalosis, and are often dehydrated.

Table 3.6 Causes of an increased anion gap.

Mechanism	Examples of causes
Plasma unmeasured anions increased with or without changes in Na^+ and Cl^-	Some causes of metabolic acidosis – renal failure, lactic acidosis, DKA, salicylate overdose, methanol ingestion
Increase in plasma Na^+	Treatment with sodium salts, e.g. salts of some high-dose antibiotics such as carbenicillin; this increases plasma unmeasured anions
Artefact	Improper handling of specimens after collection, causing loss of CO_2

Treatment of acid–base disturbances

A thorough clinical assessment is the basis on which the results of acid–base analyses are interpreted and treatment initiated. When the nature of an acid–base disturbance has been defined, treatment should aim to correct the primary disorder and assist the physiological compensatory mechanisms. In some cases, more active intervention may be necessary (e.g. treatment with $NaHCO_3$). It is often possible to correct an acid–base disturbance by treatment aimed only at the causative condition (e.g. DKA is usually corrected without the administration of $NaHCO_3$). Where active treatment of the acid–base disturbance is necessary, it is usually for metabolic disturbances.

In metabolic acidosis, treatment with HCO_3^- is usually not indicated unless H^+ concentration is very high (e.g. >90 nmol/L), except for patients with proximal renal tubular acidosis, who lose HCO_3^- because of the primary defect.

In metabolic alkalosis, many patients inappropriately retain HCO_3^- because of volume depletion, potassium depletion or mineralocorticoid excess, perpetuating the alkalosis. These patients respond to the administration of isotonic saline. Nonresponders include patients with mineralocorticoid excess, either due to primary adrenal hyperfunction or due to those causes of secondary adrenal hyperfunction that are not due to hypovolaemia and ECF depletion. These include renal artery stenosis, magnesium deficiency and Bartter's syndrome. Treatment of these is directed at the primary disorder.

Oxygen transport

Oxygen delivery to tissues depends on the combination of their blood supply and the arterial O_2 content. In turn the O_2 content depends on the concentration of Hb and its saturation. Tissue hypoxia can therefore be caused not just by hypoxaemia, but also by impaired perfusion (e.g. because of reduced cardiac output or vasoconstriction), anaemia and the presence of abnormal Hb species. The full characterisation of the oxygen composition of a blood sample requires measurement of P_{O_2}, Hb concentration and percentage oxygen saturation. Hb measurements are widely available, and P_{O_2} is one of the measurements automatically performed by most blood gas analysers as part of the full acid–base assessment of patients. Hb saturation is measured using an oximeter within the laboratory, or using a pulse oximeter at the bedside. This comprises a probe which is attached to the patient's finger or earlobe.

Measurements of P_{O_2} in arterial blood (reference range 12–15 kPa) are important, and are often valuable in assessing the efficiency of oxygen therapy, when high P_{O_2} values may be found. Above a P_{O_2} of

CASE 3.6

The junior doctor first on call for the A&E department examined a 22-year-old woman who was having an acute attack of asthma. The patient was very distressed, so the doctor treated her with a nebulised bronchodilator immediately and returned 10 min later to examine her, when she was more settled and was breathing air. He decided to check the patient's arterial blood gases, the results of which were as follows:

Blood gas analysis	Result	Reference ranges (adult female)
H^+	44	37–45 nmol/L
P_{O_2}	6.0	4.27–6.00 kPa
HCO_3^-	27.0	21–29 mmol/L
P_{O_2}	10.2	11.1–14.4 kPa

The doctor asked the A&E consultant whether he could send the patient home. Would you consider that these results suggested that it would be safe to do so?

Comments: It would not be safe to send this patient home. In a moderately severe asthmatic attack, the ventilatory drive from hypoxia and from mechanical receptors in the chest normally results in a P_{CO_2} at or below the lower end of the reference range. A P_{CO_2} greater than this is a serious prognostic sign, indicative either of extensive 'shunting' of blood through areas of the lung that are underventilated because of bronchoconstriction or plugging with mucus, or of the patient becoming increasingly tired. A rising P_{CO_2} in an asthmatic attack is an indication for ventilating these patients.

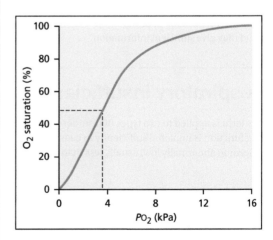

Figure 3.4 The oxygen dissociation curve of Hb. It is important to note that, above a P_{O_2} of approximately 9 kPa, Hb is over 95% saturated with O_2. Also shown in the figure is the value of the P_{O_2}, 3.8 kPa, that corresponds to 50% saturation with O_2; this value is called the P_{50} value.

10.5 kPa, however, Hb is almost fully saturated with O_2 (Figure 3.4), and further increases in P_{O_2} do not result in greater O_2 carriage. Conversely, as P_{O_2} drops, initially there is little reduction in O_2 carriage on Hb, but when it falls below about 8 kPa, saturation starts to fall rapidly. In addition, results of P_{O_2} measurements may be misleading in conditions where the oxygen-carrying capacity of blood is grossly impaired, as in severe anaemia, carbon monoxide poisoning and when abnormal Hb derivatives (e.g. methaemoglobin) are present. Measurement of both the blood Hb and the percentage oxygen saturation are required in addition to P_{O_2} under these circumstances.

Indications for full blood acid–base and oxygen measurements

The main indications for full acid–base assessment, coupled with P_{O_2} or oxygen saturation measurements, are in the investigation and management of patients with pulmonary disorders, severely ill patients in ICUs and patients in the operative and peri-operative periods of major surgery who may often be on assisted ventilation. Other important applications include the investigation and management of patients with vascular abnormalities involving the shunting of blood.

Full acid–base assessment is less essential in patients with metabolic acidosis or alkalosis, for whom measurements of plasma total CO_2 on venous blood may give sufficient information.

Respiratory insufficiency

This term is applied to two types of disorder in which lung function is impaired sufficiently to cause the P_{O_2} to become abnormally low, usually less than 8.0 kPa.

Type I: low P_{O_2} with normal or low P_{CO_2}

Hypoxia without hypercapnia occurs in patients in whom there is a preponderance of alveoli that are adequately perfused with blood, but inadequately ventilated. It occurs, for example, in emphysema, pulmonary oedema and asthma. Type II respiratory insufficiency can also occur in some of these conditions, if they are sufficiently severe.

In type I respiratory insufficiency, there is, in effect, a partial right-to-left shunt, bringing unoxygenated blood to the left side of the heart. Increased ventilation of the adequately perfused and ventilated alveoli is able to compensate for the tendency for the P_{CO_2} to rise. It cannot, however, restore the P_{O_2} to normal, since the blood perfusing the normal alveoli conveys Hb that is already nearly saturated with O_2.

Type II: low P_{O_2} with high P_{CO_2}

This combination means that there is hypoventilation. The cause may be central in origin, or due to airways obstruction, or it may be neuromuscular. There may be altered ventilation/perfusion relationships, with an excessive number of alveoli being inadequately perfused; this causes 'wasted' ventilation and an increase in 'dead space'.

Chronic obstructive airways disease is an important cause of type II respiratory insufficiency. It also occurs with mechanical defects in ventilation (e.g. chest injuries, myasthenia gravis). In severe asthma, if serial measurements show a rising P_{CO_2} and falling P_{O_2}, more intensive treatment is urgently needed.

Oxygen therapy

The most recent British guidelines for the administration of emergency oxygen emphasise that oxygen is a treatment for hypoxaemia, not breathlessness, since oxygen has not been shown to have any effect on the sensation of breathlessness in nonhypoxaemic patients. They stress the importance of oxygen saturation, measured by pulse oximetry, recommending that oxygen is administered to patients whose oxygen saturation falls below target ranges. These are 94–98% for most acutely ill patients, and 82–92% for patients at risk of hypercapnic respiratory failure. Oxygen therapy should be adjusted to achieve saturations within these target ranges, rather than using fixed doses. Most therapy will use nasal cannulae rather than masks.

 FURTHER READING

British Thoracic Society Emergency Oxygen Guideline Group (2008) Guidelines for emergency oxygen use in adult patients. *Thorax* **63** (Suppl VI), vi1–vi68.

4

Renal disease

Learning objectives

To understand:

✔ the means and limitations of assessments of glomerular function;

✔ the assessment of renal tubular function;

✔ the definitions and further investigation of acute kidney injury and chronic kidney disease.

Introduction

The kidneys are paired retroperitoneal organs each comprising about 1 million nephrons, which act as independent functional units. They have multiple physiological functions, which can be broadly categorised as the excretion of waste products, the homeostatic regulation of the ECF volume and composition, and endocrine. In order to achieve these functions, they receive a rich blood supply, amounting to about 25% of the cardiac output.

The excretory and homeostatic functions are achieved through filtration at the glomerulus and tubular reabsorption. The glomeruli act as filters which are permeable to water and low molecular weight substances, but impermeable to macromolecules. This impermeability is determined by both size and charge, with proteins smaller than albumin (68 kDa) being filtered, and positively charged molecules being filtered more readily than those with a negative charge. The filtration rate is determined by the differences in hydrostatic and oncotic pressures between the glomerular capillaries and the lumen of the nephron, by the nature of the glomerular basement membrane and by the total glomerular area available for filtration. The total glomerular area available reflects the total number of functioning nephrons. The total volume of the glomerular filtrate amounts to about 170 L/day (12 times the typical ECF volume), and has a composition similar to plasma except that it is almost free of protein.

The renal tubules are presented with this volume of water, most of which needs to be reabsorbed, containing a complex mixture of ions and small molecules, some of which have to be retained and some in a regulated manner; small amounts of small proteins which are reabsorbed and catabolised; and metabolic waste products such as urea, creatinine and sulphate ions, which are excreted. The proximal convoluted tubule is responsible for the obligatory reabsorption of much of the glomerular filtrate, with further reabsorption in the distal convoluted tubule being subject to homeostatic control mechanisms. In the proximal tubule, energy-dependent mechanisms reabsorb about 75% of the filtered Na^+ and all of the K^+, HCO_3^-, amino acids and glucose, with an iso-osmotic amount of water. In the ascending limb of the loop of Henle, Cl^- is pumped out into the interstitial fluid, generating the medullary hypertonicity on which the ability to excrete concentrated urine depends. This removal of Na^+ and Cl^- in the ascending limb results in the delivery to the distal convoluted tubule of hypotonic fluid containing only 10% of the filtered Na^+ and 20% of the filtered water. The further reabsorption of Na^+ in the distal convoluted tubule is under the control of aldosterone, and generates an electrochemical gradient which promotes the secretion of K^+ and H^+.

Clinical Biochemistry Lecture Notes, Tenth Edition. Peter Rae, Mike Crane and Rebecca Pattenden.
© 2018 John Wiley & Sons Ltd. Published 2018 by John Wiley & Sons Ltd.
Companion website: www.lecturenoteseries.com/clinicalbiochemistry

The collecting ducts receive the fluid from the distal convoluted tubules and pass through the hypertonic renal medulla. In the absence of vasopressin, the cells lining the ducts are impermeable to water, resulting in the excretion of dilute urine. Vasopressin stimulates the incorporation of aquaporins into the cell membranes. Water can then be passively reabsorbed under the influence of the osmotic gradient between the duct lumen and the interstitial fluid, and concentrated urine is excreted.

The endocrine functions of the kidney include the ability to synthesise hormones (e.g. renin, erythropoietin, calcitriol), to respond to them (e.g. aldosterone, parathyroid hormone (PTH)) and to inactivate or excrete them (e.g. insulin, glucagon). All of these functions may be affected by renal disease, with local or systemic consequences.

Many diseases affect renal function. In some, several functions are affected; in others, there is selective impairment of glomerular function or of one or more tubular functions. In this chapter, we discuss the use of chemical tests to investigate glomerular and tubular function. In general, chemical tests are mainly of value in detecting the presence of renal disease by its effects on renal function, and in assessing its progress. They are of less value in determining the causes of disease.

Impaired renal function

It is convenient to subdivide the causes of impaired renal function into pre-renal, renal and post-renal.

- *Pre-renal causes* may develop whenever there is reduced renal perfusion, and are essentially the result of a physiological response to hypovolaemia or a drop in blood pressure. This causes renal vasoconstriction and a redistribution of blood such that there is a decrease in GFR, but preservation of tubular function. Stimulation of vasopressin secretion and of the renin–angiotensin–aldosterone system causes the excretion of small volumes of concentrated urine with a low Na content. Renal blood flow also falls in congestive cardiac failure, and may be further reduced if such patients are treated with potent diuretics. If pre-renal causes are not treated adequately and promptly by restoring renal perfusion, there can be a progression to intrinsic renal failure.
- *Renal causes* may be due to acute kidney injury or chronic kidney disease, with reduction in glomerular filtration.

- *Post-renal causes* occur due to outflow obstruction, which may occur at different levels (i.e. in the ureter, bladder or urethra), due to various causes (e.g. renal stones, prostatism, genitourinary cancer). As with pre-renal causes, this may in turn cause damage to the kidney.

 CASE 4.1

An elderly man was struck by a car while crossing the road, and received multiple injuries. He was admitted to a hospital, where he underwent emergency surgery. After 24 h, he was observed to be clinically dehydrated, hypotensive and only to have passed 400 mL of urine. Results of biochemical investigations were as follows:

Serum	Result	Reference ranges (adult male)
Urea	23.2	2.5–6.6 mmol/L
Creatinine	225	64–111 µmol/L
Na$^+$	143	135–145 mmol/L
K$^+$	4.8	3.6–5.0 mmol/L

Urine	Result	Reference ranges
Urea	492	170–600 mmol/24 h
Na$^+$	6	mmol/24 h (dependent on intake)
Osmolality	826	mmol/kg (interpret in context of serum result)

Comments: The patient has pre-renal impairment of his renal function due to inadequate fluid replacement. He has passed a small volume of concentrated urine that is low in sodium. This is a normal physiological response by the kidney to impaired perfusion, due in this case to hypovolaemia. The urea concentration has increased relatively more than the creatinine due to passive tubular reabsorption, and possibly also due to increased tissue catabolism as part of the response to trauma.

The biochemical features that distinguish pre-renal from renal causes are listed in Table 4.4, although in practice there may be some overlap. The prerequisite for using these values is the presence of oliguria, when the presence of concentrated low-sodium urine is a reliable indication of pre-renal causes. Dilute sodium-containing urine is not only characteristic of intrinsic renal failure in the presence of oliguria, but is also found in well-hydrated healthy individuals. The biochemical values for making this distinction are all invalidated by the use of diuretics, and osmolalities are invalidated by the use of X-ray contrast media.

Tests of glomerular function

The GFR depends on the net pressure across the glomerular membrane, the physical nature of the membrane and its surface area, which in turn reflects the number of functioning glomeruli. All three factors may be modified by disease, but, in the absence of large changes in filtration pressure or in the structure of the glomerular membrane, the GFR provides a useful index of the numbers of functioning glomeruli. It gives an estimate of the degree of renal impairment by disease.

Accurate measurement of the GFR by clearance tests requires determination of the concentrations, in plasma and urine, of a substance that is filtered at the glomerulus, but which is neither reabsorbed nor secreted by the tubules; its concentration in plasma needs to remain constant throughout the period of urine collection. It is convenient if the substance is present endogenously, and important for it to be readily measured. Its clearance is given by

$$\text{Clearance} = UV/P,$$

where U is the concentration in urine, V is the volume of urine produced per minute and P is the concentration in plasma. When performing this calculation manually, care should be taken to ensure consistency of units, especially for the plasma and urine concentrations.

Inulin (a complex plant carbohydrate) meets these criteria, apart from the fact that it is not an endogenous compound, and needs to be administered by IV infusion. This makes it completely impractical for routine clinical use, but it remains the original standard against which other measures of GFR are assessed.

In routine laboratory practice most assessments of GFR are based on measurements of creatinine, measurement of which is simple and cheap, but which has some well-known limitations. Urea measurements have historically been part of panels of tests of renal function, but suffer from even more limitations. Assessment of GFR using cystatin C may offer a number of advantages, but is not in widespread use since its measurement is considerably more expensive.

Measurement of creatinine clearance

Creatine is synthesised in the liver, kidneys and pancreas, and is transported to its sites of usage, principally muscle and brain. About 1–2% of the total muscle creatine pool is converted daily to creatinine

through the spontaneous, nonenzymatic loss of water. Creatinine is an end-product of nitrogen metabolism, and as such undergoes no further metabolism, but is excreted in the urine. Creatinine production reflects the body's total muscle mass.

Creatinine meets some of the criteria for use as a measure of glomerular filtration mentioned above. Plasma creatinine concentration may not remain constant over the period of urine collection but it is filtered freely at the glomerulus. A small amount of this filtered creatinine undergoes tubular reabsorption. A larger amount, up to 10% of urinary creatinine, is actively secreted into the urine by the tubules. Its measurement in plasma is subject to analytical overestimation. In practice, the effects of tubular secretion and analytical overestimation tend to cancel each other out at normal levels of GFR, and creatinine clearance is a reasonable approximation to the GFR. As the GFR falls, however, creatinine clearance progressively overestimates the true GFR.

Estimation of creatinine clearance

A number of formulae exist for predicting creatinine clearance (or GFR, see Chapter 4: Estimation of glomerular filtration rate) from plasma creatinine and other readily available information, such as age, sex and weight. The best known of these is that of Cockcroft and Gault (1976):

$$\text{Creatinine clearance} =$$
$$\frac{(140 - \text{age}) \times wt \times (0.85 \text{ if patient is female})}{0.814 \times \text{serum creatinine}}$$

(creatinine clearance in mL/min, age in years, weight in kg, creatinine in μmol/L).

This equation has been shown to be as reliable an estimate of creatinine clearance as its actual measurement, since it avoids the inaccuracies inherent in timed urine collections. However, since it estimates creatinine clearance (not GFR), it suffers from the same overestimation of GFR as creatinine clearance when renal function declines. This calculation should not be used when serum creatinine concentration is changing rapidly, when the diet is unusual, in extremes of muscle mass (malnutrition, muscle wasting, amputations) or in obesity.

The dosage of a number of potentially toxic chemotherapeutic agents is stratified by creatinine clearance calculated using the Cockcroft–Gault or a similar equation, so these calculations remain in use in pharmacy practice.

Plasma creatinine

If endogenous production of creatinine remains constant, the amount of it excreted in the urine each day becomes constant and the plasma creatinine concentration will then be inversely proportional to creatinine clearance. The reference range for serum creatinine in adults is 64–111 µmol/L in males and 50–98 µmol/L in females. However, individual subjects maintain their creatinine concentration within much tighter limits than this. The consequence of this and the form of the relationship between creatinine concentration and creatinine clearance is that a raised plasma creatinine is a good indicator of impaired renal function, but a normal creatinine does not necessarily indicate normal renal function (Figure 4.1). If a patient's 'personal' reference range is low within the overall population reference range, creatinine may not be elevated until the GFR has fallen by as much as 50%. However, a progressive rise in serial creatinine measurements, even within the reference range, indicates declining renal function, and is part of the definition of acute kidney injury (see Chapter 4: Acute kidney injury).

Creatinine clearance or plasma creatinine?

Measurement of plasma creatinine is more precise than measurement of creatinine clearance, as there are two extra sources of imprecision in clearance measurements – timed measurement of urine volume and urine creatinine. Accuracy of urine collections is very dependent on the care with which the procedure has been explained or supervised and patients' cooperation. The combination of these errors causes an imprecision (1 SD) in the creatinine clearance of about 10%

under ideal conditions with 'good' collectors; this increases to 20–30% under less ideal conditions. This means that large changes in apparent creatinine clearance may not reflect any real change in renal function.

Creatinine clearance measurements are therefore cumbersome and potentially unreliable. They have been superseded by calculation of the eGFR (see Chapter 4: Estimation of glomerular filtration rate).

Low plasma creatinine concentration

A low creatinine is found in subjects with a small total muscle mass (Table 4.1). Plasma creatinine is therefore lower in children than in adults, and values are, on average, normally lower in women than in men. Abnormally low values may be found in wasting diseases and starvation, and in patients treated with corticosteroids, due to their protein catabolic effect. Creatinine synthesis is increased in pregnancy, but this is more than offset by the combined effects of the retention of fluid and the physiological rise in GFR that occurs in pregnancy, so plasma creatinine is usually low.

High plasma creatinine concentration

Plasma creatinine concentration tends to be higher in subjects with a large muscle mass (Table 4.1). Other nonrenal causes of increased plasma creatinine include the following:

- A high meat intake can cause a temporary increase.
- Transient, small increases may occur after vigorous exercise.

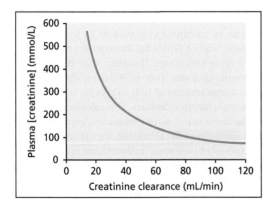

Figure 4.1 Relationship between plasma creatinine concentration and creatinine clearance.

Table 4.1 **Causes of an abnormal plasma creatinine concentration.**

Reduced plasma creatinine concentration	
• Physiological	Pregnancy
• Pathological	Reduced muscle mass (e.g. starvation wasting diseases, steroid therapy)
Increased plasma creatinine concentration	
• No pathological significance	Increased muscle mass, high meat intake, strenuous exercise Drug effects (e.g. salicylates) Analytical interference (e.g. due to cephalosporin antibiotics)
• Pathological	Renal causes, i.e. any cause (acute or chronic) of a reduced GFR

- Some analytical methods are not specific for creatinine. For example, plasma creatinine will be overestimated by some methods in the presence of high concentrations of acetoacetate or cephalosporin antibiotics.
- Some drugs (e.g. salicylates, cimetidine) compete with creatinine for its tubular transport mechanism, thereby reducing tubular secretion of creatinine and elevating plasma creatinine.

If nonrenal causes can be excluded, an increased plasma creatinine indicates a fall in GFR, which can be due to pre-renal, renal or post-renal causes, as follows:

- Impaired renal perfusion (e.g. reduced blood pressure, fluid depletion, renal artery stenosis).
- Loss of functioning nephrons (e.g. acute and chronic glomerulonephritis).
- Increased pressure on the tubular side of the nephron (e.g. urinary tract obstruction due to prostatic enlargement).

It is worth emphasising that any of these causes of a raised creatinine will result in the calculation of a low eGFR.

Plasma urea

Urea is formed in the liver from ammonia released by deamination of amino acids. Over 75% of nonprotein nitrogen is excreted as urea, mainly by the kidneys; small amounts are lost through the skin and the GI tract. Urea measurements are widely available, and have come to be accepted as offering a measure of renal function. However, as a test of renal function, plasma urea is inferior to plasma creatinine, since 50% or more of urea filtered at the glomerulus is passively reabsorbed through the tubules, and this fraction increases if urine flow rate decreases, such as in dehydration. It is also more affected by diet than creatinine.

Low plasma urea concentration

Less urea is synthesised in the liver if there is reduced availability of amino acids for deamination, as in the case of starvation or malabsorption (Table 4.2).

However, in extreme starvation, plasma urea may rise, as increased muscle protein breakdown then provides the major source of fuel. In patients with severe liver disease (usually chronic), urea synthesis may be impaired leading to a fall in plasma urea.

Plasma urea may fall as a result of water retention associated with inappropriate vasopressin secretion or dilution of plasma with IV fluids.

High plasma urea concentration

Causes of high urea largely overlap with causes of impaired renal function and can likewise be considered under the headings of pre-renal, renal and post-renal causes (Table 4.2).

- Increased production of urea in the liver occurs on high protein diets, or as a result of increased protein catabolism (e.g. due to trauma, major surgery, extreme starvation). It may also occur after haemorrhage into the upper GI tract, which gives rise to a 'protein meal' of blood.
- Plasma urea increases relatively more than plasma creatinine in pre-renal impairment of renal function. This is because the reduced urine flow in turn causes increased passive tubular reabsorption of urea whereas relatively little reabsorption of creatinine occurs. Thus shock, due to burns, haemorrhage or loss of water and electrolytes (e.g. severe diarrhoea), may lead to a disproportionately increased plasma urea in comparison with creatinine.
- Back-pressure on the renal tubules enhances back-diffusion of urea, so that plasma urea rises disproportionately more than plasma creatinine.

Table 4.2 **Causes of an abnormal plasma urea concentration.**

Reduced plasma urea concentration	Low protein diet, severe liver disease, water retention
Increased plasma urea concentration	
• Pre-renal causes	High protein diet, GI haemorrhage ('meal' of blood)
	Any cause of increased protein catabolism (e.g. trauma, surgery, extreme starvation)
	Any cause of impaired renal perfusion (e.g. ECF losses, cardiac failure, hypoproteinaemia)
• Renal causes	Any cause (acute or chronic) of a reduced GFR
• Post-renal causes	Any cause of obstruction to urine outflow (e.g. benign prostatic hypertrophy, malignant stricture or obstruction, stone)

Cystatin C

Cystatin C is a small protein produced at a constant rate by all nucleated cells. It is relatively freely filtered at the glomerulus and reabsorbed and broken down in the proximal tubule. It has no other route of elimination. It fulfills many of the requirements of a marker of the GFR. Studies have shown that it accurately reflects GFR throughout life, including in children and the elderly. It is not affected by dietary meat intake, but may be influenced by thyroid status and obesity. It is stable in blood samples and readily measured by immunoassay. Cystatin C has been repeatedly confirmed as being superior to creatinine as a marker of GFR.

The widespread adoption of cystatin C as a measure of GFR in routine clinical practice has been hampered by its measurement being much more expensive than that of creatinine, and this will be multiplied by the large number of such measurements that a laboratory might expect to make every day.

Estimation of glomerular filtration rate

A number of large studies of renal function have allowed the derivation of equations for calculating an estimate of the GFR from more readily measured parameters. These equations get around some of the problems associated with creatinine (see Chapter 4, High plasma creatinine concentration) by incorporating age and sex in the calculation.

One such formula for eGFR was developed from a large study of patients with renal impairment (the Modification of Diet in Renal Disease (MDRD) study). A number of equations were derived in this study, but the four-variable MDRD equation is widely used in clinical laboratories. It uses creatinine, age, sex and ethnic origin (for African-Caribbean people the eGFR should be multiplied by 1.212). This equation is not valid in people less than 18 years old, in acute kidney injury, when creatinine concentration is changing rapidly, pregnancy, muscle wasting diseases, malnutrition or amputees. Estimated GFR (eGFR) is now widely reported on laboratory report forms. The eGFR suffers from significant imprecision, and as GFR increases, the precision and accuracy of eGFR decrease. Most laboratories therefore report eGFR >60 mL/min/1.73 m^2 as such, rather than as an exact number. The eGFR is the basis for detecting and staging chronic kidney disease.

Other equations, including versions incorporating cystatin C, are available. The cystatin C equations offer at best a modest improvement in accuracy over creatinine based equations, but they may offer some advantages in predicting poorer outcomes.

Tests of tubular function

Specific disorders affecting the renal tubules may affect the ability to concentrate urine or to excrete an appropriately acidic urine, or may cause impaired reabsorption of amino acids, glucose, phosphate, etc. In some conditions, these defects occur singly; in others, multiple defects are present. Renal tubular disorders may be congenital or acquired, the congenital disorders all being very rare. Chemical investigations are needed for specific identification of these abnormalities and may include amino acid chromatography, or investigation of calcium and phosphate metabolism (Chapter 5), or an oral glucose tolerance test (see Chapter 6: Oral glucose tolerance test (OGTT)). The functions tested most often are renal concentrating power and the ability to produce an acid urine.

The healthy kidney has a considerable reserve capacity for reabsorbing water, and for excreting H$^+$ and other ions, only exceeded under exceptional physiological loads. Moderate impairment of renal function may reduce this reserve, and this is revealed when loading tests are used to stress the kidney. Tubular function tests are only used when there is reason to suspect that a specific abnormality is present.

Urine osmolality and renal concentration tests

Urine osmolality varies widely in health, between 50 and 1250 mmol/kg, depending upon the body's requirement to produce a maximally dilute or a maximally concentrated urine.

The failing kidney loses its capacity to concentrate urine at a relatively late stage. A patient with polyuria due to chronic kidney disease is unable to produce either a dilute or a concentrated urine. Instead, urine osmolality is generally within 50 mmol/kg of the plasma osmolality (i.e. between about 240 and 350 mmol/kg). This has important implications. To excrete the obligatory daily solute load of about 600 mmol requires approximately 2 L of water at a maximum urine osmolality of 350 mmol/kg, compared with 500 mL of the most concentrated urine achieved by the normal kidney. Hence, patients with CKD require a daily water intake of at least 2 L to maintain their water balance. On the other hand, a large intake of water can lead to dangerous hyponatraemia, since water excretion is limited by the inability to produce a sufficiently dilute urine.

Urine osmolality is directly proportional to the osmotic work done by the kidney, and is a measure of concentrating power. Urine specific gravity, which can be estimated using urinalysis dipsticks, is usually directly proportional to osmolality, but gives spuriously high results if there is significant glycosuria or proteinuria.

Renal concentration tests are not normally required in patients with established chronic kidney disease, and indeed may be dangerous. However, the tests may be indicated in patients with polyuria in whom common causes (e.g. diabetes mellitus) have first been excluded. In a number of conditions, the kidney loses its ability to maintain medullary hyperosmolality, and hence to excrete a concentrated urine, but these should have been excluded before renal concentration tests are performed. Causes of failure to concentrate urine are shown in Table 4.3.

In patients with polyuria, measurement of the osmolality of early morning urine specimens should be made before proceeding to formal concentration tests. If urinary osmolality greater than 800 mmol/kg is observed in any specimen, as should be the case in most patients who can concentrate urine

normally, there is no need to perform further tests of concentrating ability.

Formal tests of renal concentrating power measure the concentration of urine produced in response either to fluid deprivation or to intramuscular (IM) injection of 1-deamino, 8-D-arginine vasopressin (DDAVP), a synthetic analogue of vasopressin. If the patient is receiving drugs that affect the renal concentrating ability (e.g. carbamazepine, chlorpropamide, DDAVP), these should be stopped for at least 48 h before testing. A fluid deprivation test is performed first. If the patient is unable to concentrate the urine adequately following fluid deprivation, then a DDAVP test follows immediately.

Fluid deprivation test

This test is effectively a bioassay of vasopressin, which is itself difficult to measure. The test can be hazardous in a patient excreting large volumes of dilute urine, and requires close supervision. There are a number of ways of performing a fluid deprivation test, differing in detail but all involving fluid deprivation over several hours, ensuring that the patient under observation takes no fluid, and that excessive fluid losses do not occur. Local directions for test performance should be followed. For instance, beginning at 10 pm, the patient is told not to drink overnight, and urine specimens are collected while the patient continues not to drink between 8 am and 3 pm the next day. During the test, the patient should be weighed every 2 h, and the test should be stopped if weight loss of 3–5% of total body weight occurs. Blood and urine specimens are collected for measurement of osmolality.

Normally, there is no increase in plasma osmolality (reference range 285–295 mmol/kg) over the period of water deprivation, whereas urine osmolality rises to 800 mmol/kg or more. A rising plasma osmolality and a failure to concentrate urine are consistent with either a failure to secrete vasopressin or a failure to respond to vasopressin at the level of the distal nephron. When this pattern of results is obtained, it is usual to proceed immediately to perform the DDAVP test.

DDAVP test

The patient is allowed to drink a moderate amount of water at the end of the fluid deprivation test, to alleviate thirst. An IM injection of DDAVP is then given, and urine specimens are collected at hourly intervals for a further 3 h and their osmolality measured.

Table 4.3 Causes of failure to concentrate urine.

Causal mechanism	Examples of causes
Insufficient secretion of vasopressin	Lesions of the supraoptic–hypothalamic–hypophyseal tract (e.g. trauma, neoplasm)
Inhibition of vasopressin release	Psychogenic polydipsia, lesions of the thirst centre causing polydipsia
Inability to maintain renal medullary hyperosmolality	Chronic kidney disease, hydronephrosis, lithium toxicity, hypokalaemia, hypercalcaemia, renal papillary necrosis (e.g. analgesic nephropathy)
Inability to respond to vasopressin	Renal tubular defects (e.g. nephrogenic diabetes insipidus, Fanconi syndrome)
Increased solute load per nephron	Chronic kidney disease, diabetes mellitus

Interpretation of tests of renal concentrating ability

These tests are of most value in distinguishing among hypothalamic–pituitary, psychogenic and renal causes of polyuria (Table 4.3).

- Patients with diabetes insipidus of hypothalamic–pituitary origin produce insufficient vasopressin; they should therefore not respond to fluid deprivation, but should respond to the DDAVP. As a rule, these patients show an increase in plasma osmolality during the fluid deprivation test, to more than 300 mmol/kg, and a low urine osmolality (200–400 mmol/kg). There is a marked increase in urine osmolality, to 600 mmol/kg or more, in the DDAVP test.
- Polyuria of renal origin may be due to inability of the renal tubule to respond to vasopressin, as in nephrogenic diabetes insipidus. In this condition, there is failure to produce a concentrated urine in response either to fluid deprivation or to DDAVP injection, the urinary osmolality usually remaining below 400 mmol/kg; in these patients, plasma osmolality increases as a result of fluid deprivation.
- Patients with psychogenic diabetes insipidus should respond to both fluid deprivation and DDAVP. In practice, however, renal medullary hypo-osmolality often prevents the urine osmolality from reaching 800 mmol/kg after fluid deprivation or DDAVP injection in these tests, as normally performed. Also, the chronic suppression of the physiological mechanism that controls vasopressin release may impair the normal hypothalamic response to dehydration. These patients have a plasma osmolality that is initially low, but which rises during the tests. However, fluid deprivation may have to be continued for more than 24h in these patients before medullary hyperosmolality is restored; only then do they show normal responses to fluid deprivation or to DDAVP injection.

Urinary acidification tests

Urine is normally acidic, compared with plasma, in healthy subjects on a meat-containing diet. An alkaline urine may be found in vegans, in patients ingesting alkali or in patients with urinary tract infections. Urinalysis using dipsticks can be used to give a rough estimate of urine pH over the range 5–9. It is important to measure urine pH on freshly voided urine specimens.

Urine acidification is a function of the distal nephron, which can secrete H^+ until the limiting intraluminal pH of approximately 5.0 or less is reached. Acidification occurs as a result of the kidney reabsorbing the large amounts of the HCO_3^- that were filtered at the glomerulus, and excreting H^+ produced

---

 CASE 4.2

A 58-year-old man, a patient with known manic depression who was being treated with lithium, was admitted to a hospital psychiatric ward with a recent history of lethargy and confusion. On examination, he was found to be very dehydrated, and the results of biochemical investigations were

Serum	Result	Reference ranges (adult male)
Urea	16.1	2.5–6.6 mmol/L
Na⁺	197	135–145 mmol/L
K⁺	3.6	3.6–5.0 mmol/L
Glucose	6.2	mmol/L

Urine	Result	Reference range
Osmolality	209	mmol/kg

Comments: The value for the calculated plasma osmolality, using the formula given in Chapter 2: Osmolality, osmolarity and tonicity is 423 mmol/kg. This high value accords with the findings on clinical examination. The kidneys would have been expected to produce a very concentrated urine, and the low urinary osmolality (lower than the plasma value) indicates either that vasopressin is not being secreted (leading to cranial diabetes insipidus), or that the kidneys are not responding to vasopressin (nephrogenic diabetes insipidus). It was not known whether or not the patient felt thirsty, but patients with any kind of diabetes insipidus, if unable or unwilling to respond to the thirst stimulus, rapidly become dehydrated.

Lithium is a known cause of nephrogenic diabetes insipidus and can also cause hypothyroidism and hypercalcaemia. Lithium has a narrow therapeutic : toxic ratio, and its dosage should be reviewed periodically and renal function, electrolytes, Ca^{2+} and thyroid function checked.

as nonvolatile acids during tissue metabolism. The amount of H$^+$ that can be secreted into the tubules before the limiting intraluminal pH is reached depends on the presence of urine buffers. The H$^+$ in urine is only partly eliminated as such, and it is mostly excreted as H$^+$ combined with buffer ions, principally inorganic phosphate (see Figures 3.1 and 3.2).

It is possible to assess the capacity of the kidney to produce an acid urine after a metabolic acidosis has been induced by administering ammonium chloride (NH$_4$Cl). In response to the NH$_4$Cl load, urine pH normally falls to below 5.3 in at least one specimen. It is essential to check that a satisfactory acidosis was induced, and this is assumed to have occurred if plasma total CO$_2$ falls by about 4 mmol/L after NH$_4$Cl ingestion. More elaborate tests of urinary acidification (e.g. determining the renal threshold for HCO$_3^-$) are needed to differentiate between proximal and distal renal tubular acidosis.

Renal tubular acidosis

At least two distinct tubular abnormalities may give rise to conditions in which there is acidosis of renal origin but little or no change in plasma creatinine, or other measures of the GFR. The impaired ability to excrete H$^+$ means that when Na$^+$ is reabsorbed in the distal tubule, there is an increased loss of K$^+$, resulting in K$^+$ depletion and hypokalaemia. This combination of metabolic acidosis and hypokalaemia is an unusual one, since hyperkalaemia is more commonly seen in acidosis.

- *Distal renal tubular acidosis* (type I) is the more common type. It is due to an inability to maintain a gradient of H$^+$ concentration across the distal tubule and collecting ducts. It is usually caused by an inherited abnormality, but may occur in certain forms of acquired renal disease. Bone disease, commonly osteomalacia, results from the buffering of H$^+$ by bone, and there is often hypercalciuria and nephrocalcinosis. Loss of Na$^+$ and K$^+$ in the urine and hypokalaemia are common. Urinary pH rarely falls below 6.0 and never below 5.3 in the ammonium chloride test of urinary acidification.
- *Proximal renal tubular acidosis* (type II) is much less common. It is due to proximal tubular loss of HCO$_3^-$ caused by a low renal threshold for HCO$_3^-$. This means that if the HCO$_3^-$ is low, HCO$_3^-$ may be completely reabsorbed, resulting in the excretion of normal amounts of acid, but at the expense of a continuing systemic acidosis. HCO$_3^-$ rarely falls below about 15 mmol/L. Occasionally, this is an isolated abnormality. More often, it occurs as one

of the features in some patients with Fanconi syndrome (see Chapter 4: Fanconi syndrome). If these patients are given enough NH$_4$Cl to reduce plasma total CO$_2$ below the renal threshold for HCO$_3^-$, urinary pH may fall below 5.3. Diagnosis requires assessment of the renal threshold for HCO$_3^-$.

Glycosuria

Glucose is most commonly found in the urine in patients with diabetes, when the plasma glucose concentration exceeds the renal threshold. Glycosuria in the presence of a normal plasma glucose occurs in proximal tubular malfunction causing a reduced renal threshold. This can be a benign isolated abnormality, may occur during pregnancy or may be part of a more generalised disorder (see Chapter 4: Fanconi syndrome).

The aminoacidurias

Amino acids can be categorised into four groups – the neutral, acidic and basic amino acids, and the imino acids proline and hydroxyproline. Each has its own specific mechanism for transport across the proximal tubular cell. Normally, the renal tubules reabsorb all the filtered amino acids except for small amounts of glycine, serine, alanine and glutamine. Aminoaciduria may be due to disease of the renal tubule (renal or low threshold type), or to raised plasma amino acids (generalised or overflow type).

Renal aminoaciduria may be due to impairment of one of the specific transport mechanisms. For example, in cystinuria there is a hereditary defect in the epithelial transport of cystine and the basic amino acids lysine, ornithine and arginine; it is a rare cause of renal (cystine) stones. Renal aminoaciduria may also occur as a nonspecific abnormality due to generalised tubular damage, together with reabsorption defects affecting glucose or phosphate, or both.

The overflow types of aminoaciduria result when the renal threshold for amino acids is exceeded, due to overproduction or to accumulation of amino acids in the body (e.g. PKU – see Chapter 22: Phenylketonuria (PKU)); acute hepatic necrosis.

Fanconi syndrome

Fanconi syndrome may be inherited (e.g. in cystinosis) or secondary to a number of other disorders (e.g. heavy metal poisoning, multiple myeloma).

The syndrome comprises multiple defects of proximal tubular function. There are excessive urinary losses of amino acids (generalised aminoaciduria), phosphate, glucose and sometimes HCO_3^-, which gives rise to a proximal renal tubular acidosis. Distal tubular functions may also be affected. Sometimes globulins of low molecular mass may be detectable in urine, in addition to the aminoaciduria.

Renal handling of sodium and potassium

Sodium excretion

The kidneys are essential for maintaining sodium balance, normally filtering about 21 000 mmol Na^+/day through the glomeruli. On a diet of 100 mmol Na^+, and in the absence of any pathological loss of Na^+, the kidney matches this intake with an excretion of 100 mmol Na^+, which represents about 0.5% of the filtered Na^+ load.

As the GFR declines in chronic renal failure, the proportion of the filtered Na^+ that is excreted needs to increase progressively to maintain Na^+ balance. The limit cannot generally exceed 20–30% of the filtered Na^+ load. Once this is reached, any further reduction in GFR, or an increase in dietary Na^+, leads to Na^+ retention. Most patients with chronic renal failure tolerate normal levels of dietary Na^+ if the GFR is more than 10 mL/min. However, if the GFR falls below this level, Na^+ retention occurs, leading to expansion of the ECF, weight gain and worsening hypertension. In the presence of other Na^+-retaining states (e.g. congestive cardiac failure or cirrhosis), Na^+ retention will be even more pronounced. Treatment depends upon Na^+ restriction and careful use of diuretic therapy.

In chronic renal failure, excessive Na^+ loss may also occur. The capacity of the kidneys to adapt to changes in Na^+ intake is limited, and a requirement to conserve Na^+ (e.g. in response to excessive use of diuretics or if the patient has severe diarrhoea) may not be met by the damaged kidneys. This leads on to a further fall in GFR. In chronic pyelonephritis and other disorders primarily affecting the renal tubules, large amounts of Na^+ may be lost in the urine, and severe Na^+ and water depletion can occur.

Potassium excretion

About 90% of K^+ in the glomerular filtrate is normally reabsorbed in the proximal tubules, the distal tubules regulating the amount of K^+ excreted in the urine. The rate of secretion of K^+ by the distal tubules is influenced by the transtubular potential and by the tubular cell K^+ concentration, and is usually maintained adequately, provided the daily urine flow rate is greater than 1 L.

In the presence of a normal GFR, about 550 mmol K^+ is filtered daily at the glomerulus. An average dietary intake of K^+ is about 80 mmol/day, and external K^+ balance is normally achieved by excreting about 15% of the filtered K^+. A reduction in GFR to about 10 mL/min requires an increase in the proportion of the filtered K^+ that is excreted to 150%. Distal tubular secretion of K^+ is needed to achieve this. Generally, the normal daily intake of K^+ can be tolerated if the GFR is 10 mL/min. At a GFR of about 5 mL/min, however, the limit of adaptation is reached, leading to K^+ retention and hyperkalaemia. The ability of the GI tract to increase excretion of K^+ helps to delay the onset of hyperkalaemia.

In chronic renal disease, excessive renal losses of K^+ are rare, but the Na^+ depletion that sometimes develops in renal disease may be associated with secondary aldosteronism, which in turn causes excessive loss of K^+.

Measurement of urinary K^+ output can prove helpful in patients suspected of losing abnormal amounts of K^+. Persistence of a relatively high urinary K^+ output in the presence of hypokalaemia strongly suggests that the kidney is unable to conserve K^+ adequately.

Acute kidney injury

Acute kidney injury is a broad clinical syndrome of abrupt onset due to intrinsic kidney diseases as well pre-renal and post-renal causes. It includes, but is not restricted to, acute renal failure. It is one of a number of acute kidney diseases, and can co-exist with other acute or chronic kidney diseases. The concept of acute kidney disorders is relatively new, and the definitions are evolving. The diagnosis of acute kidney injury, and staging of its severity, are based on changes in serum creatinine and urine output. Acute kidney injury is defined by any of the following.

- increase in serum creatinine by 26.5 μmol/L or more within 48 hours;
- increase in serum creatinine to 1.5 or more times baseline, which is known or presumed to have occurred within the previous 7 days;
- urine output of less than 0.5 mL/kg/h for 6 hours.

Acute kidney failure is then a stage of acute kidney injury defined by a GFR <15 mL/min per 1.73 m² body surface area, or the requirement for renal replacement therapy (i.e. dialysis or transplantation). By definition, this is renal disease of acute onset, severe enough to cause failure of renal homeostasis. Often oliguric, diuretic and recovery phases can be recognised, although a few patients maintain a normal urine output throughout the course of the illness. Chemical investigations help to determine the severity of the disease and to follow its course, but do not help much in determining the cause. eGFR calculations are not valid in acute renal failure or when creatinine is changing rapidly. Proteinuria is present, and haem pigments from the blood may make the urine dark.

Oliguric phase

In this phase, less than 400 mL of urine is produced each day; if the renal failure is due to outflow obstruction, there may be anuria. The oliguria is mainly due to a fall in GFR. The urine that is formed usually has an osmolality similar to plasma and a relatively high Na^+, since the composition of the small amount of glomerular filtrate produced is little altered by the damaged tubules.

Plasma Na^+ concentration is usually low due to a combination of factors, including intake of water in excess of the amount able to be excreted, increase in metabolic water from increased tissue catabolism and possibly a shift of Na^+ from ECF to ICF. Plasma K^+, on the other hand, is usually increased due to the impaired renal output and increased tissue catabolism, which is aggravated by the shift of K^+ out of cells that accompanies the metabolic acidosis that develops due to failure to excrete H^+ and also due to the increased formation of H^+ from tissue catabolism.

Retention of urea, creatinine, phosphate, sulphate and other waste products occurs. The rate at which plasma urea rises is affected by the rate of tissue catabolism; this, in turn, depends on the cause of the acute renal failure. In renal failure due to trauma (including renal failure developing after surgical operations), plasma urea tends to rise more rapidly than in patients with renal failure due to medical causes such as acute glomerulonephritis.

To differentiate the low urinary output of suspected acute renal failure from that due to severe circulatory impairment with reduced blood volume, the tests summarised in Table 4.4 may be helpful. However, none of these tests can be completely relied upon to make the important and urgent distinction between renal failure and hypovolaemia. Careful assessment of the patient's fluid status, possibly including measurement of the central venous pressure, is also required.

For monitoring patients in the oliguric phase of acute renal failure, plasma creatinine and K^+ concentrations are particularly important, and need to be determined at least once daily. Decisions to use haemodialysis are reached at least partly on the basis of the results of these tests. The volume of urine and its electrolyte composition (and the volume and composition of any other measurable sources of fluid loss) should also be assessed in order to determine fluid and electrolyte replacement requirements.

Diuretic phase

With the onset of this phase, urine volume increases, but the clearance of urea, creatinine and other waste products may not improve to the same extent. Plasma urea and creatinine may therefore continue to rise, at least at the start of the diuretic phase. Large losses of electrolytes may occur in the urine and require to be replaced orally or parenterally. Measurement of these losses is needed so that correct replacement therapy can be given; this requires urine collections, for urine Na^+ and K^+ measurement, and calculation of daily outputs.

Plasma K^+ tends to fall as the diuretic phase continues, due to the shift of K^+ back into the cells and to marked losses in urine resulting from impaired conservation of K^+ by the still-damaged tubules. Usually, Na^+ deficiency also occurs, due to failure of renal conservation. Throughout the diuretic phase, therefore, it is important to measure plasma creatinine and both plasma Na^+ and K^+ at least once daily, and to monitor the output of Na^+ and K^+ in the urine.

Table 4.4 Investigation of low urinary output.

Investigation	Simple hypovolaemia	Acute renal failure
Urine osmolality	Usually >500 mmol/kg	Usually <400 mmol/kg
Urine urea: plasma urea	Usually >10	Usually <5
Urine Na^+	Usually <20 mmol/L	Usually >40 mmol/L

CASE 4.3

A previously healthy 32-year-old bricklayer was admitted to a hospital in shock, with severe crush injuries to his legs caused by the collapse of a wall under which he had been trapped for several hours. The following results were obtained on specimens collected 3 days later:

Serum	Result	Reference ranges (adult male)
Urea	42	2.5–6.6 mmol/L
Na⁺	131	135–145 mmol/L
K⁺	6.8	3.6–5.0 mmol/L
Total CO₂	12	22–30 mmol/L
Osmolality	330	280–296 mmol/kg

Urine	Result	Reference ranges
Volume	36	mL/24 h
Urea	280	170–600 mmol/24 h
Na⁺	62	mmol/24 h (dependent on intake)
Osmolality	330	mmol/kg (interpret in context of serum result)

Comments: This man has developed acute kidney injury as a result of his crush injury. The combination of hypovolaemia with the release of myoglobin from the crushed muscles has caused acute impairment of renal function, with a high plasma urea. The plasma K^+ is increased as a result of the acute renal failure; there might also be significant K^+ leakage from damaged cells contributing to this increase. The low plasma total CO_2 reflects the metabolic acidosis that is a feature of acute renal failure.

The urine volume is very low, as glomerular filtration has almost completely ceased. This low volume is accompanied by a urine with a composition inappropriate for someone who is severely volume depleted, i.e. it is dilute and contains a relatively high Na⁺. Vasopressin and aldosterone levels would both be expected to have been high in this patient, leading to urine that was both concentrated and low in Na⁺.

In general terms, the formation of a urine that is both dilute and containing relatively high Na⁺, in a patient with an acute increase in plasma urea, favours an acute failure of renal function rather than pre-renal causes (where renal function may be intrinsically normal). A urine osmolality >500 mmol/kg and a urine Na⁺ <20 mmol/L would tend to favour a pre-renal (reversible) cause, whereas a urine osmolality <400 mmol/kg and a urine Na⁺ >40 mmol/L would tend to favour a renal cause for the acute kidney injury.

Chronic kidney disease

Most of the functional changes seen in chronic renal impairment can be explained in terms of a full solute load falling on a reduced number of normal nephrons. The GFR is invariably reduced, associated with retention of urea, creatinine, urate, various phenolic and indolic acids, and other organic substances. The progress and severity of the disease are usually monitored by measuring plasma creatinine and by calculating the eGFR.

Chronic kidney disease (CKD) affects up to 10% of the population and is often asymptomatic until renal function is severely reduced. Furthermore, mild CKD is a significant risk factor for cardiovascular disease. Detection of asymptomatic progressive CKD could allow patients to be actively treated to preserve renal function and reduce cardiovascular risk. Creatinine concentration gives an indication of GFR and is readily performed, but can be misleading. In particular, creatinine is influenced by muscle mass (and hence by sex and age) as well as by GFR. A small elderly woman could lose a large proportion of her GFR and still have a creatinine within the population reference range and less than that of a young more muscular man, so a 'normal' creatinine can be misleading in such a patient. By incorporating age and sex into its calculation, the eGFR circumvents these problems, although it is not always applicable (see Chapter 4: Tests of glomerular function).

eGFR is the basis for the detection and classification of CKD (Table 4.5). It should be emphasised that an eGFR >60 mL/min/1.73 m² should be regarded as normal in the absence of any other indication of kidney disease. This can be structural, such as polycystic kidney disease, or a urine abnormality, such as proteinuria or haematuria.

Sodium, potassium and water

The renal handling of Na⁺, K⁺ and water by normal kidneys and in chronic renal failure has already been

Table 4.5 **Classification of CKD.**

Stage	eGFR mL/min/1.73 m²	Description	Treatment stage
1*	90+	Normal kidney function	Observation Control blood pressure
2*	60–89	Mildly impaired kidney function	Observation Control blood pressure and risk factors
3A 3B	45–59 30–44	Moderately impaired kidney function	Observation Control blood pressure and risk factors
4	15–29	Severely impaired kidney function	Planning for end-stage renal failure
5	<15	Established kidney failure	Treatment choices for renal replacement therapy

*In addition to eGFR results, the diagnosis of stage 1 or 2 CKD requires a structural abnormality of the kidneys (such as polycystic kidney disease) or a functional abnormality (such as persistent proteinuria or haematuria). In the absence of these an eGFR between 60 and 89 is not abnormal.

considered above (see Chapter 4: Renal handling of sodium and potassium).

Acid–base disturbances

The total excretion of H⁺ is impaired, mainly due to a fall in the renal capacity to form NH_4^+. Metabolic acidosis is present in most patients, but its severity remains fairly stable in spite of the reduced urinary H⁺ excretion. There may be an extrarenal mechanism for H⁺ elimination, possibly involving buffering of H⁺ by calcium salts in bone; this would contribute to the demineralisation of bone that often occurs in chronic kidney disease.

Calcium and phosphate

Plasma calcium concentration tends to be low, often due, at least partly, to reduced plasma albumin. Plasma phosphate is high, mainly due to the reduction of GFR.

Virtually all patients with the later stages of chronic kidney disease have secondary or, much less often, tertiary hyperparathyroidism, and they may develop osteitis fibrosa. Plasma calcium, which is decreased or close to the lower reference value in patients with secondary hyperparathyroidism, increases later if tertiary hyperparathyroidism develops. Many patients with a low plasma calcium have reduced activity of renal cholecalciferol 1α-hydroxylase, the enzyme responsible for the synthesis of the most active form of vitamin D. They can potentially develop osteomalacia or rickets, but this would be uncommon in adequately treated patients. A few patients show a third type of bone abnormality: increased bone density (osteosclerosis). It is not clear why any particular one of these various types of renal osteodystrophy should develop in an individual patient (see Chapter 5: Renal osteodystrophy).

Other laboratory abnormalities

Other findings in chronic kidney disease may include impaired glucose tolerance (IGT) and raised plasma magnesium. These may need appropriate treatment, but are of no particular diagnostic significance. Impaired renal erythropoietin synthesis contributes to the anaemia which is often present in patients with chronic kidney disease. Biosynthetic erythropoietin can be used to treat this.

Proteinuria

Glomerular filtrate normally contains about 30 mg/L protein; this corresponds to a total filtered load of about 5 g/24 h. Since less than 200 mg of protein is normally excreted in the urine each day (half of which is Tamm–Horsfall mucoprotein, secreted by tubular cells), tubular reabsorption and catabolism are very efficient in health.

Proteinuria is described as glomerular proteinuria if the glomerulus becomes abnormally leaky, or as tubular proteinuria when tubular reabsorption of protein becomes defective. Abnormally large amounts of some plasma proteins may lead to an overflow proteinuria. Protein may also enter the urinary tract distal to the kidneys (e.g. due to inflammation), leading to post-renal proteinuria; if post-renal proteinuria is suspected, urine microscopy (including cytology) and culture should be carried out. Electrophoresis of a concentrated urine specimen may help to distinguish these forms of proteinuria, although this is not often necessary. In tubular proteinuria, the proteins are mainly of low molecular weight, having been filtered through the glomerulus but not reabsorbed. In glomerular proteinuria, larger proteins that have filtered through the defective glomeruli are also present.

Dipstick testing of urine for protein should be part of the full clinical examination of every patient. These tests detect albumin at concentrations greater than 200 mg/L, but are less sensitive to other proteins, and in particular fail to detect the Bence Jones proteins that may be excreted in multiple myeloma. If the presence of proteinuria is confirmed, it should be quantified as a protein : creatinine ratio, or in a timed (usually 24 h) urine collection, and simple tests of renal function performed. If the renal function tests are normal and the protein excretion is less than about 500 mg/24 h, it is probably not necessary to subject the patient to further investigation, although follow-up should be arranged. If the protein excretion is greater than this, or renal function is impaired, further investigation is necessary, and may include imaging techniques and biopsy.

CASE 4.4

A 62-year-old man visited his GP and complained of malaise, tiredness and weight loss over the previous 6 months. His only other complaint was of passing more urine than usual, especially at night, when he had to get up three or four times. He appeared pale and was hypertensive, with a blood pressure of 182/114. Urinalysis revealed protein, but no glucose.

The results of simple initial investigations were as follows:

Serum or blood	Result	Reference ranges (adult male)
Urea	38.2	2.5–6.6 mmol/L
Creatinine	635	64–111 µmol/L
Sodium	129	135–145 mmol/L
Potassium	5.4	3.6–5.0 mmol/L
Total CO_2	17	22–30 mmol/L
Glucose	5.2	mmol/L
Calcium	1.88	2.2–2.6 mmol/L
Phosphate	2.38	0.8–1.4 mmol/L
Alkaline phosphatase (ALP)	226	40–125 U/L
Hb	92	135–180 g/L

Comments: The lengthy history suggests the onset of a slowly progressive illness, rather than an acute one. The symptoms of weight loss, tiredness and polyuria might suggest the onset of diabetes, but the lack of glycosuria, backed up by the normal random glucose, rules this out. The results are typical of chronic renal failure. This is supported by the anaemia and the raised ALP (due to renal osteodystrophy), neither of which is a specific finding, but which are more consistent with chronic kidney disease than with acute kidney injury. Chronic kidney disease is also supported by the presence of hypertension, and by the finding of small kidneys if the patient goes on to receive an abdominal ultrasound examination.

Overflow proteinuria

Several conditions may give rise to abnormal amounts of low molecular mass proteins (i.e. less than about 70 kDa) in plasma and in urine. These proteins are filtered at the glomerulus and may then be neither reabsorbed nor catabolised completely by the renal tubular cells. The principal examples are listed in Table 4.6.

Glomerular proteinuria

Table 4.7 classifies glomerular proteinuria separately from tubular proteinuria, but many patients show features of both glomerular and tubular protein loss. Where quantitative measurements of urine protein loss are required (e.g. when monitoring treatment for the nephrotic syndrome), side-room tests are insufficiently precise; laboratory measurements are required.

Some patients, typically with protein excretion rates of less than 1 g/24 h, have benign or functional proteinuria. This probably results from blood flow changes through the glomeruli, and is found in association with exercise, fever and congestive cardiac failure. Amongst these conditions, it is particularly important to recognise orthostatic proteinuria.

Nephrotic syndrome

In the nephrotic syndrome, large amounts of protein are lost in the urine, and hypoproteinaemia and oedema (due to the low albumin and secondary hyperaldosteronism) develop. Usually, the protein losses in the urine are over 5 g/24 h. More than this is filtered at the glomerulus, but most is catabolised

Table 4.6 **Overflow proteinuria.**

Protein	Molecular mass (kDa)	Cause
Amylase	45	Acute pancreatitis
Bence Jones protein	44	Multiple myeloma
Hb	68	Intravascular haemolysis
Lysozyme	15	Myelomonocytic leukaemia
Myoglobin	17	Crush injuries

Table 4.7 **Glomerular and tubular proteinuria.**

Classification	Examples of causes
Glomerular proteinuria	
• May or may not be of pathological significance	Orthostatic proteinuria, effort proteinuria, febrile proteinuria
• Of pathological significance	Glomerulonephritis, all forms; pathological causes of altered haemodynamics (e.g. renal artery stenosis)
Tubular proteinuria	Chronic nephritis and pyelonephritis, acute tubular necrosis, renal tubule defects (e.g. renal tubular acidosis), heavy metal poisoning, renal transplantation

 CASE 4.5

A 6-year-old boy developed marked oedema over a period of a few days, and his parents had noted that his urine had become frothy. His GP detected proteinuria and arranged admission to a hospital where the following results were obtained:

Serum	Result	Age-related reference ranges
Urea	3.4	2.5–6.6 mmol/L
Creatinine	48	20–44 μmol/L
Sodium	131	132–144 mmol/L
Potassium	4.0	3.3–4.7 mmol/L
Total CO$_2$	27.0	19–27 mmol/L
Calcium	1.65	2.2–2.7 mmol/L
Albumin	14	28–45 g/L
Total protein	34	39–73 g/L
Cholesterol	11	mmol/L
Triglyceride	15	<1.7 mmol/L
24-h urine protein	12	0–0.3 g/24 h

Comments: The nephrotic syndrome is the combination of oedema, hypoproteinaemia and proteinuria, as seen in this child. The oedema is the consequence of the hypoproteinaemia causing a redistribution of ECF from the vascular compartment to the interstitial fluid, often exacerbated by a consequent secondary hyperaldosteronism causing sodium retention and potassium depletion. Proteins other than albumin are also depleted, including antithrombin III, immunoglobulins (Igs) and complement. Conversely, some large proteins are present in high concentrations, fibrinogen and apolipoproteins being examples. These changes can predispose patients to infection and to venous thrombosis.

In nephrotic syndrome, the GFR may be low, normal or high. In the age group of this patient, the most common cause of nephrotic syndrome is minimal change nephropathy. The GFR is often high, as reflected by the observed low urea and creatinine. These patients usually respond satisfactorily to steroids, and the prognosis is good.

in the tubules and is therefore lost from the circulation, but does not appear in the urine. The amount of proteinuria does not correlate well with the severity of the renal disease. Patients with nephrotic syndrome may also have a secondary hyperlipidaemia.

Causes of nephrotic syndrome include glomerulonephritis, systemic lupus erythematosus and diabetic nephropathy.

Glomerulonephritis

This is the most common group of causes of persistent proteinuria. Plasma proteins escape in varying amounts, depending on their molecular mass, on the amount of glomerular damage and on the capacity of the renal tubule cells to reabsorb or metabolise the proteins that have passed the glomerulus.

The degree of proteinuria does not provide an index of the severity of renal disease. However, it is convenient to distinguish mild or moderate proteinuria, in which the loss is not sufficient to cause protein depletion, from severe proteinuria, in which the protein loss exceeds the body's capacity to replace losses by synthesis (usually 5–10 g/24 h). Severe, persistent proteinuria is one feature of the nephrotic syndrome, in which urinary protein loss is sometimes more than 30 g/24 h.

Orthostatic proteinuria

This is usually a benign condition that affects children and young adults, who exhibit proteinuria only after they have been standing up. For orthostatic (or postural) proteinuria to be diagnosed, protein is not detectable in an early morning urine specimen when tested by normal side-room methods (i.e. urine contains <100 mg/L). The patient is instructed to empty the bladder just before going to bed, and the test for protein is performed on a specimen of urine passed the following morning, collected immediately after getting up.

Orthostatic proteinuria is usually observed in only some of the urine specimens passed when up and about, and for these individuals the prognosis is good. It is less so for those in whom proteinuria is always detected.

Tubular proteinuria

This may be due to tubular or interstitial damage resulting from a variety of causes. The proteinuria is due to failure of the tubules to reabsorb some of the plasma proteins filtered by the normal glomerulus, or possibly due to abnormal secretion of protein into the urinary tract. The proteins excreted in tubular proteinuria mostly have a low molecular mass, for example β_2-microglobulin (11.8 kDa) and lysozyme (15 kDa). The loss of protein is usually mild, rarely more than 2 g/24 h.

Urinary β_2-microglobulin excretion is normally very small (<0.4 mg/24 h). Its measurement has been used as a sensitive test of renal tubular damage. However, the test is of limited value for this purpose if there is evidence of impaired renal function, for example increased plasma creatinine.

Renal stones

Physicochemical principles govern the formation of renal stones, and are relevant to the choice of treatment aimed at preventing progression or recurrence. Stones may cause renal damage, often progressive.

The solubility of a salt depends on the product of the activities of its constituent ions. Frequently, the solubility product in urine is exceeded without the formation of a stone, provided there is no 'seeding' by particles present in urine, such as debris or bacteria, which promote crystal formation. Formation of stones can also be prevented by inhibitory substances that are normally present in the urine, such as citrate, which can chelate calcium, keeping it in solution.

People living or working in hot conditions are liable to become dehydrated, and show a greater tendency to form renal stones, as the urine becomes more concentrated. There are also several metabolic factors that can cause stones to form in the renal tract. However, in many patients, no cause can be found to explain why stones have formed. The main types of renal stones are listed in Table 4.8.

Hypercalciuria

Stones in the upper renal tract occur in 5–10% of adults in western Europe and the USA. These are mostly either pure calcium oxalate or a mixture of calcium oxalate and phosphate. However, not every patient with renal stones has hypercalciuria, since there is considerable overlap between the 24-h urinary calcium excretion of healthy individuals on their normal diet (up to 12 mmol/24 h) and the urinary calcium excretion of stone-formers.

Increased urinary calcium excretion may be associated with hypercalcaemia, for instance in primary hyperparathyroidism (see Chapter 5: Primary hyperparathyroidism), vitamin D overdosage and hypersensitivity to vitamin D (see Chapter 5: Other causes of hypercalcaemia) or with normocalcaemia, as in idiopathic hypercalciuria, prolonged immobilisation and renal tubular acidosis. In many patients with what was previously considered to be 'idiopathic' hypercalciuria, the underlying disorder is an increase in intestinal calcium absorption.

Up to 10% of renal calculi, depending on the series, have been attributed to primary hyperparathyroidism

Table 4.8 Renal stones.

Type of stone	Frequency in UK (%)	Metabolic cause or relevant factors
Calcium oxalate stones and mixed (calcium oxalate and phosphate stones)	80–55	Hypercalciuria (see text), excessive absorption of dietary oxalate, primary hyperoxaluria
Triple phosphate stones	5–10	Urinary tract infection (fall in H^+)
Urate stones	5–10	Gout, myeloproliferative disorders, high protein diet, uricosuric drugs
Cystine stones	~1	Cystinuria
Xanthine stones	<1	Xanthinuria

(see Chapter 5: Primary hyperparathyroidism). It is important to investigate patients with recurrent renal calculi for primary hyperparathyroidism, as this condition can be cured.

Oxalate, cystine and xanthine excretion

The majority of urinary calculi contain oxalate, but excessive excretion of oxalate is primarily responsible for the formation of stones in only a small percentage of cases. Other occasional causes of stone formation include cystinuria and xanthinuria.

Primary hyperoxaluria is a rare condition in which there is increased excretion of oxalate and of glyoxylate, the latter due to deficiency of the enzyme responsible for converting glyoxylate to glycine. Patients with disease of the terminal ileum may have an increased tendency to form oxalate stones, due to the hyperoxaluria caused by increased absorption of dietary oxalate.

Chemical investigations on patients with renal stones

Stones should be analysed for some or all of the constituents listed in Table 4.8, as this can be helpful.

The following tests may also be helpful in reaching a diagnosis:

- Plasma calcium, albumin, phosphate, total CO_2 and urate concentrations, and ALP activity. Full acid–base assessment is rarely needed.
- Urine dipstick testing (pH and protein), and measurement of 24-h excretion of calcium, phosphate and urate. Occasionally, assessment of urinary excretion of oxalate, cystine or xanthine may be required, or urinary acidification tests.
- Renal function tests (plasma creatinine, eGFR and/or plasma urea).

In addition to chemical tests, microbiological examination of urine is usually performed. Radiological investigations of the urinary tract will be required to localise the stone.

 FURTHER READING

Cockcroft, D.W. and Gault, M.H. (1976) Prediction of creatinine clearance from serum creatinine. *Nephron* **16**, 41.

KDIGO (2012) Clinical Practice Guideline for Acute Kidney Injury. *Kidney International Supplements* **2**, 2; doi:10.1038/kisup.2012.2

5

Disorders of calcium, phosphate and magnesium metabolism

Learning objectives

To understand:

✔ the regulation of calcium homeostasis;

✔ the differential diagnosis of hyper- and hypocalcaemia;

✔ the clinical biochemistry of metabolic bone disease;

✔ disturbances in phosphate and magnesium homeostasis.

Calcium is the most abundant mineral in the body, there being about 25 mol (1 kg) in a 70 kg man. Approximately 99% of the body's calcium is present in the bone, mainly as the mineral hydroxyapatite, where it is combined with phosphate. About 85% of the body's phosphate content is in the bone.

In this book, 'calcium' is used as a composite term that embraces ionised calcium, protein-bound calcium and complexed calcium, whereas 'Ca^{2+}' means that only calcium ions are being considered. The total concentration of calcium in serum or urine is shown as serum or urine calcium, whereas plasma Ca^{2+} refers specifically (and solely) to the concentration of ionised calcium.

Both hypercalcaemia and hypocalcaemia are relatively common biochemical abnormalities, as are abnormalities in serum phosphate. Abnormal serum calcium measurements often arise from alterations in serum albumin, the major calcium-binding protein in serum. Other cases result from an increase or decrease in the unbound or ionised calcium. It is important to identify the latter group because pathological levels of ionised calcium may

be life threatening and the conditions themselves are amenable to treatment.

In this chapter, the hormonal regulation of plasma Ca^{2+} is described, followed by a consideration of the causes of hypercalcaemia and hypocalcaemia and their investigation. Abnormalities in serum phosphate and magnesium are also briefly discussed.

Calcium homeostasis

Calcium balance

In adults, calcium intake and output are normally in balance (Figure 5.1). External balance is largely achieved through the body matching net absorption over 24 h closely with the corresponding 24-h urinary excretion; this varies with the diet. On a normal diet, urinary calcium excretion in healthy adults may overlap with the output in some patients who are renal stone-formers. In infancy and childhood, there is

---

Clinical Biochemistry Lecture Notes, Tenth Edition. Peter Rae, Mike Crane and Rebecca Pattenden.
© 2018 John Wiley & Sons Ltd. Published 2018 by John Wiley & Sons Ltd.
Companion website: www.lecturenoteseries.com/clinicalbiochemistry

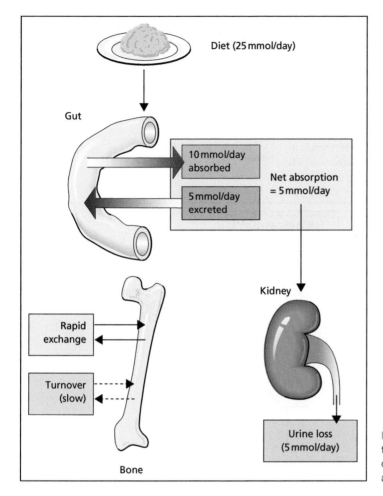

Figure 5.1 Summary of the typical daily movements of calcium between ECF, gut, bone and kidney.

usually a positive balance, especially at times of active skeletal growth. In older age, calcium output may exceed input, and a state of negative balance then exists; this negative external balance is particularly marked in women after the menopause, and is important in the development of post-menopausal osteoporosis. In women, calcium is lost during pregnancy to the foetus, and by lactation during breastfeeding.

Biological function of calcium

Calcium is a major mechanical constituent of the bone. Bone itself is a specialised mineralised connective tissue containing cellular elements (bone-forming osteoblasts and bone-resorbing osteoclasts), organic matrix (type I collagen, proteoglycan, etc.) and the calcium-containing mineral hydroxyapatite. Calcium salts in bone have a mechanical role, but are not metabolically inert. There is a constant state of turnover in the skeleton associated with deposition of calcium in sites of bone formation and release at sites

of bone resorption (~5% per year of the adult skeleton is remodelled). Calcium in the bone also acts as a reservoir that helps to stabilise ECF Ca^{2+}.

Maintenance of extracellular Ca^{2+} within narrow limits is necessary for normal excitability of nerve and muscle. An increase in Ca^{2+} raises the threshold for the nerve action potential, and vice versa. The ion is also required in the activation of the clotting and complement cascades.

While the ECF Ca^{2+} is approximately 1 mmol/L $(10^{-3} M)$, cytosolic Ca^{2+} is much lower, approximately 100 nmol/L $(10^{-7} M)$. Cells possess a number of transport mechanisms for Ca^{2+} that allow maintenance of this large gradient across the cell membrane.

An increase in cytosolic Ca^{2+} serves as a signal for several cell processes, which include cell shape change, cell motility, metabolic changes, secretory activity and cell division. Many intercellular signals, including several hormones, bring about an increase in cytosolic Ca^{2+} by opening plasma membrane Ca^{2+} channels, or by releasing intracellular stores of Ca^{2+}, or by a combination of these effects.

Control of calcium metabolism

Calcium is present in plasma in three forms (Table 5.1), in equilibrium with one another. Plasma Ca^{2+} is the physiologically important component, and is closely regulated in humans by PTH and 1,25-dihydroxycholecalciferol (DHCC): both act to increase plasma Ca^{2+} and hence plasma calcium. The body's responses to a fall in plasma Ca^{2+}, in terms of changes in PTH and 1,25-DHCC production, are shown in Figure 5.2. Growth hormone (GH), glucocorticoids

Table 5.1 The components of calcium in plasma.

Calcium component	Percentage of plasma calcium
Ionised calcium, Ca^{2+}	50–65
Calcium bound to plasma proteins – mainly albumin	30–45
Calcium complexed with citrate, etc.	5–10

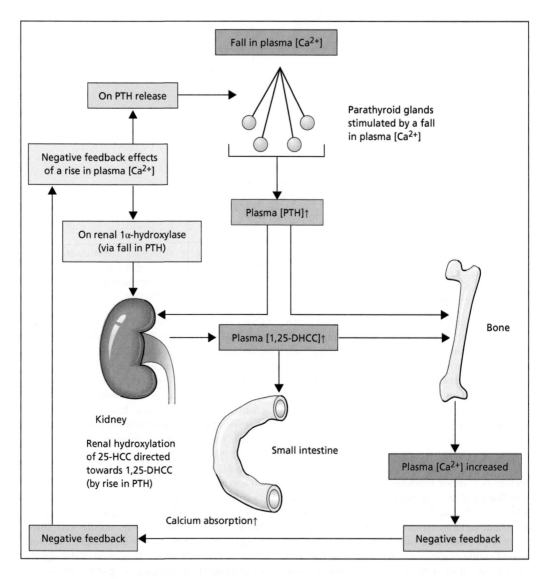

Figure 5.2 Calcium homeostasis in man showing the main hormonal responses to a fall in plasma Ca^{2+}, and indicating the places where the negative feedback mechanism operates if plasma Ca^{2+} becomes high. The effect of PTH on the renal tubules, causing increased reabsorption of calcium, is not shown.

(e.g. cortisol), oestrogens, testosterone and thyroid hormones (thyroxine (T4) and tri-iodothyronine (T3)) also influence calcium metabolism.

Parathyroid hormone (PTH)

PTH is the principal acute regulator of plasma Ca^{2+}. Plasma PTH levels exhibit a diurnal rhythm, being highest in the early hours of the morning and lowest at about 9 am. The active hormone is secreted in response to a fall in plasma Ca^{2+}, and its actions are directed to increase plasma Ca^{2+}. An increase in plasma Ca^{2+} suppresses PTH secretion.

- *In bone*, PTH stimulates bone resorption by osteoclasts, with a requirement for osteoblasts to mediate this effect. Biochemical measures of both increased osteoblast activity (e.g. increased serum ALP activity) and increased osteoclast activity (e.g. raised urinary hydroxyproline and deoxypyridinoline excretion) may be evident. In severe hyperparathyroidism, radiological demineralisation may be seen, including subperiosteal resorption of the terminal phalanges, bone cysts and pepper skull.
- *In the kidney*, PTH increases the distal tubular reabsorption of calcium. It also reduces proximal tubular phosphate reabsorption and promotes activity of the 1α-hydroxylation of calcidiol (see next section). Renal loss of HCO_3^- also increases, which may lead to a mild metabolic acidosis. Formation of 1,25-DHCC indirectly increases the absorption of calcium from the small intestine.

1,25-Dihydroxycholecalciferol (1,25-DHCC, or calcitriol)

Most vitamin D_3 (cholecalciferol) is synthesised by the action of ultraviolet light on the vitamin D precursor 7-dehydrocholesterol in the skin. Vitamin D_3 is also present naturally in food (a rich source is fish oils), while vitamin D_2 (ergosterol) is added to margarine.

Endogenous synthesis of vitamin D_3 is important. Vitamin D deficiency can develop if exposure to sunlight is inadequate, or because of inadequate dietary intake, but is usually a result of the combined effects of these two factors. In the body, vitamin D_3 and vitamin D_2 undergo two hydroxylation steps before attaining full physiological activity (Figure 5.3):

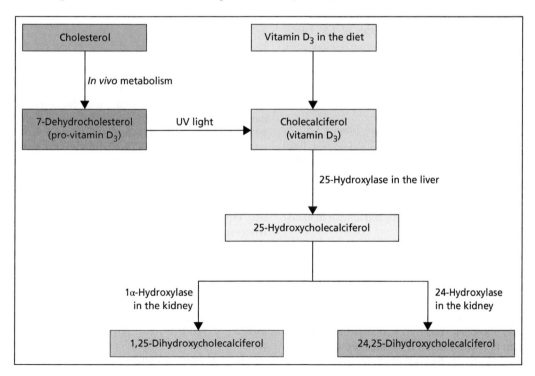

Figure 5.3 The formation of 1,25-DHCC, the most active form of vitamin D_3, from pro-vitamin D_3 (normally the main source of the vitamin in man) and from dietary vitamin D_3. Vitamin D_2 (ergosterol) undergoes similar hydroxylations. By the action of ultraviolet (UV) light, pro-vitamin D_3 is converted in the dermis into pre-vitamin D_3 (not shown) in which the B-ring of the steroid skeleton has been opened; pre-vitamin D_3 then rearranges spontaneously to give vitamin D_3. The factors that influence the hydroxylation of 25-HCC in the direction of 1,25-DHCC or 24,25-DHCC are described in the text.

- *25-Hydroxylation:* This occurs in the liver, with the production of 25-hydroxycholecalciferol (25-HCC, or calcidiol). Other inactive metabolites are formed, but are excreted in the bile. The main form of vitamin D circulating in the plasma is 25-HCC, bound to a specific transport protein; it is carried to the kidney for further metabolism. Plasma 25-HCC is the vitamin D metabolite routinely measured; it shows marked seasonal variation, with levels highest in summer.
- *1α-Hydroxylation of 25-HCC:* This takes place in the kidney, with the production of 1,25-DHCC, biologically the most active naturally occurring derivative of vitamin D. The kidney also contains other hydroxylases, such as 24-hydroxylase, which converts 25-HCC to 24,25-DHCC. Renal 1α-hydroxylation is increased by low plasma phosphate, high PTH and where there is a tendency to hypocalcaemia, whatever the cause. The reverse circumstances direct metabolism of 25-HCC towards the formation of 24,25-DHCC, which has no clearly established physiological function.

The principal action of 1,25-DHCC is to induce synthesis of a Ca^{2+}-binding protein in the intestinal epithelial cell necessary for the absorption of calcium from the small intestine. Deficiency of 1,25-DHCC leads to defective bone mineralisation. Maintenance of both ECF Ca^{2+} and ECF phosphate by 1,25-DHCC may be a key factor in normal mineralisation.

Calcitonin

Although calcitonin can decrease plasma Ca^{2+} by reducing osteoclast activity and decreasing renal reabsorption of calcium and phosphate, its actions are transient, and chronic excess or deficiency is not associated with disordered calcium or bone metabolism. Its use as a tumour marker is discussed elsewhere (Chapter 17: Malignancy and tumour markers/Calcitonin).

Investigation of abnormal calcium metabolism

Measurement of serum calcium and albumin, inorganic phosphate and ALP, and sometimes magnesium, PTH and vitamin D metabolites underlies the diagnosis of most disorders of calcium metabolism.

Serum calcium (reference range 2.20–2.60 mmol/L)

Because of technical difficulties associated with the measurement of Ca^{2+}, clinical biochemistry laboratories only measure serum calcium routinely, despite the physiologically important fraction being plasma Ca^{2+}.

Effects of serum albumin

Because albumin is the principal binding protein for calcium, a fall in serum albumin will lead to a fall in bound calcium and a decrease in total calcium (and vice versa). Under these circumstances, the unbound plasma Ca^{2+}, the physiologically important fraction, will be maintained at normal levels by PTH. Modest but potentially misleading increases in serum calcium may also result from abnormal calcium binding, due to raised serum albumin. This is often due to incorrect or nonstandardised venepuncture technique (Chapter 16: Albumin). To avoid misdiagnosis of hypocalcaemia or hypercalcaemia, serum albumin should always be measured at the same time as serum calcium. The serum calcium (in mmol/L) can be 'adjusted' to take account of an abnormal albumin (in g/L) using a formula such as

$$\text{'Adjusted'}[calcium] = measured[calcium] + 0.02 \times (40 - [albumin])$$

Effects of plasma H^+

In acidosis, the protonation of albumin reduces its ability to bind calcium, leading to an increase in unbound Ca^{2+}, and vice versa, without any change in total calcium. Thus, hyperventilation with respiratory alkalosis can reduce plasma Ca^{2+}, with the development of tetany. In chronic states of acidosis or alkalosis, PTH acts to readjust the plasma Ca^{2+} back to normal.

Serum phosphate (reference range 0.8–1.4 mmol/L)

Serum phosphate shows considerable diurnal variation, especially following meals; the reference range relates to the fasting state. Different ranges should be used for different age groups. About 85% of serum phosphate is free and 15% protein bound.

Alkaline phosphatase (ALP)

Reference ranges for serum ALP activity are method dependent. For physiological reasons, there are also considerable variations in this enzyme's activity in childhood, adolescence and pregnancy. The bone isoenzyme of ALP activity is increased in serum from patients with diseases in which there is increased osteoblastic activity, for example hyperparathyroidism, Paget's disease, rickets and osteomalacia, and carcinoma with osteoblastic metastases.

Hypercalcaemia

Increased plasma Ca^{2+} is a potentially serious problem that can lead to renal damage, cardiac arrhythmias and general ill-health. The clinical features are listed in Table 5.2. The most common causes (Table 5.3) are primary hyperparathyroidism and malignant disease, although the likelihood of these diagnoses will vary depending on the patient population. In asymptomatic ambulatory patients with hypercalcaemia, primary hyperparathyroidism may account for up to 80% of cases whereas in sick hospitalised hypercalcaemic patients, malignancy-associated hypercalcaemia is more likely.

Table 5.2 Clinical consequences of high Ca^{2+}.

- Neurological symptoms (inability to concentrate, depression, confusion)
- Generalised muscle weakness
- Anorexia, nausea, vomiting, constipation
- Polyuria with polydipsia
- Nephrocalcinosis, nephrolithiasis
- ECG changes (shortened Q–T interval), with bradycardia, first-degree block
- Pancreatitis, peptic ulcer

Primary hyperparathyroidism

Autonomous overproduction of PTH occurs typically from a single, parathyroid adenoma. Diffuse hyperplasia (involving all four glands) or, rarely, parathyroid carcinoma may be responsible.

The excess PTH leads to a raised Ca^{2+}, with the potential for clinical problems (Table 5.2). Both serum calcium and albumin should be measured, and may need to be repeated, since the hypercalcaemia can be intermittent. Serum phosphate is sometimes low as a result of the phosphaturic effect of PTH, though this is not a reliable finding. A mild metabolic acidosis may be present, since PTH increases urinary HCO_3^- losses. Some patients develop bony problems as a consequence of the high plasma PTH, especially if the problem becomes chronic. Markers of increased osteoblast and osteoclast activity may be increased (Chapter 5: Markers of bone turnover). Table 5.4 summarises the results of first-line chemical tests for the investigation of suspected hyperparathyroidism.

PTH assay

The single most important test in the differential diagnosis of hypercalcaemia is the measurement of serum PTH (Figure 5.4). Immunometric ('sandwich') assays that measure serum intact PTH are now in widespread use. They have a high diagnostic

Table 5.3 The causes of hypercalcaemia.

Category	Examples
Common	
• Parathyroid disease	Hyperparathyroidism, primary and tertiary; multiple endocrine neoplasia syndromes, MEN I and MEN IIa
• Malignant disease	Lytic lesions in bone: myeloma, breast carcinoma PTHrP: carcinoma of lung, oesophagus, head and neck, renal cell, ovary and bladder Ectopic production of 1,25-DHCC by lymphomas
Uncommon	
• Endogenous production of 1,25-DHCC	Sarcoidosis and other granulomatous diseases
• Excessive absorption of calcium	Vitamin D overdose (including self-medication); milk–alkali syndrome
• Bone disease	Immobilisation
• Drug induced	Thiazide diuretics, lithium
Miscellaneous (mostly rare)	Familial hypocalciuric hypercalcaemia Hypercalcaemia in childhood Thyrotoxicosis Addison's disease
• Artefact	Poor venepuncture technique (excessive venous stasis)

PTHrP = PTH-related protein.

Table 5.4 'First-line' biochemical tests for investigating suspected hyperparathyroidism.

Plasma or serum	Comments
Calcium	Increased serum calcium supports the diagnosis
Albumin	Should be performed as a check on serum calcium
Phosphate (fasting)	Decreased serum phosphate supports the diagnosis
ALP	Increased enzymic activity supports the diagnosis
Total CO$_2$	If decreased, supports the diagnosis
Creatinine and/or urea	Simple tests of renal function, needed in all patients with suspected abnormalities of calcium metabolism
PTH	See Figure 5.4

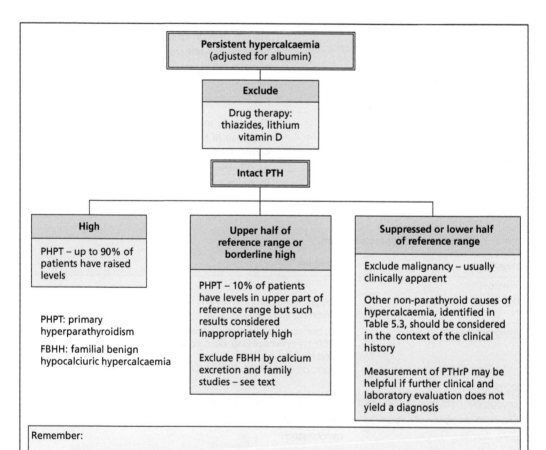

Figure 5.4 Biochemical investigation of persistent hypercalcaemia.

sensitivity, and up to 90% of patients with primary hyperparathyroidism have an elevated level. Approximately 10% of patients with primary hyperparathyroidism may have serum intact PTH in the upper part of the reference range. However, in the setting of persistent hypercalcaemia, such levels are considered to be inappropriately high since serum intact PTH should be suppressed if hypercalcaemia is unrelated to increased parathyroid activity. If serum intact PTH is within reference limits or is only marginally elevated in an asymptomatic hypercalcaemic patient, the diagnosis of familial benign hypocalciuric hypercalcaemia (FBHH) should also be considered (see Figure 5.4).

Sometimes PTH assays are required for the investigation of patients who also require urgent therapeutic intervention to reduce marked hypercalcaemia. Under these circumstances, it is important to obtain a sample for PTH analysis before treatment is initiated, since an acute fall in plasma Ca^{2+} may trigger a rebound in PTH secretion and complicate the interpretation of the result.

Occasionally, in patients with proven hyperparathyroidism who have undergone an unsuccessful neck exploration, PTH assay on samples collected during selective venous catheterisation may be used to localise the source of PTH. A sestamibi parathyroid imaging scan may also be useful in this setting.

Management of primary hyperparathyroidism

In view of the technical difficulty often associated with parathyroid surgery, it is not unusual for the operation to be deferred in patients with asymptomatic hyperparathyroidism if their serum calcium is less than 3.0 mmol/L. As symptoms may develop insidiously, these patients must be followed up with regular further measurements of serum calcium and careful clinical reassessment. Indications for parathyroidectomy include (1) the presence of clearcut symptoms; (2) a urine calcium excretion over 9 mmol/24 h; (3) cortical radial bone density over 2 SD below normal; (4) reduced creatinine clearance (if no other cause identified); and (5) age under 50 years. In general, it is advisable to proceed to parathyroidectomy early rather than late.

After parathyroidectomy, serum calcium falls rapidly, and it should be measured several times on the

---

 CASE 5.1

A 47-year-old secretary was admitted as an emergency with left-sided ureteric colic. She had had one similar episode 3 years before, when she had passed a small calculus spontaneously. In addition, she had been receiving treatment with cimetidine for the previous 6 months, for dyspepsia. Physical examination only revealed slight tenderness in the left loin and on palpating the abdomen. Side-room tests on urine showed a trace of blood, and a plain X-ray of the abdomen showed a small opacity in the line of the left ureter. Blood investigations were performed, with the following results:

Serum	Result	Reference range
Creatinine	150	50–98 μmol/L
Na⁺	141	135–145 mmol/L
K⁺	4.2	3.6–5.0 mmol/L
Total CO_2	20	22–30 mmol/L
Urea	8.1	2.5–6.6 mmol/L
Albumin	40	36–47 g/L
Calcium	3.49	2.20–2.60 mmol/L
Phosphate	0.60	0.8–1.4 mmol/L
ALP activity	160	40–125 U/L

What was the likely cause of this patient's urinary calculi? What further chemical investigations would you have requested in order to confirm the diagnosis? What treatment would you have instituted after initiating these further investigations?

Comments: The most likely diagnosis is primary hyperparathyroidism; the history of recurrent renal calculi and peptic ulceration is highly suggestive and strongly supported by the results for the serum calcium, phosphate and ALP measurements, and by the presence of a mild metabolic acidosis.

The diagnosis in this patient was confirmed by measuring serum PTH; results for this analysis are most readily interpreted if the blood specimen is collected at a time when the serum calcium is increased, i.e. before any calcium-lowering treatment is instituted. This patient's serum calcium was sufficiently high to warrant urgent attempts to lower it, after an IV urogram had been performed to make sure that the calculus was not causing obstruction. Treatment would consist of fluids to correct dehydration, and might require a loop diuretic (frusemide). This patient then proceeded to parathyroidectomy for removal of a solitary adenoma.

first post-operative day and at least daily for the next few days. If the serum calcium falls below normal, calcium gluconate should be given and treatment with 1,25-DHCC or 1α-HCC should be started.

Multiple endocrine neoplasia (MEN) syndromes

Primary hyperparathyroidism may be one of the abnormalities in the so-called MEN syndrome. Three types of MEN syndrome have been described, all of them familial. Further details are discussed elsewhere (Chapter 17: Malignancy and tumour markers/Calcitonin).

Hypercalcaemia of malignancy

Several factors are responsible for the hypercalcaemia of malignancy. These vary, depending on the type of tumour and on whether or not there are bone metastases:

- Solid tumours that have metastasised to bone may cause hypercalcaemia by paracrine activation of osteoclasts. The tumour cells may also increase bone resorption directly.
- Some solid tumours (e.g. carcinoma of the lung, head and neck), in the absence of bony metastases, may give rise to hypercalcaemia. An important factor in this humoral hypercalcaemia of malignancy is PTHrP, a peptide with marked sequence homology with PTH that also acts through the PTH receptor. PTHrP may also be secreted by some tumours that metastasise to bone, so that humoral and local osteolytic mechanisms may combine to produce hypercalcaemia. True ectopic production of PTH appears to be rare.
- In multiple myeloma, hypercalcaemia appears to result from the release of local cytokines that promote local bone resorption. Lymphomas may also cause hypercalcaemia.
- Serum intact PTH is usually suppressed in patients with malignancy-associated hypercalcaemia, although it sometimes falls within the lower part of the reference range. Assays for PTHrP are available in specialist laboratories and may occasionally be helpful in the investigation of patients with unexplained hypercalcaemia.

Other causes of hypercalcaemia

The history of the patient's illness, the findings on clinical examination and various investigations as suggested by the provisional diagnosis will usually mean that the other conditions (Table 5.3) can be recognised. These will be briefly considered here.

Vitamin D excess

Increased serum 1,25-DHCC and hypercalcaemia may result from excessive vitamin D intake or if overdosage with 25-HCC, 1α-HCC or 1,25-DHCC occurs. Measurement of serum 25-HCC or 1,25-DHCC confirms the diagnosis.

Drugs

A mild degree of hypercalcaemia may develop during treatment with thiazide diuretics; these interfere with renal calcium excretion. Long-term lithium therapy may also be a cause, possibly by stimulating PTH secretion. Serum calcium should be monitored on a regular basis in patients receiving lithium therapy.

Sarcoidosis

About 10–20% of patients with sarcoidosis may have hypercalcaemia, often only intermittently. More often, they have hypercalciuria. The unregulated conversion of 25-HCC to 1,25-DHCC (and consequently increased intestinal absorption of calcium) by sarcoid tissue macrophages is responsible. Hypercalcaemia may show seasonal variation in parallel with the production of vitamin D_3 in the skin in response to sunlight.

Tertiary hyperparathyroidism

This description refers to the development of parathyroid hyperplasia as a complication of previously existing secondary hyperparathyroidism. This diagnosis needs to be considered in patients with renal failure or intestinal malabsorption if they develop hypercalcaemia that is not attributable to treatment with vitamin D or one of its hydroxylated derivatives (usually 1α-HCC or 1,25-DHCC). Serum calcium is almost always increased and serum PTH inappropriately high. Unlike primary hyperparathyroidism, however, fasting serum phosphate may be increased, especially if tertiary hyperparathyroidism develops in a patient with renal failure.

Familial benign hypocalciuric hypercalcaemia (FBHH)

This is an autosomal dominant disorder that is usually asymptomatic and may have a population prevalence of up to 1:16 000. It arises from an inactivating mutation in the calcium-sensing receptor gene in the parathyroid gland, kidney and other organs, and results in a high plasma Ca^{2+} that is sensed as 'normal', with normal or marginally elevated plasma PTH. It is important that FBHH is distinguished from primary hyperparathyroidism since parathyroidectomy does not reduce plasma Ca^{2+}, and no active treatment is indicated. While there is no single biochemical test that can always distinguish, unequivocally, FBHH from primary hyperparathyroidism, in patients with FBHH urinary calcium is usually low and serum magnesium tends to be high normal. Therefore, a combination of family studies and the measurement of calcium excretion together with serum magnesium is helpful in identifying the condition. Calcium excretion is measured on a second void spot urine and blood sample obtained after an overnight fast, and is calculated by multiplying the urine calcium : creatinine ratio (both in mmol/L) by the serum creatinine (in μmol/L). Calcium excretion $\leq$14μmol/L of glomerular filtrate suggests FBHH whereas calcium excretion $\geq$0.27μmol/L suggests PHPT. If uncertainty remains after these initial investigations, testing for mutations in the calcium-sensing receptor gene may be performed.

Endocrine disorders

Hypercalcaemia has been reported occasionally in association with hypoadrenalism, phaeochromocytoma and thyrotoxicosis.

Milk–alkali syndrome

Milk consumption may be excessive in patients with symptoms of peptic ulceration; calcium intake is correspondingly increased. If this is accompanied by excessive intake of alkali (e.g. $NaHCO_3$), as an antacid, hypercalcaemia may develop. The alkali is thought to reduce urinary calcium excretion and to be important in the pathogenesis of the condition.

Other bone-related causes

Causes other than malignant disease include Paget's disease in association with immobilisation.

Hypocalcaemia

If potentially misleading hypocalcaemia due to either contamination of the sample with EDTA (from a full blood count tube) or decreased serum albumin is first excluded, then the hypocalcaemia must be pathological and must result from a decrease in plasma Ca^{2+}.

Tetany is the symptom that classically suggests the presence of a low plasma Ca^{2+}. It may occur in any of the pathological conditions listed in Table 5.5, and may also be caused by a rapid fall in plasma H^+ (e.g. acute respiratory alkalosis produced by hyperventilation or IV infusion of $NaHCO_3$). Occasionally it is due to a low plasma Mg^{2+} in the absence of low plasma Ca^{2+}, and rarely it is due to a sudden increase in plasma phosphate. Neuropsychiatric symptoms and cataract are other possible consequences of hypocalcaemia (Table 5.6).

This section considers the underlying pathological processes that may lead to the development of hypocalcaemia.

Vitamin D deficiency

The most common pathological cause of hypocalcaemia is defective calcium absorption due to inadequate

---

Table 5.5 **The causes of hypocalcaemia.**

Category	Examples
Artefact	EDTA contamination of sample
Hypoproteinaemia	Low serum albumin
Renal disease	Hydroxylation of 25-HCC impaired
Inadequate intake of calcium	Deficiency of calcium or vitamin D, or of both; intestinal malabsorption
Magnesium depletion	See below
Hypoparathyroidism	Autoimmune, post-surgical, magnesium deficiency, infiltrative disease
Pseudohypoparathyroidism	Target organ resistance to PTH
Neonatal hypocalcaemia	
Acute pancreatitis	Calcium soaps in the abdominal cavity?
Critical illness	Mixed pathology – not clearly defined

Table 5.6 **Clinical consequences of hypocalcaemia.**

- Enhanced neuromuscular irritability (positive Chvostek's sign and Trousseau's sign); tetany
- Numbness, tingling (fingers, toes, circumoral)
- Muscle cramps (legs, feet, lower back)
- Seizures
- Irritability, personality changes
- ECG changes (prolonged Q–T interval)
- Basal ganglia calcification; subcapsular cataracts (especially with low PTH)

plasma levels of 1,25-DHCC. Deficiency of 1,25-DHCC may result from lack of vitamin D or failure at any stage in its conversion to 1,25-DHCC (Figure 5.3); rarely, the action of 1,25-DHCC is defective at the receptor level. In malnutrition, the effects of vitamin D deficiency are accentuated by inadequate dietary calcium.

Defective absorption of calcium ultimately leads to a low plasma Ca^{2+} accompanied by increased PTH secretion in response to the low ECF Ca^{2+} (i.e. secondary hyperparathyroidism). Serum phosphate is often low, partly through impaired absorption, but also as a result of the secondary hyperparathyroidism (renal disease is an exception). Serum ALP activity is often increased, reflecting increased osteoblastic activity. However, its measurement is of limited diagnostic value in childhood because of the marked physiological variations in activity that normally occur in this age group. Urinary calcium excretion is nearly always low or very low.

Confirmation of the diagnosis of vitamin D deficiency depends on measurement of serum 25-HCC or (less widely available) serum 1,25-DHC. Serum 25-HCC assays provide a reasonable indication of the overall vitamin D status of the patient if renal function is normal and renal 1α-hydroxylase activity can be assumed to be normal. There is a seasonal variation in serum 25-HCC that can make interpretation of single results difficult.

The main causes of hypocalcaemia due to lack of vitamin D or disturbances of its metabolism will be briefly considered here.

- *Nutritional deficiency of vitamin D* Poor diet, inadequate exposure to sunlight or a combination of these can lead to vitamin D deficiency with development of hypocalcaemia and osteomalacia (see Chapter 5: Metabolic bone disease). This has largely been eliminated in developed countries with vitamin D supplementation of food, but the elderly are still at risk (as they may be immobile indoors with an inadequate diet). Cultural and geographical factors are probably important in the susceptibility to vitamin D deficiency of the immigrant Asian community in Northern Europe.
- *Malabsorption of vitamin D* This may be due to coeliac disease, or may occur as a result of fat malabsorption due to pancreatic disease, biliary obstruction or as a complication of gastric or intestinal surgery (e.g. intestinal bypass or resection). Biliary obstruction is much more likely to lead to vitamin D deficiency (through malabsorption) than the theoretical possibility of 25-HCC deficiency in parenchymal liver disease.
- *Renal disease* Destruction of the renal parenchyma leads to loss of 1α-hydroxylase activity, reduced formation of 1,25-DHCC and consequent malabsorption of calcium. Serum phosphate is likely to be high in renal failure, and this may interfere with the 1α-hydroxylation step.
- Specific deficiency of 1α-hydroxylase may be the cause of hypocalcaemia in vitamin D-resistant rickets, type I, a rare inherited disorder. In vitamin D-resistant rickets, type II, there is end-organ unresponsiveness to 1,25-DHCC.

Hypoparathyroidism

Primary hypoparathyroidism is rare. The combination of a reduced serum calcium and an increased serum phosphate in a patient who does not have renal disease suggests the diagnosis of hypoparathyroidism; serum ALP activity is usually normal. Measurement of intact PTH confirms the diagnosis; levels are reduced and are sometimes undetectable even by the most sensitive assays.

Failure to secrete PTH may be a secondary complication of thyroid or parathyroid surgery, or it may be familial or sporadic in origin. Also, the parathyroid glands may be destroyed by an autoimmune process, or as a result of infiltration by carcinoma of the thyroid or other neoplasms.

- *Secondary hypoparathyroidism* may occasionally be observed in patients with magnesium deficiency (see Chapter 5: Hypomagnesaemia and magnesium deficiency).
- *Pseudohypoparathyroidism* is a rare but interesting condition in which the end-organ receptors in the bone and kidneys fail to respond normally to PTH. Patients with pseudohypoparathyroidism have increased serum PTH.

Other causes of hypocalcaemia are listed in Table 5.5.

Metabolic bone disease

Generalised defects in bone mineralisation, frequently associated with abnormal calcium or phosphate metabolism, are sometimes grouped together under the term 'biochemical or metabolic bone diseases'. The most common are osteoporosis, rickets and osteomalacia, and Paget's disease.

In many examples of metabolic bone disease, patients show features of two or more of these conditions, and it can be difficult to define the pathological process fully, even with the aid of radiological examination and bone biopsy. Results of biochemical investigations (Table 5.7) must be interpreted in relation to all the available evidence. For example, in renal osteodystrophy, a combination of osteomalacia, hyperparathyroidism and other metabolic abnormalities contributes to the metabolic bone disease. Various other conditions, often rare, may produce generalised bone disease, with or without biochemical changes.

Markers of bone turnover

Biochemical markers of bone turnover can be divided into those that reflect bone formation and those that reflect bone resorption (Table 5.8). The formation markers include enzymes and peptides released by the osteoblast at the time of bone formation, whereas the resorption markers are typically a measure of the breakdown products of type I collagen. While bone markers cannot reveal how much bone is present in the skeleton and cannot substitute for the measurement of bone mineral density, they have the potential to be used in the assessment of fracture risk and may be used to monitor the response of patients with osteoporosis to anti-resorptive and anabolic therapies. However, the clinical utility of routine bone marker measurements has not yet been fully established and these assays remain available in specialist centres only.

Rickets and osteomalacia

Patients who have vitamin D deficiency or disturbed metabolism of vitamin D are all liable to suffer from the bone disease osteomalacia or, in children, from rickets. These patients have bone pain, with local tenderness, and may have a proximal myopathy. Skeletal deformity may be present, particularly in rickets. Mineralisation of osteoid is defective, with absence of the calcification front.

Other causes of rickets or osteomalacia, unrelated to vitamin D deficiency or defects in its metabolism, have also been described. An inherited defect in the tubular reabsorption of phosphate, hypophosphataemic vitamin D-resistant rickets, leads to similar bone deformities, but without muscle weakness; there is a low serum phosphate and phosphaturia. In Fanconi syndrome (Chapter 4: Fanconi syndrome), tubular phosphate loss may also lead to low serum phosphate associated with rickets or osteomalacia.

Hypophosphatasia is a hereditary disease in which vitamin D-resistant rickets is the most prominent

Table 5.7 Metabolic bone disease: biochemical investigations on blood specimens.

Diagnosis	Calcium	Phosphate (fasting)	PTH	Alkaline phosphatase	Ca²⁺
Hyperparathyroidism					
Primary	↑ (or N)	↓ or N	↑ or N*	N or ↑	↑ (or N)
Secondary	↓ or N	↑ or N	↑	↑ or N	N
Tertiary	↑ or N	↑ or N	↑	↑ or N	↑
Rickets and osteomalacia					
Deficient intake	↓ or N	↓ or N	↑ (or N)	↑	N (or ↓)
Renal failure	↓ or N	↑ or N	↑	↑	N
Fanconi syndrome†	↓ or N	↓ or N	N	↑	N
Osteoporosis	N	N	N	N	N
Paget's disease	N (or ↑)	N	N	↑	N

N = normal; ↑ = increased; ↓ = decreased. N* indicates that plasma PTH is sometimes within the upper reference range, i.e. it is inappropriately high in primary hyperparathyroidism and not suppressed, as would normally be expected, in the presence of hypercalcaemia. † Included as an example of proximal renal tubular defects.

Table 5.8 The most sensitive biochemical markers of bone turnover.

Formation	Resorption
Serum	
• Bone alkaline phosphatase	C-telopeptide cross-links (CTX)
• Osteocalcin	
• Procollagen type 1 N-terminal propeptide (P1NP)	
Urine	N-telopeptide cross-links (NTX)
	Deoxypyridinoline

finding. Tissue and serum ALP activities are usually low, and excessive amounts of phosphoryl ethanolamine are present in the urine.

Osteoporosis

This is a very common disorder that affects about one in four women. It is characterised by low bone mass and susceptibility to vertebral, forearm and hip fractures in later life. Results of routine chemical investigations are usually all normal.

Table 5.9 lists some of the risk factors for the development of osteoporosis. The diagnosis should exclude primary hyperparathyroidism, thyrotoxicosis, corticosteroid excess, multiple myeloma and hypogonadism.

Table 5.9 Risk factors for osteoporosis.

Unmodifiable
- Age (1.4- to 1.8-fold increase per decade)
- Genetic (Caucasians and Orientals > Blacks and Polynesians)
- Sex (female > male)

Modifiable (environmental)
- Nutritional calcium deficiency
- Physical inactivity
- Smoking
- Alcohol excess; drugs (e.g. glucocorticoids, anti-convulsants)

Modifiable (endogenous)
- Endocrine (oestrogen or androgen deficiency, hyperthyroidism)
- Chronic diseases (gastrectomy, cirrhosis, rheumatoid arthritis)

 CASE 5.2

A 64-year-old retired shop assistant with Crohn's disease (regional ileitis) had had her condition well controlled by means of oral prednisolone until 2 or 3 months before her regular follow-up outpatient appointment. Latterly, she had had severe pain in the back, and radiological examination showed a compression fracture of the fourth lumbar vertebra. Biochemical investigations on a blood specimen gave the following results:

Serum	Result	Reference range
Albumin	26	36–47 g/L
Calcium	1.72	2.20–2.60 mmol/L
Phosphate, fasting	0.8	0.8–1.4 mmol/L
ALP activity	170	40–125 U/L
Total protein	50	60–80 g/L
Creatinine	110	64–111 µmol/L
Urea	5.8	2.5–6.6 mmol/L
Na$^+$	136	135–145 mmol/L
K$^+$	3.5	3.6–5.0 mmol/L
Total CO$_2$	21	22–30 mmol/L

Comment on these results. What further investigations might be indicated?

Comments: The long-term use of steroids may lead to the development of osteoporosis. However, in uncomplicated osteoporosis, the serum calcium would be expected to be normal. In this patient the serum calcium is low, and lower than can be accounted for in terms of the low serum albumin. The combination of a low serum calcium with a low normal serum phosphate and elevated ALP activity is consistent with a diagnosis of osteomalacia. The low serum total protein and albumin, and the low total CO$_2$, indicative of a mild metabolic acidosis, suggest that chronic diarrhoea with intestinal malabsorption could be the cause of the osteomalacia.

A diagnosis of osteomalacia can be confirmed by bone biopsy. However, this is seldom required if the history is suggestive and the results of chemical investigations and radiological examination (generalised rarefaction of bones, Looser's zones) are characteristic. Measurement of 25-HCC in serum might be considered worthwhile, and responses to a therapeutic trial of vitamin D might be helpful as a means of making a diagnosis of osteomalacia retrospectively.

Paget's disease

This is a common disorder of the bone, affecting up to 5% of the population over 55 years old in the UK. Bone turnover is focally increased, with disordered bone remodelling. Serum calcium and phosphate are usually normal, although hypercalcaemia can develop, especially as a result of immobilisation. The increased bone turnover leads to a high serum ALP activity and an increase in indices of osteoclast activity.

Renal osteodystrophy

Renal osteodystrophy is the alteration in bone morphology in patients with chronic kidney disease. The pathophysiology is complex and is illustrated in Figure 5.5. The bone changes are varied, and derive from one or more of the following mechanisms:

- *Vitamin D metabolism* There is ineffective conversion of 25-HCC to 1,25-DHCC due to loss of renal 1α-hydroxylase. This causes defective calcium absorption and osteomalacia in adults or rickets in children. It may be corrected by treatment with 1α-HCC or 1,25-DHCC.
- *Phosphate retention* There is increased plasma phosphate, and this, by complexing with Ca^{2+} and combined with defective calcium absorption, tends to make plasma Ca^{2+} fall. This leads to secondary hyperparathyroidism, which tends to restore plasma phosphate and plasma calcium towards normal. Phosphate retention can further

inhibit the renal 1α-hydroxylase. Osteitis fibrosa, if it develops, may require parathyroidectomy.
- *Dialysis fluid composition* The fluid calcium must be carefully controlled; if it is too low, osteoporosis often develops. If fluid calcium is too high, extraskeletal calcification may occur. Care is also needed to ensure that dialysis fluid aluminium is sufficiently low.
- In order to control and treat these various abnormalities, all patients with chronic renal failure require biochemical monitoring. Serum creatinine, urea, Na^+, K^+, total CO_2, albumin, calcium and phosphate concentrations and ALP activity should all be measured regularly. The main objective of treatment with 1α-HCC or 1,25-DHCC is to increase plasma calcium to normal and to reverse bone disease due to parathyroid overactivity. If treatment is successful, serum PTH falls to normal. When treatment is first started, it may be difficult to adjust the dose of 1α-HCC or 1,25-DHCC satisfactorily, and hypercalcaemia, possibly with extraskeletal calcium deposition, may occur if too much is given.

Phosphate metabolism

Eighty-five per cent of body phosphorus is located in the mineral phase of bone. The remainder is present outside bone, largely in an intracellular location as phosphate compounds. In the ECF, phosphate is mostly inorganic, where it exists as a mixture of HPO_4^{2-}

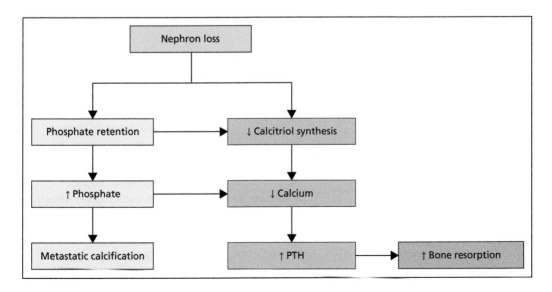

Figure 5.5 Pathophysiology of renal osteodystrophy.

and $H_2PO_4^-$ at physiological pH. Intracellular phosphate has vital functions in macromolecular structure (e.g. in DNA), energy metabolism (e.g. energy-rich phosphates such as ATP), cell signalling and enzyme activation by phosphorylation. Intracellular phosphate is largely organic as a component of phospholipids, phosphoproteins, nucleic acids and nucleotides (e.g. ATP).

Hypo- and hyperphosphataemia

Phosphate and calcium homeostasis are inextricably linked, and several of the factors that influence serum phosphate have already been discussed earlier in this chapter. The causes of hypophosphataemia and hyperphosphataemia are summarised in Table 5.10.

A serum phosphate below 0.4 mmol/L may be associated with widespread cell dysfunction and even death. Muscle pain and weakness, including respiratory muscle weakness, associated with a raised CK, are possible. Urgent phosphate supplementation is required. Dietary deficiency is unusual (phosphate occurs widely in food), but antacids may bind phosphate. Movement of phosphate into the cell occurs with metabolic and respiratory acidosis. Hypophosphataemia in DKA may be worsened when insulin is administered (insulin promotes cellular uptake of glucose and phosphate). Hyperalimentation or re-feeding starved patients is also accompanied by cellular utilisation of phosphate and the potential for serious hypophosphataemia in the absence of appropriate supplementation.

Magnesium metabolism

Magnesium is the second most abundant intracellular cation. It is essential for the activity of many enzymes, including the phosphotransferases. Bone contains about 50% of the body's magnesium; a small proportion of the body's content is in the ECF.

Dietary intake of magnesium is normally about 12 mmol (300 mg) daily. Green vegetables, cereals and meat are good sources. Significant amounts are contained in gastric and biliary secretions. Factors concerned with the control of magnesium absorption have not been defined, but may involve active transport across the intestinal mucosa by a process involving vitamin D. Renal conservation of magnesium is at least partly controlled by PTH and aldosterone. When the dietary intake is restricted, renal conservation mechanisms are normally so efficient that depletion, if it develops at all, only comes on very slowly.

Plasma magnesium is normally kept within narrow limits, which implies close homeostatic control. Marked alterations in the body's content can occur with little or no change detectable in serum magnesium. In this respect, magnesium is very much like potassium. The serum magnesium may be normal although a state of intracellular depletion exists.

Table 5.10 Causes of hyperphosphataemia and hypophosphataemia.

Hyperphosphataemia		Hypophosphataemia	
Increased intake	IV therapy	Decreased intake/absorption	Vitamin D deficiency
	Phosphate enemas		Malabsorption
	Oral (laxatives)		Oral phosphate binders
Reduced excretion	Acute/chronic renal failure	Increased excretion	Primary PTH excess
	Low PTH or resistance to PTH		Secondary PTH excess (e.g. vitamin D deficiency)
	Vitamin D toxicity		Post-renal transplant
Redistribution	Tumour lysis	Redistribution	Re-feeding starved patients
	Rhabdomyolysis		Hyperalimentation
			Recovery from diabetic ketoacidosis
	Heat stroke		Alkalosis (respiratory)
Genetic causes	X-linked hypophosphataemic rickets	Genetic causes	Pseudohypoparathyroidism

CASE 5.3

A 25-year-old woman was admitted to hospital with chest pain and numbness of her hands and feet. Examination was unremarkable other than an increased respiratory rate of 32/min. Results of initial biochemical investigations were as follows:

Blood	Result	Reference range
H^+	30	37–45 nmol/L
P_{CO_2}	3.6	4.27–6.00 kPa
P_{O2}	16.0	11.1–14.4 kPa
HCO_3^-	26	21–29 mmol/L

Describe the acid–base disturbance.

What further investigations would you suggest to determine the cause?

Comments: The blood gas results are consistent with a respiratory alkalosis. Additional tests revealed significant hypophosphataemia (phosphate=0.35 mmol/L), which is often associated with acute respiratory alkalosis as a result of redistribution.

 CASE 5.4

The following results were obtained from a 47-year-old lady with known chronic renal failure:

Serum	Result	Reference range
Urea	16.7	2.5–6.6 mmol/L
Creatinine	362	50–98 μmol/L
Na^+	142	135–145 mmol/L
K^+	4.6	3.6–5.0 mmol/L
Calcium	1.95	2.20–2.60 mmol/L
Albumin	38	36–47 g/L
Phosphate	1.76	0.8–1.4 mmol/L
PTH	220	1.6-6.9 pmol/L

How do you interpret the results obtained?

Comments: The high phosphate seen in patients with renal failure is due to the decreased renal excretion. Loss of renal 1α-hydroxylase results in ineffective conversion of 25-HCC to 1,25-DHCC and defective calcium absorption. These two factors result in hypocalcaemia, resulting in secondary hyperparathyroidism.

Hypomagnesaemia and magnesium deficiency

Magnesium deficiency (Table 5.11) rarely occurs as an isolated phenomenon. Usually it is accompanied by disorders of potassium, calcium and phosphorus metabolism. It may therefore be difficult to identify signs and symptoms that can be specifically attributed to magnesium deficiency. However, muscular weakness, sometimes accompanied by tetany, cardiac arrhythmias and CNS abnormalities (e.g. convulsions), may all be due to magnesium deficiency.

Normal levels of magnesium are not only necessary for PTH release but may also be required to ensure an adequate end-organ response to PTH. Therefore, magnesium deficiency should be suspected in patients who present with hypocalcaemia and/or hypokalaemia without an obvious cause or who fail to respond to treatment of these abnormalities. Serum magnesium is usually below 0.5 mmol/L in patients with symptoms directly attributable to magnesium deficiency; its level

Table 5.11 Magnesium deficiency.

Causes	Examples
Abnormal losses	
• GI tract	Prolonged aspiration, persistent diarrhoea, malabsorptive disease, fistula, jejuno-ileal bypass, small-bowel resection
• Urinary tract	
Renal disease	Renal tubular acidosis, chronic pyelonephritis, hydronephrosis, inherited renal tubular defects (e.g. Gitelman's, Bartter's syndrome)
Extrarenal	Conditions that modify renal function (e.g. primary and secondary hyperaldosteronism, diuretics, osmotic diuresis) Conditions affecting transfer of magnesium from cells to bone (e.g. primary and tertiary hyperparathyroidism, ketoacidosis)
Reduced intake	Alcoholism, malnutrition, total parenteral nutrition
Mixed aetiology	Chronic alcoholism, hepatic cirrhosis, proton pump inhibitors
Redistribution	Re-feeding syndrome, treatment of DKA

CASE 5.5

A 73-year-old man with no significant medical history was admitted as an emergency. He had been unwell over the past 2 weeks and there had been episodes of vomiting and diarrhoea. On admission he was confused and clinically dehydrated. His diet had been poor for some time and he regularly consumed half a bottle of whisky a day. The results of initial biochemical investigations were as follows:

Serum	Result	Reference range
Urea	18.3	2.5–6.6 mmol/L
Creatinine	150	64–111 μmol/L
Na$^+$	141	135–145 mmol/L
K$^+$	2.3	3.6–5.0 mmol/L
Total CO$_2$	35	22–30 mmol/L
Calcium	1.10	2.20–2.60 mmol/L
Albumin	30	36–47 g/L
Phosphate	0.9	0.8–1.4 mmol/L
ALP activity	106	40–125 U/L

Comment on these results. What further investigations are indicated?

Comments: These data reveal significant disturbances in renal function and in calcium and potassium homeostasis. The modest increase in serum urea, which is disproportionately greater than the increase in serum creatinine, is consistent with a moderate degree of renal impairment in a dehydrated patient.

The marked reduction in serum calcium is not due to specimen contamination with EDTA (from a full blood count tube) because the serum potassium would be increased under these circumstances. After adjustment of the serum calcium for the low serum albumin, the adjusted calcium remains very low at 1.30 mmol/L. Consideration of the clinical history suggested that the hypocalcaemia was likely to relate to magnesium depletion and the serum magnesium was subsequently shown to be <0.10 mmol/L. Magnesium depletion may develop following long-term alcohol abuse as a result of a renal leak of magnesium and poor nutritional intake, and in this patient losses in diarrhoea fluid may have been a contributing factor. Patients with magnesium deficiency develop secondary hypoparathyroidism and end-organ resistance to the effects of PTH. Serum intact PTH on admission was subsequently shown to be 63 ng/L (reference range 10–55 ng/L). Although elevated, the observed value was much lower than expected in such a markedly hypocalcaemic patient. In view of the poor nutritional history, 25OH vitamin D$_3$ was also measured and found to be undetectable, indicating that vitamin D deficiency may have contributed to the hypocalcaemia. The reduction of serum potassium may have been related to poor intake, vomiting with an associated mild alkalosis suggested by the increased serum bicarbonate and to magnesium depletion which induces renal potassium loss.

The patient was treated with IV fluids containing magnesium and potassium, together with oral calcium supplements. On the day after admission, the serum magnesium had risen to 0.9 mmol/L and the intact PTH to 320 ng/L. Within 5 days, all biochemical parameters had returned to normal.

should be measured before treatment with magnesium salts is instituted.

Serum magnesium may not reflect the true state of the body's reserves, particularly in chronic disorders. Other tests have been advocated (e.g. erythrocyte magnesium, muscle magnesium, magnesium loading tests), but there is no general agreement on the best test to use. Urinary excretion of magnesium is relatively easy to measure, and it is useful in distinguishing renal losses of magnesium from the other causes of hypomagnesaemia and magnesium deficiency. Renal excretion of magnesium often falls below 0.5 mmol/24 h in nonrenal causes of magnesium deficiency.

Hypermagnesaemia

This is most often due to acute renal failure or the advanced stages of chronic renal failure. Its presence is readily confirmed by measuring serum magnesium. There may be no symptoms. However, if serum magnesium exceeds 3.0 mmol/L, nausea and vomiting, weakness and impaired consciousness may then develop, but these symptoms may not necessarily be caused solely by the hypermagnesaemia.

Hypermagnesaemia may rarely be caused by IV injection of magnesium salts, and adrenocortical hypofunction may cause a slight increase in serum magnesium.

6

Diabetes mellitus and hypoglycaemia

Learning objectives

To understand:

✔ more about diabetes, the most common metabolic disorder, whose incidence is increasing;

✔ the biochemical measurements that are particularly important in diagnosing diabetes, monitoring its control and treating its metabolic complications;

✔ more about hypoglycaemia, which occurs in insulin-treated diabetic patients and which, though otherwise rare, can have serious consequences;

✔ how to diagnose hypoglycaemia and its underlying cause.

Glucose homeostasis

Blood glucose concentration is maintained within a narrow range, imposed at the lower limit by the undesirable effects of hypoglycaemia and at the upper limit by the potential for loss in the urine if the renal threshold is exceeded. The liver plays a key role in maintaining blood glucose. After a carbohydrate-containing meal, it removes about 70% of the glucose load that is delivered via the portal circulation. Some of the glucose is oxidised and some is converted to glycogen for use as a fuel under fasting conditions. Glucose in excess of these requirements is partly converted by the liver to fatty acids and triglycerides, which are then incorporated into very low density lipoproteins (VLDLs) and transported to adipose tissue stores.

In the fasting state, blood glucose is maintained by glycogen breakdown in the liver in the short term, while glycogen stores last, and then by gluconeogenesis (from glycerol, lactate and pyruvate and from the gluconeogenic amino acids), occurring mostly in the liver but also in the kidneys. Glucose is spared, under fasting conditions, by the ability of muscle and other tissues to adapt to the oxidation of fatty acids, and by the ability of the brain and some other organs to utilise ketone bodies that are formed under these conditions.

The hormones mainly concerned with regulating glucose metabolism in the fed and fasting states are insulin, glucagon, GH, adrenaline and cortisol. Of these, insulin has the most marked effects (Table 6.1) and is the only hormone that lowers blood glucose. Glucagon, GH, adrenaline and cortisol all tend, in general, to antagonise the actions of insulin (Table 6.2).

Clinical Biochemistry Lecture Notes, Tenth Edition. Peter Rae, Mike Crane and Rebecca Pattenden.
© 2018 John Wiley & Sons Ltd. Published 2018 by John Wiley & Sons Ltd.
Companion website: www.lecturenoteseries.com/clinicalbiochemistry

Table 6.1 **The effects of insulin on cellular metabolism.**

Tissue	Processes activated by insulin	Processes inhibited by insulin
Liver	Uptake of amino acids and glycerol Synthesis of glycogen, proteins, triglycerides and VLDLs	Glycogenolysis Gluconeogenesis Ketone body formation
Muscle	Uptake of glucose and amino acids Synthesis of glycogen	Triglyceride utilisation Lipolysis
Adipose	Uptake of chylomicrons and VLDLs and of glucose Utilisation of glucose	

Table 6.2 **The effects on glucose metabolism of hormones that antagonise the actions of insulin.**

| Tissue and hormone | Effects of the various hormones on glucose metabolism | | | |
	Gluconeogenesis	Glycogenolysis	Glycolysis	Glucose uptake
Liver				
• Adrenaline	Increased	Increased	Decreased	
• Cortisol	Increased			Decreased
• Glucagon	Increased	Increased		
• Growth hormone		Increased	Increased	Decreased
Muscle				
• Adrenaline		Increased	Increased	
• Cortisol				Decreased
• Growth hormone				
Short term			Increased	
Long term			Decreased	
Adipose				
• Cortisol			Decreased	

Insulin secretion

Insulin is synthesised in the β-cells of the islets of Langerhans in the pancreas. It is formed as prepro-insulin, which is rapidly cleaved to pro-insulin. The pro-insulin is packaged into secretory granules in the Golgi apparatus and cleaved to insulin and C peptide. Insulin and C peptide are later released into the circulation in equimolar amounts.

A rise in blood glucose is the main stimulus for insulin secretion. Some amino acids (e.g. leucine), fatty acids and ketone bodies also promote insulin secretion, as does vagal stimulation. The release of insulin in response to hyperglycaemia is enhanced by the presence of incretin hormones released from the gastrointestinal tract (glucagon-like polypeptide-1 (GLP-1) and glucose-dependent insulinotropic polypeptide (GIP)). Incretins explain the larger release of insulin that occurs in response to an oral glucose load, compared with the same dose of glucose given intravenously. GLP-1 and GIP are inactivated in the circulation by the enzyme dipeptidyl peptidase-4 (DPP-4). Some new drugs for the treatment of type 2 diabetes enhance glucose-dependent endogenous insulin secretion by targeting this system. Both GLP-1 agonists and DPP-4 inhibitors are available.

The insulin receptor is located on the cell surface and is internalised after insulin binding. Within different organs, target enzymes have been identified that serve to explain the known effects of insulin on intermediary metabolism. For instance, activation of glucose transport, induction of hexokinase (or glucokinase) and activation of phosphofructokinase, pyruvate kinase and pyruvate dehydrogenase in the liver are all consistent with the actions of insulin in promoting increased glucose uptake and glycolytic breakdown. Stimulation of glycogen synthase accords with the effects of insulin on glycogen formation in the liver.

Diabetes mellitus

Diabetes is common, affecting 1–2% of Western populations, and population screening programmes reveal that many patients are previously unrecognised. It results in chronic hyperglycaemia, usually accompanied by glycosuria and other biochemical abnormalities, expressed as a wide range of clinical presentations ranging from asymptomatic patients with relatively mild biochemical abnormalities to patients admitted to hospitals with severe metabolic decompensation of rapid onset that has led to coma. Long-term complications may develop, including retinopathy, neuropathy and nephropathy. It is a major risk factor for cardiovascular disease.

Diabetes may be a secondary consequence of other diseases. For example, in diseases of the pancreas, such as pancreatitis or haemochromatosis, there is a reduction in insulin secretion. In some endocrine disorders, such as acromegaly or Cushing's syndrome, there is antagonism of insulin action by abnormal secretion of hormones with opposing activity. Several drugs adversely affect glucose tolerance. Table 6.3 summarises these different causes. Secondary diabetes is, however, not common.

Most cases of diabetes are not associated with other conditions but are primary and fall into two distinct types. In type 1 diabetes, there is essentially no insulin secretion, whereas in type 2 diabetes insulin is secreted, but in amounts that are inadequate to prevent hyperglycaemia, or there is resistance to its action.

- *Type 1 diabetes* usually presents acutely over a period of days or a few weeks in young non-obese subjects, but can occur at any age. In addition to polyuria, thirst and glycosuria, there is often marked weight loss and ketoacidosis. Insulin is required for its treatment. Type 1 diabetes is an autoimmune condition with genetic and environmental precipitating factors in its pathogenesis. Islet-cell antibodies that react with the β-cells of the pancreas have been demonstrated in serum from over 90% of patients with newly diagnosed type 1 diabetes. They have also been demonstrated occasionally in serum several years before clinical and biochemical features of diabetes have developed. Most of the islet-cell antibodies are directed against the enzyme glutamic acid decarboxylase (GAD). Individuals with certain human leucocyte antigens (HLAs) have been shown to have a particularly high risk of developing type 1 diabetes. There is a well-recognised association between type 1 diabetes and other autoimmune endocrinopathies, such as hypothyroidism and Addison's disease, and also with pernicious anaemia.
- *Latent autoimmune diabetes of adults* presents more insidiously than 'normal' type 1 diabetes. Patients are often thought to have type 2 diabetes and are started on oral hypoglycaemic agents, but progress relatively rapidly to needing insulin treatment, often within months. These patients often have GAD antibodies.
- *Type 2 diabetes* generally presents in a less acute manner in older (>40 years) patients who are obese; many patients have clearly had the condition for some time (even years) before diagnosis. Type 2 diabetes is rare in younger patients, but is increasing with the increased prevalence of obesity in this age group. Measurable levels of insulin are present, and the metabolic defect appears to lie either in defective insulin secretion or in insulin resistance. In general, insulin administration is not required for the prevention of ketosis, as these patients are relatively resistant to its development. However, insulin may be needed to correct abnormalities of blood glucose. There appears to be no association between type 2 diabetes and either the HLA system or the development of autoimmunity. However, there is a strong genetic element to the disorder. Type 2 diabetes is a progressive condition that requires intensification of treatment over time to maintain glycaemic control. The distinction

Table 6.3 **Examples of causes of secondary diabetes or of IGT.**

Category of cause	Examples
Drugs	Oestrogen-containing oral contraceptives, corticosteroids, salbutamol and some other catecholaminergic drugs, thiazide diuretics
Endocrine disorders	Acromegaly, Cushing's syndrome and Cushing's disease, glucagonoma, phaeochromocytoma, prolactinoma, thyrotoxicosis (occasionally)
Insulin receptor abnormalities	Autoimmune insulin receptor antibodies, congenital lipodystrophy
Pancreatic disease	Chronic pancreatitis, haemochromatosis, pancreatectomy

Table 6.4 Distinction between type 1 and type 2 diabetes.

Type 1 diabetes	Type 2 diabetes
Younger age	Older age
Rapid onset	Obesity
Significant weight loss	Asian origin
Ketonaemia/ketonuria	Features of the metabolic
GAD antibodies	syndrome – hypertension, high triglycerides, low HDL

 CASE 6.1

A 27-year-old man was referred to the local diabetes clinic. He had been diagnosed as having type 2 diabetes 3 years previously and his control was poor (HbA$_{1c}$ 9.6%) despite being on an optimal dose of metformin. The GP was wondering whether this man needed to start on insulin. Several close family members also had diabetes. The man was slightly overweight with a BMI of 26, and he was normotensive.

Comments: In view of the strong family history of diabetes and the fact that he did not fit the typical phenotype of type 2 diabetes (he was relatively young, not obese and normotensive) the possibility of maturity onset diabetes of the young (MODY) was raised. Genotyping revealed a mutation in the *HNF1α* gene. Metformin was stopped and he achieved excellent control on a low dose of gliclazide.

between type 1 and type 2 diabetes is usually obvious, and can be guided by relatively simple clinical and laboratory criteria which make one or the other possibility more likely (Table 6.4).

- *Gestational diabetes* is a term describing carbohydrate intolerance of variable severity that is either first recognised or has its onset during pregnancy. It can therefore include patients with previously unrecognised type 1 or type 2 diabetes. In these patients and in established diabetic patients who become pregnant, poor blood glucose control is associated with a higher incidence of intrauterine death and foetal malformation, and urgent treatment is needed. This term also describes women with abnormal glucose tolerance that reverts to normal after delivery. Trials have shown that these pregnancies have a high rate of large for gestational age infants and perinatal morbidity, and that intervention to manage blood glucose is effective in reducing these risks. The best strategy for screening and diagnosing gestational diabetes remains controversial. In early pregnancy an important aim of screening is to identify previously undiagnosed type 2 diabetes, and women with risk factors such as a high body mass index, a family history of diabetes, or previous gestational diabetes should have HbA$_{1c}$ or fasting blood glucose measured. If results diagnostic of diabetes (see Chapter 6: Diagnosis) are obtained they should be regarded as having pre-existing diabetes. Women with intermediate results should be assessed for the need for home glucose monitoring. All women with risk factors should undergo an oral glucose tolerance test (see Chapter 6: Oral glucose tolerance test (OGTT)) at 24–28 weeks. In this test the criteria for the diagnosis of frank diabetes are the same as those in non-pregnant individuals. The internationally agreed criteria for gestational diabetes differ from these, and are a fasting plasma glucose of 5.1 mmol/L or more, or a one hour value of 10 mmol/L or more, or a two hour value of 8.5 mmol/L or more.

Monogenic forms of diabetes may account for 1–2% of cases of diabetes. Clinical features may overlap with those of type 1 or type 2 diabetes. Forms include:

- *Neonatal diabetes* is diabetes diagnosed within the first 6 months of life and may be transient or permanent. Up to 60% of patients with permanent neonatal diabetes have a mutation in one of the potassium channel genes, which results in failure of insulin production. This is an important diagnosis because 90% of these patients can stop insulin and achieve good control on sulphonylureas.
- *Maturity onset diabetes of the young (MODY)* may be better called familial diabetes and may be suspected in a patient with a strong family history of diabetes or when apparent type 2 diabetes occurs at a relatively young age, or in the absence of typical type 2 features such as insulin resistance. Patients may be on insulin. A number of subtypes are recognised, the more common ones being caused by mutations in:
  - Glucokinase (MODY2). This often causes mild asymptomatic hyperglycaemia typically only picked up during screening. Diabetic complications are very unusual and treatment can usually be stopped.
  - Hepatic nuclear factor 1 alpha (HNF-1α) (MODY3). This is the most common cause of MODY. Glucose concentration increases with age and becomes symptomatic in adolescence or young adulthood. Diabetic complications occur, so treatment is

needed. Low dose sulphonylureas achieve excellent glucose control and in patients less than 45 years old may even replace insulin if that has been started before the correct diagnosis was made.

Diagnosis

The diagnosis of diabetes mellitus has serious consequences. It confers a risk of long-term diabetic complications, including blindness, renal failure and amputations, as well as an increased risk of cardiovascular disease. It also means a lifetime of dietary restriction and medications and can seriously curtail lifestyle and employment prospects. The diagnosis may be suggested by the patient's history, or by the results of dipstick tests for glucose on urine specimens. However, urine glucose measurements by themselves are inadequate for diagnosing diabetes. They potentially yield false-positive results in subjects with a low renal threshold for glucose, and in a patient with diabetes they may yield false-negative results if the patient is fasting. A provisional diagnosis of diabetes mellitus must always be confirmed by laboratory measurements on blood specimens.

Criteria for the diagnosis of diabetes mellitus were laid down by the World Health Organization (WHO) in 2006. It is likely that the precise requirements for the diagnosis of diabetes and the states of impaired glucose regulation will continue to evolve as knowledge of the relationship between glucose regulation and the future development of complications accumulates. Separate criteria are described depending on whether venous or capillary whole blood, or venous or capillary plasma specimens are used. In practice, results for this important diagnosis will usually come from a clinical laboratory and use venous plasma. According to the criteria, a random venous plasma glucose of 11.1 mmol/L or more, or a fasting plasma glucose of 7.0 mmol/L or more, establishes the diagnosis. A single result is sufficient in the presence of typical hyperglycaemic symptoms of thirst and polyuria. In their absence, a venous plasma glucose in the diabetic range should be detected on at least two separate occasions on different days. Where there is any doubt, an OGTT should be performed (see Chapter 6: Oral glucose tolerance test (OGTT)), and if the fasting or random values are not diagnostic, the 2-h value should be used. In practice, the diagnosis is often obvious clinically, and glucose is only needed for confirmation and is unequivocally high. The diagnosis should never be made on the basis of a single test in a patient without symptoms.

At the time the WHO criteria were published, a raised glycated haemoglobin (HbA_{1c}) was not recommended for making a diagnosis of diabetes because of poor analytical standardisation, and because HbA_{1c} is influenced by red cell lifespan as well as by glucose concentration. However, improvements in standardisation (see Chapter 6: Glycated haemoglobin) have resulted in the WHO and the American Diabetes Association (ADA) changing their stance on the use of HbA_{1c} for the diagnosis of diabetes. HbA_{1c} can now be used as a diagnostic test provided that stringent quality assurance tests are in place and assays are standardised to criteria aligned to the international reference values, and there are no conditions present which preclude its accurate measurement. The introduction of HbA_{1c} for the diagnosis of diabetes does not invalidate the use of glucose measurements. HbA_{1c} is a more convenient test than an oral glucose tolerance test, for both the patient and health care providers. However, its cost means that it not widely available in lower income countries. There are also a number of situations where its use is inappropriate, primarily when diabetes may be developing relatively rapidly (Table 6.5).

An HbA_{1c} of 48 mmol/mol (6.5%) is recommended as the cut-point for diagnosing diabetes. However, a value less than this does not exclude diabetes diagnosed using glucose tests. In patients without symptoms the test should be repeated. If the second result is <48 mmol/mol the patient should be considered to be at high diabetes risk and the test should be repeated in 6 months or sooner if symptoms develop.

Table 6.5 Situations where HbA_{1c} is not appropriate for the diagnosis of diabetes.

- Children and young people
- Patients of any age suspected of having type 1 diabetes
- Patients with symptoms of diabetes for less than two months
- Patients at high diabetes risk who are acutely ill
- Patients taking medication that may cause rapid glucose rise, e.g. steroids
- Patients with acute pancreatic damage
- Pregnancy
- Presence of genetic, haematologic and illness-related factors that influence HbA_{1c} and its measurement

Source: Diabetes UK (2011) *Care Recommendations: New Diagnostic Criteria for Diabetes*, January.

Blood and plasma glucose

Most laboratory instruments measure plasma glucose, but some use whole blood. Plasma glucose concentration is 10–15% higher than whole blood glucose, because red cells contain less water per unit volume than plasma. The discrepancy can be greater than this if glucose changes rapidly, because glucose will not have reached equilibrium across the red cell membrane. Plasma, therefore, yields more reliable results. At normal plasma glucose levels, there is little difference between results obtained on capillary and venous blood. However, at hyperglycaemic levels, capillary plasma glucose may be significantly higher than venous plasma glucose. These factors are important in the interpretation of glucose tolerance tests.

If there is likely to be any delay in measuring glucose in blood specimens, it is essential either to separate the plasma immediately or to use a tube containing an inhibitor of glycolysis to stabilise the glucose. Sodium fluoride is often used for this purpose, but is not as effective as used to be thought. Measurements of blood glucose that are to be performed using a 'stick' test must be carried out without delay on specimens that do not contain sodium fluoride.

Oral glucose 'tolerance test (OGTT)

The OGTT retains a place in the diagnosis of diabetes despite the introduction of HbA_{1c} for this purpose, and despite being cumbersome. It should be performed when random glucose concentration falls into a range where the diagnosis is uncertain. Several precautions must be taken in preparing for and performing the test. It should not be performed on patients suffering from an intercurrent infection or the effects of trauma, or those recovering from a serious illness. Drugs such as corticosteroids and diuretics may impair glucose tolerance and should be stopped before the test if possible. The patient should have been on an unrestricted diet containing at least 150 g of carbohydrate/day for at least 3 days, and should not have indulged in unaccustomed amounts of exercise. The patient must not smoke before or during the test, nor eat or drink anything other than as specified as follows.

An OGTT is usually performed after an overnight fast, although a fast of 4–5 h may be enough. The patient is allowed to drink water during the fast. A standard dose of glucose (82.5 g of glucose monohydrate or 75 g of anhydrous glucose) dissolved in 250–300 mL of water is given by mouth over a 5-min period. Smaller amounts of glucose (1.92 g of glucose monohydrate or 1.75 g of anhydrous glucose/kg body weight) are given to children. During the test, the patient should be sitting up or lying down on the right side so as to facilitate rapid emptying of the stomach. Blood specimens are collected before giving the glucose load and after 2 h.

Table 6.6 summarises the criteria for identifying healthy adults, patients with diabetes mellitus and individuals with IGT for blood and plasma glucose, and for venous and capillary specimens.

Impaired fasting glucose (IFG) and impaired glucose tolerance (IGT)

The current WHO criteria define two conditions of impaired glucose homeostasis intermediate between normality and diabetes. These are the states of IFG and IGT. They cannot be considered as distinct clinical entities but in both there is an increased risk of development of cardiovascular (macrovascular) disease, but not the microvascular complications of diabetes. Both also increase the risk of developing diabetes in the future.

Monitoring the treatment of diabetic patients

There is now excellent evidence that, in both type 1 and type 2 diabetes, the incidence of long-term complications such as retinopathy can be reduced by achieving tight control, albeit at the expense of an increased frequency of hypoglycaemic episodes. This level of control requires meticulous monitoring of glycaemic control.

Home blood glucose monitoring

In order to achieve this level of control in type 1 patients, insulin doses need to be frequently and carefully adjusted on the basis of multiple daily blood glucose measurements. In patients in whom this level of control is unrealistic or is not needed, this requirement can be relaxed. In such patients, and in patients with type 2 diabetes, less frequent blood glucose measurements can be made, preferably covering different times of the day, although the frequency should be increased at times of illness or when control appears to have deteriorated.

Glycated haemoglobin

Blood glucose measurements made at the clinic only indicate the glucose concentration at that time, and may be unrepresentative of overall control. Measurement of

Table 6.6 Diagnostic criteria for diabetes mellitus and their dependence on the nature of the specimens collected for analysis. Clinical laboratory analysis will usually give results for venous plasma (bold).

	Glucose concentration (mmol/L)		
	Fasting		2h post-75g glucose
Normal individuals			
• Venous plasma	**<6.1**		**<7.8**
• Venous blood	<5.6		<6.7
• Capillary blood	<5.6		<7.8
Diabetes mellitus			
• Venous plasma	**≥7.0**	**or**	**≥11.1**
• Venous blood	≥6.1	or	≥10.0
• Capillary blood	≥6.1	or	≥11.1
IGT			
• Venous plasma	**<7.0**	**and**	**≥7.8 and <11.1**
• Venous blood	<6.1	and	≥6.7 and 10.0
• Capillary blood	<6.1	and	≥7.8 and 11.1
IFG			
• Venous plasma	**≥6.1 and <7.0**		**<7.8**
• Venous blood	≥5.6 and <6.1		<6.7
• Capillary blood	≥5.6 and <6.1		<7.8

the extent of the nonenzymatic glycation of Hb allows assessment of diabetic control over a longer period.

Glucose reacts spontaneously and nonenzymatically with free amino groups on proteins to form covalent glycated proteins. The extent of glycation depends on the average glucose to which the protein is exposed and on the half-life of the protein. Thus, long-lived structural proteins (e.g. lens protein) may be damaged as a result of the abnormal increase in protein glycation found in diabetics. Indeed, it has been suggested that glycation of structural proteins might be responsible for some of the long-term complications of diabetes. Shorter half-life proteins such as Hb also undergo excessive glycation in diabetes.

Several glycated derivatives of Hb exist, derived from the reaction of Hb with glucose, glucose-6-phosphate, etc. These are collectively known as HbA_1. The principal complex is the one formed with glucose itself, HbA_{1c}, which normally forms about 5% of circulating Hb.

Once formed, the HbA_{1c} stays within the red cell for its lifetime. The half-life of the red cell is about 60 days, thus the HbA_{1c} value reflects the average level of blood glucose concentration over the previous 1–2 months, with higher levels indicating poor diabetic control. The reliable interpretation of HbA_{1c} levels does however depend on the red cell half-life being normal. Artefactually low results will be obtained in any condition where the lifespan of the red cell is shortened. These conditions include haemolytic and some other anaemias, some haemoglobinopathies and repeated venesection, for example in the treatment of haemochromatosis.

A number of landmark trials have established the association between better glycaemic control, lower HbA_{1c} and lower incidence of diabetic complications. These trials have demonstrated that achieving lower levels of HbA_{1c}, ideally towards or into the non-diabetic range, reduces the incidence of micro- and macrovascular complications. However, this is at the expense of an increase in episodes of hypoglycaemia. For an individual patient, the balance between preventing future complications and avoiding hypoglycaemia will determine the goals of treatment, as judged by the HbA_{1c} achieved. In a young patient with type 1 diabetes and no pre-existing complications, the goal will be low and as close to the normal range as possible, or even into it, with the hope of achieving many years of complication-free survival. In an elderly patient with type 2 diabetes and multiple other problems, the aim of treatment may simply be the avoidance of symptoms of hyperglycaemia, and the HBA_{1c} goal will be correspondingly higher.

Standardisation of HbA_{1c} assays has been a problem in the past because of the lack both of a gold standard reference method and of preparations of absolutely known concentration to use as calibrators. Both of these issues have been solved on behalf of the International Federation for Clinical Chemistry (IFCC). Assays calibrated against these new standards give results slightly lower than previously, since there is a lack of interference from other species. International agreement was reached that from 2009 the new 'IFCC' HbA_{1c} was reported alongside the old HbA_{1c} for a period, before the old HbA_{1c} was phased out (in 2011 in the UK). In order to avoid potential confusion the units were changed from % to mmol/mol.

Glycated plasma proteins

Measurement of glycated plasma proteins (the major component of these proteins being albumin) can also be used to monitor diabetic control. The shorter half-life of albumin means that this test reflects control of blood glucose over the previous 10–15 days. Plasma fructosamine is a measure of glycated plasma proteins, but the widespread adoption of HbA_{1c} as the accepted marker of glycaemic control means that fructosamine measurements are not widely available. Fructosamine measurement has a use in patients with haemoglobinopathies, in whom HbA_{1c} can be difficult to measure and interpret.

Microalbumin

Urinary 'microalbumin' is a term that refers to urinary albumin loss that is greater than normal, but which remains below the threshold of detection by the urinalysis dipstick tests widely used for detecting the presence of urinary protein. The more sensitive tests required to detect 'microalbuminuria' are usually performed in the laboratory, although dipstick tests are also available. There is no analytical difficulty in measuring these low levels of albumin, but there is some variation in the type of sample to use and how best to express the results. Overnight timed urine collections are possibly most satisfactory, but random urine samples are usually used for convenience. Results are expressed on timed collections as an albumin excretion rate, or on a random sample as an albumin : creatinine ratio.

Up to 50% of type 1 diabetics may develop nephropathy, and the detection of microalbuminuria has been shown to signal an eventual progression to diabetic nephropathy. With the benefit of the early warning provided by the detection of microalbuminuria, there is some evidence that meticulous control of diabetes and hypertension, and the use of ACE inhibitors, delays the progress of the nephropathy.

Metabolic complications of diabetes mellitus

Patients with diabetes can develop severe metabolic derangements potentially leading to coma.

The causes can be classified as follows:

- hyperglycaemia, with or without ketoacidosis;
- lactic acidosis, with or without hyperglycaemia;
- hypoglycaemia, due to insulin excess;
- uraemia, for example due to diabetic nephropathy.

Diabetic ketoacidosis (DKA)

Diabetic ketoacidosis may be the presenting feature in a patient not previously recognised as having diabetes. In a patient with known diabetes, it may be precipitated by omitting insulin doses, or by the insulin dose becoming inadequate because of an increase in hormones with opposing action, due to intercurrent infection, trauma, or unusual physical or psychological stress. The clinical features are dehydration, ketosis and hyperventilation ('air hunger'). The degree of hyperglycaemia does not correlate with the severity of the metabolic disturbance in DKA, and in some patients it may not be very high (e.g. in children, pregnant women, malnourished or alcoholic patients).

Ketoacidosis is due to insulin deficiency, accompanied by raised plasma concentrations of the counter-regulatory hormones (adrenaline, cortisol, GH and glucagon). The changes in these circulating hormones result in hyperglycaemia and in mobilisation of free fatty acids from adipose tissue, and subsequent increased ketone body production in the liver (Figure 6.1).

The major metabolic abnormalities result from hyperglycaemia or ketoacidosis, or both. Hyperglycaemia causes extracellular hyperosmolality, which in turn leads to intracellular dehydration as well as to an osmotic diuresis. The osmotic diuresis causes loss of water, Na^+, K^+, calcium and other inorganic constituents, and leads to a fall in circulating blood volume. Ketone bodies stimulate the chemoreceptor trigger zone, so vomiting may exacerbate all these effects. The increased production of ketone bodies causes a metabolic acidosis with associated hyperkalaemia. Lactic acidosis and pre-renal uraemia may also be present.

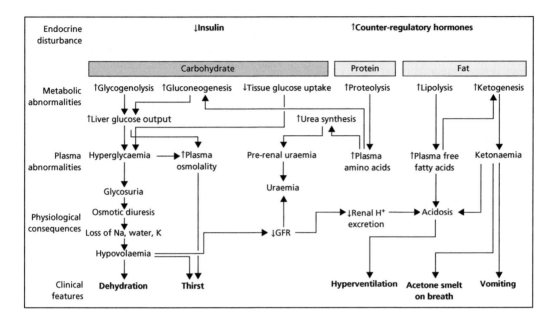

Figure 6.1 Metabolic and clinical abnormalities in DKA.

The introduction of the sodium-glucose cotransporter 2 (SGLT2) inhibitors as a new class of hypoglycaemic agent for the treatment of diabetes has caused a problem in the diagnosis of DKA. These drugs promote glucose loss in the urine, totalling up to 50–100 g/d, and are used primarily in the treatment of type 2 diabetes, but also increasingly (off label) in the treatment of type 1 diabetes. DKA appears to be a rare side effect of the SGLT2 inhibitors in both type 1 and type 2 diabetes, with predisposing factors including a reduction in insulin dose, dehydration, low food intake, weight loss and infection. Because of their mode of action the plasma glucose concentration may be unremarkably raised. Diagnosis then relies on a high index of clinical suspicion and the detection of ketonuria or ketonaemia.

Ketone bodies

Acetoacetate, β-hydroxybutyrate and acetone are collectively described as the 'ketone bodies', although β-hydroxybutyrate is not in fact a ketone. They are most commonly found in the blood in excessive amounts in uncontrolled diabetes. The levels of ketone bodies also increase during starvation, since ketone bodies form an important energy source for many tissues when carbohydrate intake or metabolism is limited. Acetoacetate is synthesised in the liver from acetyl-coenzyme A (CoA), itself derived from the oxidation of free fatty acids.

The acetoacetate may then be reduced to β-hydroxybutyrate or decarboxylated with the formation of acetone and CO_2. β-Hydroxybutyrate is the predominant ketone in DKA, and a major contributor to the acidosis.

Acetoacetic acid and 3-hydroxybutyric acid production give rise to metabolic acidosis, because the liver and other tissues cannot, in general, completely metabolise the increased amounts of these ketone bodies that are being formed. The acidosis is partly compensated by hyperventilation, with reduction in P_{CO_2}. The acidosis causes H^+ to move into cells and K^+ to move out. Increased plasma K^+ often results from the combined effects of the acidosis and the lack of insulin action that normally promotes K^+ entry into cells.

'Ketones' can be detected in serum or urine using a number of semi-quantitative point of care stick tests, and on some point of care testing glucose meters. The urine stick tests that have been most widely used in fact detect acetoacetate and do not react with β-hydroxybutyrate. This means that they may underestimate the presence of ketones in DKA. Furthermore, as DKA resolves, 3-hydroxybutyrate is oxidized to acetoacetate so urine stick testing may falsely suggest that the ketoacidosis is not improving. Laboratory assays and point of care testing meters specific for β-hydroxybutyrate are now available.

Laboratory assessment and management of diabetic ketoacidosis

An initial diagnosis is usually made on the basis of the history, clinical examination and dipstick testing of urine for glucose and ketone bodies, and measurement of blood glucose. Laboratory-based tests on blood are needed to evaluate the severity of the condition more precisely, and to monitor progress during treatment. It is rarely necessary, and indeed may be positively dangerous, to wait for laboratory results before starting emergency treatment. However, further treatment should be based on regular clinical assessment and on laboratory measurements.

Plasma glucose, urea, Na^+ and K^+ concentrations are measured on venous blood. Plasma Na^+ may be normal or low initially. Plasma K^+ is usually increased, but may be normal. Plasma urea is usually increased due to dehydration. Acid–base status is assessed by measurement of venous total CO_2 or by measurement of arterial 'blood gases' (H^+, P_{CO_2}, HCO_3^- and P_{O_2}). Plasma total CO_2 is nearly always reduced, often being less than 5 mmol/L in severe cases. Results of blood gas analysis indicate a metabolic acidosis with compensatory reduction in P_{CO_2}.

Treatment aims to replace fluid and electrolyte deficits, and to correct the metabolic abnormality by infusion of insulin. Knowledge of the fluid and electrolyte deficits likely to be present helps in planning appropriate therapy. The deficits may be as much as 5–10 L of water, 500 mmol of Na^+, 250–800 mmol of K^+ and 300–500 mmol of base (e.g. HCO_3^-) in patients with severe acidosis. Fluid replacement is usually given initially as isotonic saline. The rate of infusion will depend on the clinical circumstances, but should usually be rapid, at least initially, with careful monitoring of fluid status, often including the use of measurement of central venous pressure.

Most hospitals will have a protocol for the treatment of DKA, and this should be followed. However, a typical infusion regimen might entail isotonic saline infused at a rate of 1 L/h for the first 2 h, then 500 mL/h for the next 2 h. Potassium replacement is usually started early, in the knowledge that the patient has almost certainly developed a large K^+ deficit, and insulin will rapidly cause K^+ to enter the cells from the ECF. Serious hypokalaemia can develop quickly in the absence of early corrective action.

Insulin is usually given as a constant IV infusion, a typical starting rate being 6 U/h. If the glucose concentration does not fall in the first hour, the rate of infusion may need to be increased. Plasma glucose is monitored, and once it has fallen to between 10 and 15 mmol/L, dextrose is added to the IV fluids (e.g. 10% dextrose at an infusion rate of 100 mL/h); it may then be possible to decrease the rate of insulin infusion to maintain euglycaemia. This is continued until it is possible to re-establish the patient on oral food and water and a conventional subcutaneous insulin regimen.

The use of $NaHCO_3$ to correct the acidosis is not required or beneficial, because restoring normal renal perfusion allows excretion of H^+ and regeneration of HCO_3^-, and the return of metabolism to normal reduces H^+ production. In very severe acidosis (arterial H^+ >100 nmol/L) that does not rapidly begin to resolve with treatment it may be considered, but remains controversial and can be hazardous. It can cause:

- hypokalaemia, as rapid correction of the acidosis augments K^+ influx into cells;
- a paradoxical rise in CSF H^+ concentration rather than a fall, because CO_2 diffuses more rapidly into the CSF than HCO_3^-;
- Na^+ overload;
- shift of the oxy-haemoglobin saturation curve to the left, impairing oxygen delivery.

The frequency and timing of repeat analyses depend on the severity and nature of the ketoacidosis, and on the method of treatment. For most patients, it is advisable to repeat some of the initial analyses, particularly plasma K^+, after 1 h and thereafter at longer intervals if treatment is progressing satisfactorily.

Hyperosmolar hyperglycaemic state (HHS)

These patients are usually older than the ketotic group and typically have type 2 diabetes. Insulin deficiency has the same effects on carbohydrate metabolism as in DKA, but the presence of at least some insulin allows suppression of ketogenesis. HHS develops more slowly than DKA, taking a period of many days, and leading to more extreme losses of water and electrolytes. Severe hyperglycaemia (often >50 mmol/L) can develop with profound dehydration and a very high plasma osmolality (>320 mosm/kg), but no ketosis and minimal acidosis. This condition is often referred to as hyperosmolar nonketotic hyperglycaemia. It should be noted that patients with ketoacidosis may also have a raised osmolality, although this is not so marked.

The mortality of the hyperosmolar hyperglycaemic state is higher than that of DKA. Treatment is similar to that of ketotic hyperglycaemic patients, with administration of fluids and insulin. Despite the hypertonicity, isotonic saline replacement is usually used to restore the circulating volume and reverse dehydration. This in itself will cause a fall in glucose, and in the absence of ketonaemia insulin administration

CASE 6.2

A 14-year-old boy was found by his mother in a drowsy and uncooperative state. When the GP arrived, the mother told her that her son had seemed to be unusually thirsty for the last 1–2 months, and she thought that he had lost weight. Recently, he had been complaining of abdominal pain and discomfort.

He was admitted to a hospital as an emergency. On examination he was semi-conscious, with deep sighing respiration, a pulse rate of 120/min, a blood pressure of 94/56 and cold extremities. Chemical investigations on blood after admission showed the following:

Serum	Result	Age related reference ranges
Urea	24.5	2.5–6.6 mmol/L
Creatinine	73	31–67 µmol/L
Na⁺	128	132–144 mmol/L
K⁺	6.9	3.3–4.7 mmol/L
Glucose	35.2	mmol/L

Blood gas analysis	Result	Age related reference ranges
H^+	82	35–43 nmol/L
P_{CO2}	2.9	4.2–5.7 kPa
HCO_3^-	7.0	19–27 mmol/L
P_{O2}	14.0	10–14 kPa

What is the probable diagnosis, and how would you confirm this quickly? What principles should guide the treatment of this patient?

Comments: The patient almost certainly has DKA with typical clinical and biochemical features. The tachycardia, hypotension and cold peripheries suggest marked depletion of ECF. The arterial sample shows that he has a metabolic acidosis, and the plasma sample contains a high concentration of glucose. The high urea is consistent with renal impairment or dehydration. Ketoacidosis was confirmed by testing a urine specimen for ketone bodies (note that only some people can smell acetone in patients' breath). The mainstays of treatment for patients with DKA are:

- Fluid and electrolyte replacement, starting with saline (150 mmol/L) and containing added potassium chloride (40 mmol/L), usually as a standard regimen (check local protocols, but one regimen would be 1 L in the first 30 min, 500 mL in the next 30 min, and then 2 L over the next 4 h, and 2 L over the next 8 h).
- Insulin infusion usually starting at a rate of 6 U/h.
- Frequent monitoring of the patient's plasma glucose and K⁺, and monitoring of the central venous pressure. As the treatment takes effect, plasma K⁺ is liable to fall rapidly due to the large whole-body K⁺ deficit, despite the initially raised plasma K⁺.

should be delayed until the glucose is no longer falling with fluids alone. Most patients are insulin sensitive and, if glucose falls rapidly prior to adequate fluid replacement, the osmolality may rapidly decrease, resulting in water transfer from the extracellular to the intracellular space and cardiovascular collapse. Once the acute illness has resolved, most patients will not require continuing insulin, but will be managed on diet, with or without oral hypoglycaemic agents. There is an increased risk of thrombotic episodes in these patients, and treatment with anti-coagulants is generally considered advisable.

Hypoglycaemia

The plasma glucose concentration at which hypoglycaemic symptoms appear is very variable, often related more to the rate of fall of blood glucose than to the absolute value observed. Arbitrarily, a venous plasma glucose below 2.2 mmol/L is the biochemical definition of hypoglycaemia. It is convenient to distinguish between the hypoglycaemia that occurs after several hours of fasting and the hypoglycaemia that is due to some other stimulus (reactive hypoglycaemia), including the stimulus of a meal. It is often possible to distinguish these two categories on the basis of the patient's history.

Fasting hypoglycaemia

Fasting hypoglycaemia only occurs after some hours without food and may be precipitated by exercise. It always indicates an identifiable underlying disease. Failure to maintain a normal blood glucose in the fasting state is a feature of a number of endocrine conditions. It may be due to drugs (e.g. insulin overdose, accidental or deliberate;

sulphonylureas) or poisons (e.g. some toad-stools), inborn errors of metabolism (e.g. galactosaemia, hereditary fructose intolerance) or alcohol. It may be brought about by excess alcohol intake. Causes of fasting hypoglycaemia are summarised in Table 6.7, subdivided into causes of enhanced glucose utilisation and defective glucose production. An alternative classification is into causes of excess insulin-like activity (including insulinomas, administration of insulin or sulphonylureas, and as a paraneoplastic phenomenon in some malignancies, see Chapter 6: Other causes of fasting hypoglycaemia) and causes of noninsulin-induced hypoglycaemia (including severe hepatic dysfunction, ethanol and deficiency of cortisol or GH).

 CASE 6.3

An elderly man was visited by his son and was found to be semi-conscious. Neighbours had last seen him about 10 days previously, when he had seemed well. He was admitted to hospital. On examination, he appeared extremely dehydrated. The results of biochemical investigations were as follows:

Serum	Result	Reference ranges (adult male)
Urea	38	2.5–6.6 mmol/L
Creatinine	132	64–111 µmol/L
Na$^+$	151	135–145 mmol/L
K$^+$	4.8	3.6–5.0 mmol/L
Total CO$_2$	18	22–30 mmol/L
Glucose	61	mmol/L
Osmolality	417	280–296 mmol/kg

Comments: There is severe hyperglycaemia, resulting in a very high osmolality. The hyperglycaemia has driven an osmotic diuresis, resulting in loss of ECF and consequent reduction in the GFR and retention of urea.

The sustained osmotic diuresis causes a loss of water in excess of sodium, explaining the hypernatraemia. The total CO$_2$ is slightly reduced due to the impaired renal function, but is not as low as would be expected in a case of ketoacidosis with results as abnormal as these. The patient was very dehydrated, but was eventually able to provide a urine sample, which gave a negative test for ketones.

He had nonketotic hyperglycaemia. This only occurs in patients with type 2 diabetes. The insulin concentration required to oppose the ketogenic actions of glucagon is lower than that required to prevent increased glucose production. These patients have sufficient circulating insulin to prevent the ketogenesis, but not enough to prevent the hyperglycaemia. Treatment is by replacement of fluid and electrolyte losses, and by insulin infusion to restore the glucose. Once the acute episode is over, insulin is unlikely to be needed.

When the patient recovered, he reported having experienced increasing thirst and polyuria over several weeks. In response to the thirst, he had been drinking several large bottles of lemonade every day.

Table 6.7 Fasting hypoglycaemia.

Cause	Examples
Enhanced glucose utilisation	
• Endogenous overproduction of insulin	Hyperinsulinism of childhood (nesidioblastosis), insulinoma, pancreatitis, pancreatic tumours (as part of MEN I syndrome)
Defective glucose production	
• Endocrine disorders	Adrenocortical insufficiency and hypothyroidism (in both cases, primary and secondary), growth hormone deficiency
• Liver disease	Severe portal cirrhosis, acute hepatic necrosis, hepatic tumours
• Renal disease	End-stage renal failure
• Miscellaneous	Severe malnutrition, starvation, inherited metabolic disorders (e.g. glycogen storage disease type 1)

Reactive or post-prandial hypoglycaemia

Reactive or post-prandial hypoglycaemia occurs 2–5 h after meals and does not occur during a fast. It may occur after meals in patients who have undergone gastric surgery, or in early, usually type 2, diabetes.

Insulinoma

This is usually a small, solitary, benign adenoma of the pancreatic islets that secretes inappropriate amounts of insulin. Occasionally, multiple pancreatic adenomas may be associated with adenomas in other endocrine organs as part of the MEN I syndrome (see Chapter 5: Multiple endocrine neoplasia (MEN) syndromes; Table 17.6). The symptoms may be bizarre, and laboratory investigations play a major part in diagnosis.

Most patients develop symptomatic hypoglycaemia after a fast of 24–36 h, but in a few the fast may have to last for up to 72 h before symptomatic hypoglycaemia develops. Blood specimens are collected when hypoglycaemic symptoms develop, or after three overnight fasts. Most patients with an insulinoma will have unequivocal hypoglycaemia in one of these specimens,

even if they were asymptomatic. The diagnostic finding in patients suspected of having an insulinoma is a fasting plasma insulin that is inappropriately high in relation to the low plasma glucose.

It can be difficult to demonstrate fasting hypoglycaemia satisfactorily in some patients. In these cases, it may still be possible to obtain support for a diagnosis of insulinoma by measuring plasma C peptide concentration during an infusion of exogenous insulin sufficient to induce hypoglycaemia. Exogenous insulin contains little or no C peptide, and continuous detection of plasma C peptide shows that endogenous insulin release is not suppressed, as it should be in response to hypoglycaemia. This finding is strongly suggestive of insulinoma.

As stated above, therapeutic insulin preparations contain little or no C peptide. Accidental or deliberate overdose of insulin, giving rise to hypoglycaemia, can therefore be distinguished from insulinoma by measuring both plasma insulin and C peptide.

Other causes of fasting hypoglycaemia

Deficiency of hormones that antagonise insulin activity is an uncommon cause of hypoglycaemia. Some

---

 CASE 6.4

A 45-year-old woman who was unable to feed, wash or dress herself because of severe multiple sclerosis was being cared for in a nursing home. About 6 h after a visit by relatives, it was found that she could not be roused. On admission to a hospital, she was found to be profoundly hypoglycaemic (glucose 1.9 mmol/L), and required repeated IV infusions of glucose to maintain plasma glucose over the next 12–24 h. A sample of blood taken on admission was stored and subsequently analysed for insulin and C peptide. The results were inappropriately raised, considering the hypoglycaemia. Over the next few days, repeated overnight fasts failed to induce further hypoglycaemia. Eventually, after a prolonged fast of 4 days, glucose dropped to 2.5 mmol/L (not a hypoglycaemic level by strict criteria), at which time insulin and C peptide were undetectable.

Comments: The results on admission were suggestive of an insulinoma, with hypoglycaemia and inappropriately elevated insulin and C peptide levels. However, it proved difficult to induce a further episode of hypoglycaemia. Most patients with an insulinoma will be

hypoglycaemic on one or more occasions after three overnight fasts, even if not symptomatic. Even a prolonged fast failed to induce true hypoglycaemia, and at that time the insulin level was appropriately low. Review of her history revealed no suggestions of previous hypoglycaemic episodes. The clinical staff were accordingly forced to reconsider the initial diagnosis.

The sample of blood taken at the time of admission was sent for toxicological analysis, and was found to contain high concentrations of the oral hypoglycaemic drugs chlorpropamide and glibenclamide. These drugs are sulphonylureas, which act by enhancing pancreatic insulin secretion in response to glucose. Both chlorpropamide and glibenclamide have long half-lives, making hypoglycaemia an occasional problem even when used therapeutically in patients with diabetes.

The patient would have been unable to obtain or take these drugs. It was likely that a relative, distressed by her condition, had administered them. The police were informed, but it was felt that there was insufficient evidence to proceed further.

nonpancreatic tumours are associated with hypogly-caemia, mainly in patients with advanced malignant disease. Some of the larger tumours may consume excessive amounts of glucose, but there is also evidence for the production of hormonal insulin-like substances, as a paraneoplastic phenomenon. One cause of this is the excessive production of a large unprocessed form of insulin-like growth factor-2 (big IGF-2) by the tumour. Because of defective binding to IGF-binding proteins in the circulation, it is able to pass across capillary walls, reach insulin target tissues and exert its insulin-like effect.

 FURTHER READING

American Diabetes Association (2010) Diagnosis and classification of diabetes mellitus. *Diabetes Care* **33**, supplement 1, S62–S69.

World Health Organization (2006) *Definition and Diagnosis of Diabetes Mellitus and Intermediate Hyperglycaemia.* WHO, Geneva.

World Health Organization (2011) *Use of Glycated Haemoglobin (HbA1c) in the Diagnosis of Diabetes Mellitus: Abbreviated Report of a WHO Consultation.* WHO, Geneva.

7

Disorders of the hypothalamus and pituitary

Learning objectives

To understand:

- ✔ what hormones are released from the anterior and posterior pituitary gland and describe what target organ function they each regulate;
- ✔ the factors that regulate the synthesis and release of pituitary hormones and hypothalamic releasing factors;
- ✔ the clinical importance of prolactin measurements and why macroprolactinaemia is an important condition to recognise;
- ✔ what investigations should be carried out in patients with suspected pituitary or hypothalamic disease and be able to interpret the results of these investigations.

Introduction

Endocrinology is the study of the biological systems in the body that communicate with each other through the release of hormones. In this chapter the endocrine systems regulated through the hypo-thalamo-pituitary axis are discussed (Figure 7.1).

The diagnosis and management of endocrine diseases rely heavily on laboratory tests, often using a blood sample taken in the basal state. Occasionally, stimulation or suppression testing may have to be performed to uncover more subtle abnormalities or confirm the diagnosis. This chapter briefly describes the mechanisms that control the release of hormones by the hypothalamus and pituitary. Investigation of pituitary and hypothalamic function is often also intimately concerned with the investigation of the peripheral target glands which they control, and here we outline the methods commonly used to investigate suspected hypothalamo-pituitary dysfunction. Further information can be found in Chapters 8–10 concerning the thyroid, the adrenal and reproductive endocrinology.

The hypothalamus

The hypothalamus is derived from forebrain tissue on either side of the third ventricle and links the nervous system to the endocrine systems through the pituitary gland. The hypothalamus is a complex region in the brain that coordinates many behavioural and circadian rhythms, in addition to enforcing homeostatic mechanisms on specific target glands. The hypothalamus must respond to many different external and internal signals by releasing a variety of factors that act on the pituitary. In order to accomplish such a complex process the hypothalamus is connected with many parts of the CNS (e.g. stress results in release of corticotrophin-releasing hormone (CRH)).

Clinical Biochemistry Lecture Notes, Tenth Edition. Peter Rae, Mike Crane and Rebecca Pattenden.
© 2018 John Wiley & Sons Ltd. Published 2018 by John Wiley & Sons Ltd.
Companion website: www.lecturenoteseries.com/clinicalbiochemistry

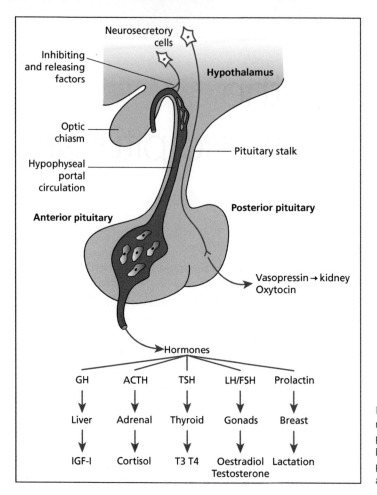

Figure 7.1 Factors which regulate the release of anterior pituitary hormones. The principal hormones released by the posterior pituitary are oxytocin and vasopressin.

Table 7.1 Factors that regulate the release of anterior pituitary hormones.

Hypothalamic stimulating hormone	Anterior pituitary hormone(s) released	Negative feedback control
CRH	ACTH	Cortisol (adrenal)
GHRH	GH	Somatostatin (hypothalamus)
GnRH	LH	Gonadal steroids (ovary and testes)
	FSH	Gonadal steroids and inhibin
TRH	TSH	FT4, FT3 (thyroid)
None identified	Prolactin	Dopamine (hypothalamus)

The hypothalamus secretes a number of hormones and other chemical agents that pass down the hypo-thalamo-hypophyseal portal blood vessels to the pituitary where they regulate the release of anterior pituitary hormones. The hormones produced by the target glands controlled by the anterior pituitary may exert negative feedback effects on the secretion of the corresponding hypothalamic or pituitary hormone. For example, plasma cortisol primarily influences the output of hypothalamic CRH, while plasma free thyroxine (FT4) primarily inhibits the release of TSH from the pituitary. Table 7.1 lists the various hypothalamic and pituitary hormones together with the factors that regulate their release. Concentrations of hypothalamic hormones in peripheral blood for the most part do not reflect hypothalamic activity, and their measurement is not considered to be of clinical relevance.

Anterior pituitary hormones

The pituitary gland comprises the embryologically and functionally distinct anterior pituitary (adenohypophysis) and posterior pituitary (neurohypophysis). The anterior pituitary hormones and their corresponding regulatory hormones/factors are described in detail in the following paragraphs.

Corticotrophin-releasing hormone and adrenocorticotrophic hormone

Hypothalamic CRH (41 amino acids) is the main stimulatory factor involved in the control of the pituitary–adrenal axis. Its release is subject to negative feedback control by cortisol released from the adrenal cortex (Figure 9.2).

ACTH is a monomeric polypeptide hormone (39 amino acids) secreted by corticotrophic cells. The biological activity of ACTH is contained in the 24 amino acids at the N-terminal end. The major activity of ACTH is the stimulation of adrenal steroid synthesis, especially that of the glucocorticoid, cortisol, but it also plays a permissive role in the synthesis of aldosterone. ACTH also stimulates melanocytes to produce melanin by a mechanism that involves further processing of the ACTH peptide to α-melanocyte stimulating hormone (α-MSH). This is the cause of the increased pigmentation seen in patients with ACTH-driven causes of Cushing's syndrome, in adrenocortical hypofunction and in Nelson's syndrome, a rare disorder arising from an ACTH-secreting pituitary macroadenoma after a therapeutic bilateral adrenalectomy. ACTH shows a marked diurnal variation, with the highest concentrations being found at approximately 8 am and the lowest at midnight. Marked increases in ACTH also occur with stress. ACTH is unstable in blood or plasma unless frozen. Blood samples should be collected in EDTA and the plasma separated within 30 min and frozen immediately.

ACTH and β-lipotrophin (β-LPH) exist next to each other at the C-terminal end of a much larger precursor molecule, pro-opiomelanocortin. In ectopic ACTH production, it seems that there may be abnormal processing of pro-opiomelanocortin which may result in the release of ACTH with a higher than normal molecular weight termed 'big ACTH'. The use of ACTH measurement in the investigation of syndromes of cortisol deficiency and excess is discussed in Chapter 9.

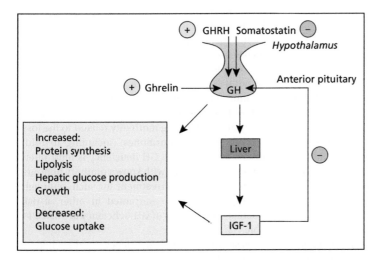

Figure 7.2 Factors which regulate the production and release of growth hormone (GH).

Gonadotrophin-releasing hormone and the gonadotrophins luteinising hormone and follicle-stimulating hormone

Gonadotrophin-releasing hormone (GnRH) is a decapeptide produced by the hypothalamus in pulses into the hypothalamic–hypophyseal portal circulation. GnRH stimulates the release of the gonadotrophins, luteinising hormone (LH) and follicle-stimulating hormone (FSH), from the gonadotroph. LH and FSH are dimeric glycopeptides and are released in pulses of approximately 90 min. This pulsatile release is essential for the gonadotrophins to exert their physiological actions. The release of GnRH is modified by oestrogens, progesterone, androgens and inhibins; these relationships are complex and are discussed in Chapter 10.

Thyrotrophin-releasing hormone and thyroid-stimulating hormone

Hypothalamic thyrotrophin-releasing hormone (TRH) is a tripeptide that controls the secretion of thyrotrophin (TSH) by the thyrotroph cells of the anterior pituitary. Free thyroid hormones inhibit the release of both TRH and TSH, but thyroid hormones exert their main negative feedback effects directly on TSH secretion (Figure 8.3).

TSH is a glycoprotein composed of an α-subunit that is common to LH, FSH and hCG, and a β-subunit specific to TSH. The place of TSH measurements in the investigation of thyroid function is discussed in Chapter 8.

Growth hormone-releasing hormone and growth hormone

The release of GH by the somatotrophs in the pituitary is stimulated by hypothalamic growth hormone-releasing hormone (GHRH), a 44 amino acid peptide, and inhibited by hypothalamic somatostatin, a 14 amino acid peptide. The peptide hormone ghrelin also stimulates the release of GH, acting in concert with GHRH to control both the timing and magnitude of GH release. Ghrelin is a 28 amino acid peptide released predominantly from epithelial cells lining the fundus of the stomach. Ghrelin also induces a feeling of hunger through action at the hypothalamus; its concentration is very high in patients with Prader–Willi

syndrome, who are typically obese and have voracious appetites. The release of GH is regulated by negative feedback of insulin-like growth factor-1 (IGF-1) and GH on the pituitary and hypothalamus. These factors modify the action of GHRH and stimulate the release of somatostatin, which in turn downregulates GH release (Figure 7.2). GH release is also suppressed by high doses of glucose, a response used in the investigation of suspected acromegaly and gigantism.

GH is a single polypeptide comprising 191 amino acids that circulates predominantly (~75%) as a 22 kDa form, with the remainder circulating as a 20 kDa form or as glycosylated and sulphated derivatives. About half of the circulating GH is bound to a GH-binding protein, which is the cleaved extracellular domain of the GH receptor; the bound fraction has a longer half-life in plasma than free GH and as such the bound fraction has prolonged bioactivity. GH is essential for normal growth, mediated in the most part by stimulating the hepatic release of IGF-1 (also known as somatomedin C). In serum, IGF-1 circulates bound to six binding proteins (IGFBPs) with IGFBP3 being the most important. There is increasing evidence to indicate that GH also promotes the release of IGF-1 locally in target tissues, which in turn act in a paracrine fashion. The GH receptor is found in many tissues in the body, including the liver, skeletal muscle and adipose tissue. Stimulation of the receptor can give rise to activation of numerous signalling pathways, which in turn allow GH to exhibit a wide variety of effects in different tissues.

Adult growth hormone deficiency

GH stimulates protein synthesis and growth, and also has metabolic effects that oppose the action of insulin, including increasing lipolysis and hepatic glucose production while decreasing tissue glucose uptake. It is now recognised that GH deficiency in the adult is associated with significant morbidity and mortality (Table 7.2). The clinical features present will depend on both the degree of GH deficiency and co-existing morbidity related to the loss of other pituitary hormones (including thyroid, adrenal and gonadal). GH deficiency is most often diagnosed in patients with known pituitary tumours or those undergoing treatment for such, although investigation may be warranted in other at-risk patients; other causes of GH deficiency are listed in Table 7.3.

Investigation of GH deficiency in the child is covered in Chapter 22.

Table 7.2 **Clinical problems associated with growth hormone deficiency.**

- Reduced bone mineral density
- Increased risk of bone fractures
- Impaired cardiac function
- Lipid abnormalities (increased LDL)
- Central obesity
- Increased insulin sensitivity
- Reduced exercise capacity
- Emotional disturbances
- Decreased quality of life
- Reduced life expectancy

Table 7.3 **Causes of adult growth hormone deficiency.**

- Pituitary tumour (± treatment)
- Cranial irradiation
- Traumatic head injury
- Idiopathic
- Sarcoidosis
- Haemochromatosis
- Lymphocytic hypophysitis

Investigation and treatment of growth hormone deficiency

Measurement of basal GH is of little value because GH is usually undetectable during the day. Although the finding of a low serum IGF-1 supports a diagnosis of GH deficiency, there is overlap between groups and normal IGF-1 does not exclude the possibility of severe GH deficiency. As a result, stimulation testing is essential to confirm the diagnosis.

GH release is stimulated by low blood glucose, exercise, stress, fasting and various pharmacological agents, which can be used to assess the GH axis. The most commonly used test to assess GH insufficiency is the insulin hypoglycaemia test (see Chapter 7: Dynamic function tests – insulin hypoglycaemia test), although arginine, GHRH, glucagon and clonidine can also be used for stimulation. Various protocols are available and local guidelines should be followed for interpretative limits. For the insulin hypoglycaemia test, a peak GH response <3 μg/L is widely considered to indicate severe GH deficiency, although there is some debate around values that constitute mild GH insufficiency, with cut-offs of 5 μg/L and 7 μg/L frequently used.

In the UK, NICE has recommended that GH treatment should only be commenced in adults with GH deficiency that is severely affecting their quality of life. To qualify for treatment, patients should meet the criteria listed in Table 7.4.

Table 7.4 **NICE criteria for treatment with recombinant GH.**

NICE Criteria for recombinant GH treatment. Patients must fulfill all criteria:

- Have a peak growth hormone response of less than 3 μg/L in the insulin hypoglycaemia test or a similar low result in another reliable test
- Have an impaired quality of life because of their GH deficiency (judged using a specific questionnaire called the 'Quality of life assessment of growth hormone deficiency in adults')
- Already be receiving replacement hormone treatment for other deficiencies of pituitary hormones, as required

Acromegaly and gigantism

These disorders are usually caused by adenomas of the anterior pituitary, or occasionally by ectopic secretion of GHRH. Gigantism results if the disorder occurs before closure of the epiphyses of the long bones, whereas acromegaly results if it occurs after their closure. Acromegaly has an insidious onset such that there is a mean delay of about 7 years prior to its diagnosis and in many cases the diagnosis is overlooked. Treatment aims to prevent the expanding tumour causing damage to the pituitary and optic nerves. Surgery is the usual first-line therapy but if this is unsuccessful, radiotherapy or medical intervention with somatostatin analogus (octreotide or lanreotide) or dopamine agonists is used. The GH antagonist pegvisomant appears to be very effective for treating the disease but requires daily injections and is very expensive.

Diagnosis

Diagnosis requires the measurement of GH and IGF-1. Random basal plasma GH is often very high in these patients, but the concentrations are too variable for accurate diagnosis and overlap with the range of GH found in some 'normal' individuals. However, a random GH below 0.5 μg/L essentially excludes a diagnosis of acromegaly *if* IGF-1 is within the reference range, whereas an elevated IGF-1 should prompt further investigation with a glucose tolerance test (see below). Reference ranges for IGF-1 are age and method specific and the local laboratory should provide these.

Glucose tolerance test

The response of plasma GH to a glucose tolerance test remains the 'gold standard' for the diagnosis of acromegaly. The patient is fasted overnight and an IV cannula is inserted. Blood samples are taken at –30, 0, 30, 60, 90 and 120 min, with glucose being given (75 g of glucose in 100 mL of water) at time 0 min. Normally, plasma GH falls to less than 0.5 µg/L at some time during this test. However, in patients with acromegaly or gigantism, GH does not fall in response to the stimulus of hyperglycaemia, and may even increase in about 30% of patients. The test is not specific for acromegaly and GH may fail to suppress in some patients who have poorly controlled diabetes mellitus, renal failure, anorexia or liver disease. In treated acromegalics, a GH of <0.5 µg/L is suggestive of cure while a GH of <1.5 µg/L indicates satisfactory control. Measurement of IGF-1 in the basal sample should also be performed.

 CASE 7.1

A 56-year-old bank manager complained to his GP of excessive sweating which was embarrassing him during meetings with clients. His GP had known him over many years, although he had not seen him recently, and thought that his facial features had become coarser over this period. Closer questioning revealed that he recently had to buy new shoes because his old ones were becoming tight, and that he had experienced problems with impotence over the past few months. Examination revealed hypertension and glucosuria. He was referred to an endocrine clinic with a presumptive diagnosis of acromegaly. Basal investigations on a sample taken at 9 am were as follows:

Serum	Result	Reference range
Cortisol	625	100–565 nmol/L
FT4	18	9–21 pmol/L
TSH	1.3	0.2–4.5 mU/L
Testosterone	7	10–30 nmol/L
LH	1.1	1.0–9.0 U/L
FSH	1.4	1.0–10.0 U/L
Prolactin	960	<500 mU/L

A GTT was performed:

Time (min)	Glucose (mmol/L)	GH (µg/L)
0	9.2	8.4
30	15.8	7.3
60	14.1	6.7
90	13.6	7.3
120	13.5	7.5

Visual fields were normal, and a magnetic resonance imaging (MRI) scan revealed the appearance of a small adenoma, confined within the pituitary gland.

Comments: The strong clinical suspicion of acromegaly is confirmed by the lack of suppression of GH during the GTT. The GTT also confirms the patient to have diabetes, due to the diabetogenic actions of GH. Abnormal glucose tolerance is seen in about a quarter of patients with acromegaly, IGT being slightly more common among these than frank diabetes.

Gonadotrophins and testosterone are low, confirming gonadal failure secondary to the pituitary lesion, rather than primary testicular failure.

The prolactin is elevated. Some GH-secreting adenomas also secrete prolactin. Alternatively, the adenoma may be interfering with the inhibitory control of prolactin secretion by dopamine.

The basal results suggest that the function of the adrenal and thyroid axes is normal.

Prolactin

Prolactin is a single polypeptide (198 amino acids) secreted by the lactotrophs of the pituitary. The lactotrophs comprise 10% of the anterior pituitary cells in men but 30% in women. Prolactin acts via specific receptors that are widely distributed, but their main location is the mammary gland where their activation by prolactin stimulates lactation and alveolar growth. Prolactin also has a role in the complex processes controlling gonadal function.

Macroprolactin is formed when normal (monomeric) prolactin combines with autoantibodies in a patient's serum to produce a prolactin–IgG complex (molecular weight 170 kDa), which is thought to be biologically inactive. The long half-life of the complex results in an apparent elevated prolactin concentration in the serum. The clinical importance of macroprolactinaemia is controversial, with a few studies reporting clinical features typically associated with hyperprolactinaemia; however, most studies suggest that there is no associated clinical disorder. In view of this controversy, it is advisable to seek an endocrine opinion if macroprolactinaemia is found in symptomatic patients. All laboratories should assess whether a persistently elevated prolactin is caused by macroprolactin. If macroprolactin is detected, the laboratory should estimate and report the concentration of monomeric prolactin.

Prolactin secretion is controlled by the inhibitory action of hypothalamic dopamine, but no hypothalamic stimulatory factor has been identified. There is a pulsatile release and diurnal rhythm of prolactin

CASE 7.2

A 30-year-old woman went to her GP with concerns about her fertility. She and her partner had been trying to have a baby for the past 7 months without success. She said she was having regular periods every 28 days.

The GP asked her to come back when she was at around day 21 of her cycle for a blood test and also to have a further blood sample taken during day 1–5 of her period. The results were as follows:

Serum	Result	Reference range
Progesterone (day 21)	43	nmol/L
Prolactin (day 3)	1400	<500 mU/L
Monomeric prolactin	250	<300 mU/L
LH (day 3)	3.0	2.0–9.0 mU/L
FSH (day 3)	3.0	2.0–10.0 mU/L
Oestradiol	120	75–140 pmol/L
TSH	2.1	0.2–4.5 mU/L
Free T4	15	9–21 pmol/L

How would you interpret these results?

Comments: The progesterone result shows that the patient is having ovulatory cycles. The prolactin is elevated but this is due to the presence of macroprolactin. Monomeric (bioactive) prolactin is within the reference range. Gonadotrophins and oestradiol are also normal. Thus there appears to be no biochemical evidence of an endocrine abnormality to explain the infertility. Further investigations may include assessing further cycles to ensure ovulation is occurring on a regular basis and also assessing her partner for infertility issues.

Table 7.5 The chief clinical problems associated with hyperprolactinaemia.

- Galactorrhoea
- Hypogonadism
- Amenorrhoea
- Breast tenderness
- Erectile dysfunction
- Decreased libido
- Gynaecomastia
- Infertility
- Osteoporosis
- Headache
- Visual field defect

Causes

There are many causes of hyperprolactinaemia including pregnancy, lactation, pituitary tumours, renal failure and the use of drugs that have dopamine agonist effects (Table 7.6).

Diagnosis

The differential diagnosis of hyperprolactinaemia requires a careful and accurate history and, where possible, drug therapy to be discontinued. Drug withdrawal may be possible if the drug is an anti-emetic or tranquilliser. It may be impossible to withdraw anti-psychotic medication, although a change to an anti-psychotic with a less profound effect on prolactin may be possible (e.g. olanzapine). The measurement should be repeated on a number of occasions to confirm that the raised level is persistent, because there is some evidence that a high result may represent a response to stress. Macroprolactinaemia should be excluded (Figure 7.3).

Pituitary tumours may secrete prolactin directly (prolactinoma) or, alternatively, a nonprolactin-secreting tumour may give rise to hyperprolactinaemia because the tumour exerts pressure on the pituitary stalk and prevents dopamine from reaching the pituitary from the hypothalamus. Prolactin is the only hormone secreted by prolactinomas, although some pituitary tumours secrete both GH and prolactin. Approximately one-third of prolactinomas are associated with only moderate increases in prolactin, in the range 700–1000 mU/L, but, if other causes are excluded, persistent basal levels of prolactin greater than 1000 mU/L strongly suggest that a tumour is present. If, in addition, radiological abnormalities are visible in the pituitary fossa, this

secretion, with the highest levels occurring during sleep and the lowest between 9 am and noon. Prolactin secretion increases in response to oestrogens, pregnancy, breastfeeding and stress. Certain drugs may also give rise to marked elevations in serum prolactin. There are male–female differences in the reference range for prolactin but often only a single range is used by laboratories.

Hyperprolactinaemia and its investigation

Features

Hyperprolactinaemia in women causes menstrual irregularities, galactorrhoea, low libido and infertility. In males low libido and erectile dysfunction are the usual early symptoms (Table 7.5).

Table 7.6 Causes of hyperprolactinaemia.

Category of cause	Examples
Physiological	Pregnancy, lactation, stress, exercise, macroprolactin
Drugs	
• Anti-psychotics	Phenothiazines, e.g. chlorpromazine Butyrophenones, e.g. haloperidol Thioxanthines, e.g. olanzapine, clozapine Risperidone Aripiprazole does not cause hyperprolactinaemia
• Anti-depressants	Tricyclics, e.g. amitriptyline SSRIs, e.g. paroxetine
• Anti-emetics	Metoclopramide, domperidone
• Cardiovascular actions	Methyldopa, reserpine, verapamil
• Histamine receptor agonists and proton pump inhibitors	Cimetidine, ranitidine Omeprazole, pantoprazole
• Monoamine oxidase inhibitors	Phenelzine
• Opiates	Morphine, methadone, etc.
• Oestrogen	Combined contraceptive pill
Pathological	Prolactinoma, pituitary macroadenoma, pituitary stalk compression, renal failure, hypothyroidism, anorexia, cirrhosis, seizures

supports the diagnosis of prolactinoma rather than functional hyperprolactinaemia in these patients. Some rare ectopic hormone-secreting tumours produce prolactin.

Hyperprolactinaemia in psychiatric patients

Hyperprolactinaemia is a common finding in psychiatric patients, particularly those taking anti-psychotic medication. A common clinical problem is to decide if anti-psychotic drug use is masking hyperprolactinaemia due to a pituitary tumour. It may be possible to address this issue by taking the blood sample just prior to a dose (e.g. olanzapine and clozapine produce levels of prolactin to around 1000 mU/L which peak 1–5 hours after taking medication). Alternatively it may be possible to change to a medication that is less likely to cause hyperprolactinaemia (e.g. aripiprazole). The need for further investigations should be guided by the degree of hyperprolactinaemia but, as can be seen from Table 7.7, there is marked overlap in the various diagnostic groups. Further investigations such as imaging may need to be performed in a few patients. It should be appreciated that patients with severe depression and those taking anti-psychotic medication often show an increase in pituitary size.

If patients are to be started on anti-psychotic medication, a protocol similar to that shown in Table 7.8 should be followed.

 CASE 7.3

A 26-year-old woman attended an outpatient clinic with a complaint of galactorrhoea for several months. Her only other medical history was of troublesome migraines since childhood, for which she had taken a variety of medications whose names she could not remember. On examination, it was possible to express milk from her breasts.

Investigations were unremarkable apart from: prolactin 1127 mU/L (reference range <500 mU/L). What might be the cause of the galactorrhoea in this patient?

Comments: Closer questioning revealed that her migraine treatment had been changed some months previously to a preparation that combined an analgesic (paracetamol) and anti-emetic (metoclopramide). Metoclopramide can cause hyperprolactinaemia through its anti-dopaminergic activity.

The patient stopped this preparation, and took paracetamol alone. The galactorrhoea and hyperprolactinaemia resolved.

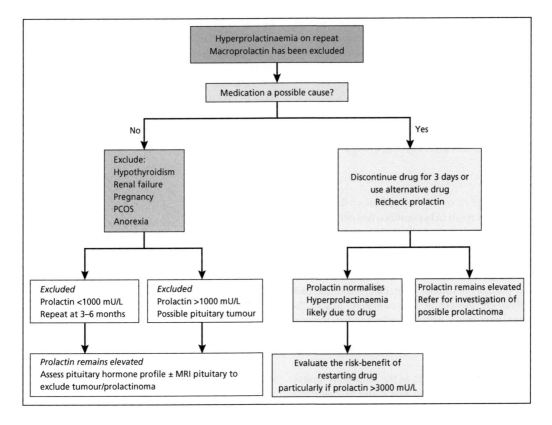

Figure 7.3 Suggested protocol for the investigation of hyperprolactinaemia.

Table 7.7 Degrees of hyperprolactinaemia in various clinical scenarios.

Prolactin (mU/L)	Clinical scenario
>6000	Macroprolactinoma
1000–3000	Microprolactinoma
500–2000	Pituitary stalk compression
Often up to 2000	Anti-psychotics
Up to 1000	Olanzapine, clozapine
Up to 5000	Thioxanthines, risperidone

Table 7.8 Monitoring patients on anti-psychotic medication for hyperprolactinaemia.

- Screen for symptoms and measure prolactin prior to starting medication
- Screen for symptoms at each visit until stable then yearly if on drug known to raise prolactin
- Check prolactin if symptoms develop. If prolactin is >3000 mU/L and does not fall on changing medication, refer for further investigation
- Choice of anti-psychotic should be tempered by history of hyperprolactinaemia
- If known osteoporosis, <25 years old or history of breast cancer, use an anti-psychotic with low risk of hyperprolactinaemia

Endocrine changes in anorexia nervosa

Anorexia nervosa results in a number of abnormal endocrine findings that are reversed once normal eating patterns and normal weight have been restored. Many of these changes arise from altered hypothalamic responses. The secretion of GnRH is often impaired in women whose BMI falls below 20 kg/m², resulting in low serum levels of LH, FSH and oestradiol. FT4 often falls to low or low normal values, while FT3 is nearly always subnormal. TSH concentrations and prolactin are usually normal. Serum cortisol is often raised as a consequence of both increased production and an increased half-life, and the usual diurnal variation is lost. GH levels are also often increased as a consequence of starvation.

Anterior pituitary disease and its investigation

Causes

A wide range of conditions can affect the anterior pituitary and result in hypopituitarism either directly or through an effect on the hypothalamus (Table 7.9). The most common cause of hypopituitarism is a pituitary tumour. Failure may be total (panhypopituitarism) or partial, in which case secretion of one or more pituitary hormones is retained. Silent microadenomas are present in approximately 20% of the normal population, with clinically apparent tumours occurring in about 2 per 100 000. Pituitary tumours are usually either nonfunctional or secrete only one hormone (Table 7.10).

Therapeutic action such as the removal of a pituitary tumour or irradiation may cause or exacerbate hypopituitarism.

Although most pituitary adenomas produce a single hormone in excess, pressure effects may decrease secretion of other pituitary hormones, so overall pituitary function should be assessed in all patients

in whom the presence of an adenoma has been established. Loss of pituitary hormones in progressive hypopituitarism usually occurs in a sequential and predictable manner. Secretion of LH, FSH and GH is usually lost first, followed by TSH and ACTH. Loss of prolactin production occurs only rarely and only when there is extensive pituitary damage. Because of this sequential loss, adults tend to have presenting symptoms that reflect loss of LH and GH (Table 7.11).

Investigation

This requires the assessment of endocrine and neuro-ophthalmological function together with

Table 7.10 Pituitary adenomas in decreasing order of frequency.

- Nonfunctional
- Prolactinoma
- GH secreting
- ACTH secreting
- TSH secreting
- LH/FSH secreting

Table 7.11 Presenting clinical features in hypopituitarism.

Features of hormone deficiency	Features of tumour process
Infertility	Headache
Menstrual disturbances	Neuro-ophthalmological defects
Decreased libido	Facial pain
Erectile dysfunction	Functional adenoma – features depend on hormone secreted, e.g. prolactinoma may present with loss of libido, amenorrhoea and galactorrhoea
Reduction in muscle bulk	
Decreased body hair	
Fatigue and cold intolerance	
Weight gain	
Polyuria and polydipsia	

Table 7.9 Causes of hypopituitarism.

Cause	Examples
Tumours	Pituitary adenoma, craniopharyngioma, cerebral tumours
Trauma	Head injury
Vascular disease	Severe hypotension, cranial arteritis, infarction (often of pre-existing tumour), post-partum necrosis (Sheehan syndrome)
Infection	Meningitis (particularly tuberculous)
Iatrogenic	Surgery, radiotherapy
Hypothalamic disorders	Tumours, functional disturbances secondary to starvation (anorexia nervosa), Cushing's syndrome
Granulomatous disease	Sarcoidosis

radiological investigations as appropriate. In many cases, the measurement of basal pituitary hormones and primary target organ hormones in serum or plasma is sufficient (Table 7.12). The investigation of suspected acromegaly (Chapter 7: Acromegaly and gigantism) and Cushing's syndrome (Chapter 9: Cushing's syndrome), however, requires the use of stimulation and/or suppression tests. Stimulation tests involving the IV administration of GnRH and TRH are now rarely used, with the exception of GnRH testing in assessing pubertal status in children.

Table 7.12 Interpretation of basal hormone measurements.

Basal hormone measurements (9am)	Interpretation
Cortisol	<100nmol/L – adrenocortical deficiency likely 100–400nmol/L – perform a Synacthen test >400nmol/L – adrenocortical deficiency unlikely
ACTH	Labile hormone; may be inconvenient to measure on first occasion. Interpret in conjunction with cortisol to identify inappropriate responses
Prolactin	Persistently >1000mU/L suggestive of a pituitary tumour if secondary causes have been excluded (Table 7.6)
TSH	Low in only 50% of cases of hypopituitarism Low also in nonthyroidal illness
Free T4	Low in all cases of secondary hypothyroidism Low values often found in nonthyroidal illness
Male LH, FSH, testosterone	Testosterone >12nmol/L with a normal LH/FSH signifies adequate function of the pituitary–gonadal axis Many elderly males have a low-normal testosterone Low LH/FSH/testosterone often found in patients with severe illness

Basal hormone measurements (9am)	Interpretation
Female LH, FSH, oestradiol	Interpretation complicated by the physiological changes that occur during the normal menstrual cycle Gonadotrophin deficiency suggested by persistently low gonadotrophins and oestradiol (if effects of oral contraceptives, stress, illness and low BMI have been excluded) The absence of a significant elevation in LH and FSH in a post-menopausal woman may raise suspicion of gonadotrophin deficiency
Osmolality (serum and urine)	Measure if there is clinical suspicion of posterior pituitary dysfunction
Growth hormone	Unhelpful – often undetectable in 'normal' individuals

Pituitary function can be assumed to be normal if the thyroid and gonadal axes and osmolalities are normal and plasma cortisol is greater than 400 nmol/L, and there are no other clinical features of pituitary disease.

Further investigations

If there is strong clinical evidence for pituitary disease or there are basal deficiencies, an insulin hypoglycaemia test can be performed to assess ACTH and GH reserve.

If thyroid and adrenal deficiencies have been identified on the basal sample, these should be treated with thyroxine (preceded by hydrocortisone therapy if required) and hydrocortisone, respectively, before any further investigation. Hypothyroidism reduces the ACTH and GH responses to an insulin hypoglycaemia test. A fluid deprivation test should be performed if symptoms or basal osmolality suggest posterior pituitary dysfunction.

CASE 7.4

A 58-year-old man saw his GP for review of his hypertension. He mentioned problems with impotence and decreased libido, which he ascribed to his anti-hypertensive medication (a β-blocker), having read the package insert containing information for patients. However, further questioning revealed that the patient was now shaving only once a week. Examination revealed pallor and loss of axillary and pubic hair. The results of baseline blood tests were as follows:

Serum	Result	Reference range
Cortisol	78	100–565 nmol/L
TSH	0.3	0.2–4.5 mU/L
FT4	8	9–21 pmol/L
Testosterone	4.2	10–30 nmol/L
LH	1.0	1.0–9.0 U/L
FSH	0.9	1.0–10.0 U/L
Prolactin	40	<500 mU/L

What do these results show? What further investigations are required?

Comments: The history, physical signs and hypofunction of multiple endocrine glands suggest hypopituitarism. In the presence of the other biochemical findings and the pallor, primary adrenal failure is unlikely to be the cause of the low plasma cortisol. This is due to ACTH deficiency. The thyroid function tests show low FT4 secondary to pituitary insufficiency, and the low gonadotrophins and testosterone confirm secondary gonadal failure.

The biochemical results are sufficiently informative and further biochemical investigation is not needed, although plasma ACTH or a Synacthen test could be used to confirm ACTH deficiency. Radiological investigation of the pituitary using computed tomography (CT) or MRI scanning is indicated. The patient can be treated with hydrocortisone and, in due course, thyroxine and testosterone. Although there is nothing in the history to suggest posterior pituitary insufficiency (diabetes insipidus), this may be unmasked by hydrocortisone treatment. The patient may need investigation using a water deprivation test.

 CASE 7.5

A 20-year-old woman presented to her GP 9 months post-partum with persistent galactorrhoea despite never having breastfed. She also complained of agitation, palpitations and weight loss. The following results were found in a random sample and confirmed in a second specimen taken 7 days later:

Serum	Result	Reference range
Cortisol	450	100–565 nmol/L
FT4	30	9–21 pmol/L
FT3	9.5	2.6–6.2 pmol/L
TSH	6.0	0.2–4.5 mU/L
LH	1.1	2.0–9.0 U/L
FSH	1.4	2.0–10.0 U/L
Prolactin	850	<500 mU/L
GH	<0.10	

There was no change in serum TSH 20 and 60 min after the injection of TRH (a TRH test).

Comment on these results.

Comments: The results are consistent with hyperthyroidism caused by a TSH secreting pituitary tumour (TSHoma) and hyperprolactinaemia due to hypothalamic disconnection causing loss of inhibitory dopamine reaching the pituitary. In end-organ resistance, the TSH response to TRH is normal or exaggerated while a flat or blunted response is seen in TSHoma. An MRI scan showed a 25 mm diameter mass arising in the pituitary fossa. The patient was treated by trans-sphenoidal surgery to remove the tumour and post-operative pituitary radiotherapy was given. This rendered the patient euthyroid with normal prolactin and a resolution of her galactorrhoea. Histopathology of the resected tumour showed pituitary tumour cells that stained positive for TSH, prolactin and α-subunit but not for gonadotrophins or ACTH. TSHoma is very rare with an incidence of 2 per 10^7, with most patients presenting with thyrotoxicosis and hyperprolactinaemia.

Treatment

Hypopituitarism is treated by giving the appropriate hormone replacement (Table 7.13). Trans-sphenoidal surgery is the usual first-line treatment for most pituitary adenomas, although for prolactinoma medical therapy with dopamine agonists is capable of successfully shrinking the tumour in more than 85% of cases.

Table 7.13 **Hormone replacement in hypopituitarism.**

Pituitary deficiency	Replacement hormone
ACTH	Hydrocortisone
TSH	Thyroxine
LH/FSH male	Testosterone
LH/FSH female	Oestrogen
GH	GH
ADH	Desmopressin
Prolactin	None required

Dynamic function tests – insulin hypoglycaemia test

The insulin hypoglycaemia test is the traditional test for the assessment of GH reserve, as well as for the HPA axis. It is also used by some for the investigation of suspected hypopituitarism in adults and children. The test is contraindicated in patients with epilepsy or heart disease, untreated hypothyroidism or those with a basal cortisol of less than 50 nmol/L.

Insulin is administered IV (typically 0.15 U/kg) to lower blood glucose to 2.2 mmol/L or less while monitoring serum cortisol and growth hormone. Samples for glucose, GH and cortisol are taken basally (before insulin) and at 30, 45, 60 and 90 min after IV insulin injection. The test requires close supervision, with glucose available for immediate IV administration if symptoms of severe hypoglycaemia develop. Failure to achieve a glucose concentration below 2.2 mmol/L invalidates the test, and repetition, with insulin incremented in steps of 0.05 U/kg, may be necessary.

Interpretation of results

Blood glucose should fall below 2.2 mmol/L or there must be a 50% or more fall in glucose concentration, and symptoms of hypoglycaemia must be present (i.e. sweating, tachycardia, etc.). Serum cortisol normally reaches its maximum at 60 or 90 min, the level reached being at least 400 nmol/L, and serum GH typically exceeds 5 μg/L. A GH response below 3 μg/L is consistent with severe GH deficiency. Patients with Cushing's syndrome, whatever the cause, do not respond normally to insulin-induced hypoglycaemia. There is often a high basal serum cortisol and usually little or no increase in serum cortisol, despite the production of an adequate degree of hypoglycaemia. The diagnosis of Cushing's syndrome is discussed further in Chapter 9.

Monitoring treatment in hypopituitarism

Following surgery or after pituitary irradiation for the treatment of a pituitary adenoma the residual pituitary function should be carefully monitored.

After surgery, transient diabetes insipidus is common. Glucocorticoid replacement is often given in the immediate post-operative period, but after 3 days the evening dose of hydrocortisone should be omitted and the morning 9 am plasma cortisol assessed. If the 9 am cortisol is less than 400 nmol/L therapy should be continued and further assessments carried out at a later period. If cortisol is more than 400 nmol/L, hydrocortisone therapy can be discontinued, but further assessment must be made at follow-up. A Synacthen test can give misleading results in the immediate post-operative period, and should not be performed until 6 weeks post-operatively. Basal FT4, TSH, LH, FSH and oestradiol in females or testosterone in males should also be assessed post-surgery and again after 6 weeks. Abnormalities in gonadotrophins and oestradiol may persist in females for 2–3 months after surgery.

After pituitary irradiation a slow decline in pituitary function may continue for many years, and long-term follow-up and monitoring is required.

Monitoring hormone replacement therapy

T4 should be given to achieve plasma FT4 in the upper third of the reference range. There is variability in practice with regards to monitoring hydrocortisone replacement, and random measurements of cortisol are of little value. Some assess serum cortisol throughout the day after each dose of hydrocortisone is given, whereas others assess the urinary free cortisol profile. If testosterone replacement is required, monitoring depends on the mode of replacement therapy given. Total testosterone should be measured a few days after an injection of testosterone ester depot followed by a repeat taken immediately before the next dose. If transdermal therapy is given, a similar protocol can be followed. For patients receiving oral testosterone undecanoate, serum testosterone can be misleading because low levels can be found when replacement is adequate; this is because of conversion of testosterone to dihydrotestosterone. Oestrogen replacement is difficult to assess biochemically because most hormone replacement pharmaceuticals for oestrogen contain synthetic or equine oestrogens that are not detected by the usual assays for oestradiol.

Posterior pituitary hormones

The posterior pituitary is an integral part of the neuro-hypophysis. It produces at least two hormones: arginine vasopressin (also known as antidiuretic hormone (ADH)) and oxytocin. Both these hormones are synthesised in the hypothalamus as larger pro-hormones that are stored in neurosecretory granules. These granules migrate by axonal flow to the nerve terminals in the posterior pituitary from where they can be released into the circulation. During this migration the pro-hormones are cleaved to produce vasopressin and oxytocin together with neurophysin I and II. Uterine contraction and milk release from the lactating breast is controlled by oxytocin. Disorders of oxytocin secretion are uncommon and are not clinically important.

Vasopressin

Vasopressin is a nonapeptide that has an important role in the control of the tonicity of the ECF and hence water balance. It increases the water permeability of the distal tubules and collecting ducts of the kidney. The major stimulus to vasopressin release is a rise in plasma osmolality sensed by the osmoreceptors. A fall in ECF volume and blood pressure (sensed by baroreceptors) or stress can also trigger vasopressin release.

SIADH is defined as the excessive secretion of vasopressin in the absence of the normal major stimuli for vasopressin secretion. SIADH is considered in more detail in Chapter 2: Hyponatraemia with normal ECF volume, and Table 2.6.

Diabetes insipidus

Deficiency of vasopressin gives rise to cranial diabetes insipidus. It is either primary (idiopathic, familial) or secondary to disease or injury in or close to the pituitary. Deficiency of vasopressin may be the sole hormonal abnormality, or there may also be disturbances of anterior pituitary hormone production in patients with secondary vasopressin deficiency. Recognition of hyposecretion of vasopressin depends on measurement of urine and plasma osmolalities and the performance of urine concentration tests (Chapter 4: Urine osmolality and renal concentration tests).

8

Abnormalities of thyroid function

Learning objectives

To understand:

- ✔ the biosynthetic pathways involved in thyroid hormone synthesis and their action;
- ✔ the mechanisms that regulate the hypothalamic–pituitary–thyroid axis;
- ✔ the causes and features of thyroid dysfunction and the investigations that should be performed when thyroid disease is suspected;
- ✔ how to interpret the results of thyroid function tests both for diagnosis and in monitoring treatment;
- ✔ the concept of subclinical thyroid disease and when treatment should be implemented in such patients;
- ✔ the mechanisms that lead to changes in thyroid function tests in nonthyroidal illness, and how to interpret results in such patients;
- ✔ the drugs that commonly give rise to abnormal thyroid function tests and the various mechanisms by which these drugs produce such an effect.

Introduction

Thyroid hormones are essential for normal growth, development and metabolism, and their production is tightly regulated through the hypothalamic–pituitary–thyroid axis.

Thyroid disease is common, particularly in women, and the prevalence rises with age such that around 10% of the population over 65 years of age may have some abnormality in thyroid function. Although primary diseases of the thyroid gland are the most common, pituitary disease and the use of certain drugs can also give rise to thyroid dysfunction. Once diagnosed, thyroid disease is easily treated, with an excellent long-term outcome for most patients.

This chapter outlines the pathways of thyroid hormone synthesis and metabolism. The tests used in diagnosis and management of thyroid disease are described, together with guidance on their interpretation.

Thyroid hormone synthesis, action and metabolism

Synthesis and metabolism

Thyroxine (T4) and small amounts of tri-iodothyronine (T3) and reverse T3 (rT3) are all synthesised in the thyroid gland (Figure 8.1) by a process involving:

Clinical Biochemistry Lecture Notes, Tenth Edition. Peter Rae, Mike Crane and Rebecca Pattenden.
© 2018 John Wiley & Sons Ltd. Published 2018 by John Wiley & Sons Ltd.
Companion website: www.lecturenoteseries.com/clinicalbiochemistry

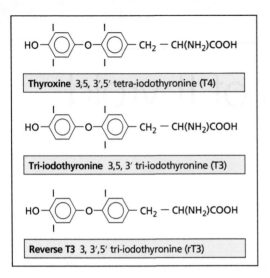

Figure 8.1 The structure of the thyroid hormones T4, T3 and reverse T3.

- Trapping of iodide from plasma by a sodium iodine symporter in the thyroid.
- Oxidation of iodide to iodine by thyroid peroxidase.
- Incorporation of iodine into tyrosyl residues on thyroglobulin in the colloid of the thyroid follicle. Mono-iodotyrosine (MIT) and di-iodotyrosine (DIT) are formed.
- Production of T4 and T3 by coupling iodotyrosyl residues in the thyroglobulin molecule.
- Splitting off T4 and T3 from thyroglobulin following its reabsorption from the colloid.
- Release of T4 and T3 into the circulation.

These stages are shown diagrammatically in Figure 8.2.

Thyroxine, a pro-hormone, is produced exclusively by the thyroid. The *biologically active hormone is T3*, and about 85% of plasma T3 is formed by outer-ring (5′) mono-deiodination of T4 in liver, kidneys and muscle (Figure 8.3). Thyroxine also undergoes inner-ring (5) mono-deiodination

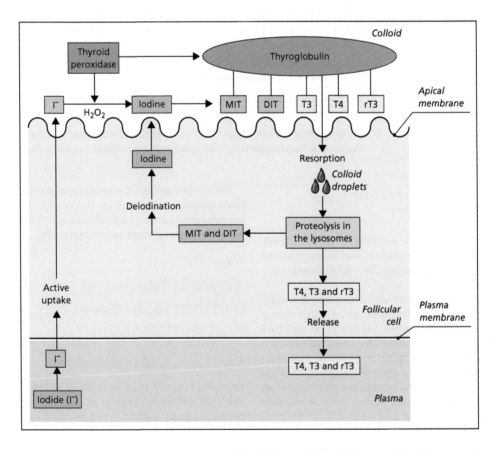

Figure 8.2 The synthesis of T3 and T4 in the thyroid gland. The metabolism of T4 is described in Figure 8.3. rT3, DIT and MIT are hormonally inactive.

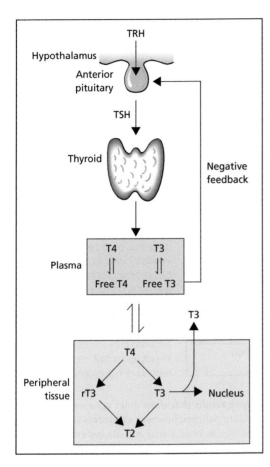

Figure 8.3 Regulation of thyroid hormone synthesis and metabolism.

in nonthyroidal tissues, with the production of metabolically inactive rT3.

Plasma transport and cellular action

Thyroid hormones are transported in plasma almost entirely bound, reversibly, to plasma proteins. Thyroxine-binding globulin (TBG) is the major binding protein, binding about 70% of plasma T4 and 80% of plasma T3. Transthyretin (also called thyroxine-binding pre-albumin) and albumin also bind thyroid hormone such that more than 99.8% of thyroid hormones circulate bound to these three proteins.

Approximately 0.05% of plasma T4 and 0.2% of plasma T3 are free (i.e. unbound to protein). Only the free fractions can cross the cell membrane and affect intracellular metabolism. After binding to high-affinity

binding sites on the plasma membrane, the hormones are actively transported into cells by specific energy-dependent transporters. In the cell T4 is metabolised to T3, which then binds to specific nuclear receptors that in turn activate T3-responsive genes. These gene products modify a wide range of cell function including basal metabolic rate and the metabolism of lipids, carbohydrates and proteins. High concentrations of thyroid hormone increase the basal metabolic rate and stimulate breakdown of protein and lipids. Low concentrations of thyroid hormone result in low metabolic rate, weight gain and poor physical and mental development in the child.

Regulation of thyroid function

The most important regulator of thyroid homeostasis is TSH (or thyrotrophin; Figure 8.3). The production of TSH is controlled by a stimulatory effect of the hypothalamic tripeptide, TRH (or thyroliberin), mediated by a negative feedback from circulating FT3 and FT4. It is thought that the hypothalamus, via TRH, sets the level of thyroid hormone production required physiologically, and that the pituitary acts as a 'thyroid-stat' to maintain the level of thyroid hormone production that has been determined by the hypothalamus. Dopamine, somatostatin and glucocorticoids also appear to be involved in inhibiting the release of TSH, and these agents together with the interleukins may be important modifiers of TSH release in nonthyroidal illness (NTI).

Investigations to determine thyroid status

Measurement of TSH and thyroid hormones should be performed to determine the patient's thyroid status. The interpretation of such results is shown in Figure 8.4.

Thyrotrophin

The measurement of TSH (reference range 0.2–4.5 mU/L) in a basal blood sample by immunometric assay provides the single most sensitive, specific and reliable test of thyroid status in both overt and subclinical thyroid disease. In primary hypothyroidism, TSH is increased, while in primary hyperthyroidism, TSH is usually undetectable (below 0.01 mU/L). There are exceptions to this, and both raised and undetectable TSH may be found in some euthyroid patients (Table 8.1).

High	Overt hyperthyroidism	TSHoma (very uncommon) or Assay interference or Thyroid-hormone resistance (uncommon)	TSHoma (very uncommon) or Assay interference or Thyroid-hormone resistance (uncommon)
Free T4 Normal	Subclinical hyperthyroidism or T3-hyperthyroidism or Nonthyroidal illness	EUTHYROID	Subclinical hypothyroidism or Recovery from nonthyroidal illness
Low	Nonthyroidal illness or Hypopituitarism (uncommon)	Nonthyroidal illness or Hypopituitarism (uncommon)	Overt hypothyroidism or Recovery from nonthyroidal illness
	Low	Normal TSH	High

Figure 8.4 Interpretation of thyroid function tests in patients being investigated for suspected thyroid disease. The lines indicate the lower and upper limits of the reference range. In cases where more than one interpretation is possible further tests may need to be performed such as T3, α-subunit, pituitary imaging. In any patient who exhibits an unusual combination of TSH/FT4 assay interference should always be excluded prior to initiating further investigations that may be expensive, e.g. imaging.

Table 8.1 Causes of an abnormal TSH in some clinically euthyroid patients.

Low TSH	High TSH
Subclinical hyperthyroidism	Subclinical hypothyroidism
Treated hyperthyroid patients (first 6 months)	Recovery phase of nonthyroidal illness
Ophthalmic Graves' disease	
Nonthyroidal illness	
Pregnancy (during the first 20 weeks)	
Treatment with dopaminergic drugs or high dose glucocorticoids	

Free T4 and free T3

Free thyroid hormone concentrations are independent of changes in the concentration and affinity of thyroid hormone-binding proteins and theoretically provide a more reliable means of diagnosing thyroid dysfunction than measurement of total hormone concentrations. The reference range for FT4 is 10–21 pmol/L and that for FT3 is 2.6–6.2 pmol/L. Several assay techniques have been developed to measure free hormone concentrations. These methods produce results that show good agreement in most ambulant patients; however, in patients with nonthyroidal illness results may not always correlate well with one another due to various assay artefacts.

Total T4 and total T3

More than 99% of T4 and T3 circulate in plasma bound to protein, thus any change in the concentration of these binding proteins, particularly TBG, will be reflected in the concentrations of total T4 and total T3 (reference ranges: total T4 70–150 nmol/L; total T3 1.2–2.8 nmol/L). However, FT4 and FT3 remain normal if pituitary–thyroid homeostasis is maintained. In practice FT4 and FT3 are more widely used than total T4 and total T3.

Selective use of thyroid function tests

Many laboratories measure only basal TSH as the initial test of thyroid function. This strategy is not infallible, but it will detect both overt and subclinical primary thyroid disease. A normal TSH concentration usually excludes primary thyroid dysfunction. If an abnormal result is obtained, thyroid hormone measurements must be made to confirm that thyroid dysfunction is present, and to determine the severity of the disease.

Table 8.2 **Situations in which first-line TSH is not ideal.**

First-line TSH not ideal	First-line TSH acceptable
Symptomatic patients – first presentation	Monitoring patients stabilised on thyroxine
Optimising treatment of hypothyroidism and hyperthyroidism – early months	Screening asymptomatic 'at risk' groups (see Table 8.3)
Screening and monitoring in pregnancy	
Diagnosis and monitoring of hypopituitarism	
Diagnosis of TSH-secreting tumour and thyroid-hormone resistance (rare)	

Initial measurement of both TSH and FT4 provides a more satisfactory method of assessing thyroid status, because in some situations a single TSH result may be misleading (Table 8.2). If this strategy is followed, a significant number of cases will arise in which one test will be abnormal while the complementary test will be normal (Figure 8.4). It is thus essential to understand and appreciate the factors that can affect the results of thyroid function tests.

Screening and surveillance for thyroid dysfunction

Screening in the healthy *asymptomatic* population is not warranted but screening should be performed in certain categories of patient who have vague symptoms or are at high risk of developing thyroid disease (Table 8.3).

Interpreting results of thyroid function tests

Figures 8.4, 8.5 and 8.6 provide guidance on the interpretation of thyroid function tests.

Hyperthyroidism

Overt primary hyperthyroidism (FT4 and/or FT3 high; TSH low)

TSH is nearly always undetectable, due to feedback inhibition on the pituitary. Free and total T4 and T3 concentrations are nearly always increased in overt hyperthyroidism. In a very small percentage of hyperthyroid patients FT4 is normal but the

Table 8.3 **Categories of patients who should have thyroid function tests performed.**

Symptomatic patient

Features of a thyroid disorder
Family history of thyroid disease
Elderly patient with nonspecific symptoms
Women presenting at menopause with nonspecific symptoms
Taking thyroxine

Patients at risk of developing thyroid disease

Presenting with diabetes	
Type 1 diabetes	annual check
Type 2 diabetes	at diagnosis
Autoimmune disease	annual check
Treated hyperthyroidism	annual check
Down's and Turner's syndrome	annual check
Post-neck irradiation	annual check
Lithium or amiodarone	before treatment and 6 monthly

Table 8.4 The main causes of hyperthyroidism.

Cause of hyperthyroidism	Pathogenesis
Graves' disease	Autoimmune – TSH receptor stimulating antibodies
Toxic multinodular goitre	Autonomously functioning nodular gland
Solitary toxic nodule	Autonomously functioning nodule
Thyroiditis	Transient phenomenon resulting from release of stored T4 from damaged thyroid gland
Iodine-induced	Chronic high iodine intake in patients with autonomously functioning thyroid gland Amiodarone (iodine-containing anti-arrhythmic)
TSHoma	Inappropriate release of TSH from pituitary tumour
Factitious	Exogenous administration of T4
Trophoblastic	Secretion of high concentration of hCG that mimics effects of TSH

concentration of FT3 is increased; this condition is known as T3 hyperthyroidism or T3 thyrotoxicosis (Figure 8.5).

The main causes of hyperthyroidism and their pathogenesis are listed in Table 8.4. In the vast majority of cases (~90%), the cause is Graves' disease or toxic multinodular goitre. Graves' disease is an autoimmune disorder characterised by diffuse thyroid enlargement, ophthalmological involvement and the presence of stimulating TSH receptor antibodies (TRAbs). Patients with toxic multinodular goitre tend to demonstrate a slowly progressive nodular goitre that becomes autonomous in function over time; this condition predominantly affects older patients (>50 years old). Patients in which the diagnosis is unclear (e.g. those with no goiter and negative TRAbs) will usually require an isotope scan (technetium [Tc]-99m pertechnetate) to identify the cause. A diffuse increased uptake of isotope is consistent with Graves' disease, whereas the presence of 'hot nodules' with surrounding areas of reduced isotope uptake is suggestive of nodular hyperthyroidism. Poor uptake of isotope across the gland is consistent with thyroiditis.

 CASE 8.1

A 30-year-old housewife attended her GP. She had lost weight (6 kg in the previous 3 months), was irritable and felt uncomfortable in the recent spell of hot weather. She was taking an oestrogen-containing oral contraceptive. On clinical examination, her palms were sweaty and she had a fine tremor of the fingers when her arms were outstretched. There was no thyroid enlargement or bruit, and no eye signs. The following results were reported for thyroid function tests:

Serum	Result	Reference range
TSH	<0.01	0.2–4.5 mU/L
FT4	19	9–21 pmol/L
FT3	12.1	2.6–6.2 pmol/L
Total T3	6.5	0.9–2.4 nmol/L

What is the diagnosis in this patient, and on which results was this diagnosis based?

Comments: The patient had T3 thyrotoxicosis, and the diagnosis was based on the increased plasma FT3 and undetectable TSH, in the presence of a normal plasma FT4. The fact that the patient was taking an oestrogen-containing oral contraceptive would account for some of the increase in total T3, since the oestrogen content in the oral contraceptive would cause an increase in plasma TBG.

In patients with thyrotoxicosis but no goitre, it is helpful to perform a thyroid isotope scan to help determine the cause of the hyperthyroidism. This patient's thyroid scan showed a diffuse and increased uptake of Tc-99m pertechnetate, and TSH receptor antibodies were detected in her serum. This patient had Graves' disease but no goitre; this is thought to arise when TRAbs are present that stimulate the pathways required for thyroid hormone synthesis, but not thyroid growth.

 CASE 8.2

A 28-year-old female office worker presented to her GP complaining she had developed what she described as a persistent sore throat following a cold she had 2 weeks earlier. The throat pain was worse when she turned her head or swallowed. She also complained of feeling very tired. There was no past medical history of note.

On examination she was pyrexial and had a fine tremor and tachycardia (90 beats/min). Her thyroid was firm but tender and appeared to be slightly enlarged.

The GP took a blood sample and the following results were found:

Haematology

The erythrocyte sedimentation rate (ESR) was markedly increased. Full blood count and blood film were unremarkable.

Biochemistry

Serum	Result	Reference range
TSH	<0.01	0.2–4.5 mU/L
FT4	40	10–21 pmol/L
FT3	10	2.6–6.2 pmol/L

The patient was referred to an endocrinologist and seen 2 weeks later. Her thyroid gland was no longer painful and repeat blood tests were performed.

The ESR remained elevated.

Serum	Result	Reference range
TSH	<0.01	0.4–4.5 mU/L
FT4	23	10–21 pmol/L
FT3	7	2.6–6.2 pmol

Anti-thyroid peroxidase and TSH-receptor antibodies were negative. The uptake of Tc-99m pertechnetate by the thyroid was found to be negligible.

What is the likely diagnosis?

Comments: The patient has viral thyroiditis (also known as de Quervain thyroiditis). This induced a transient hyperthyroidism.

The very low uptake of radioiodine is due to the low TSH (TSH is required to trap iodine) and the fact that thyroid follicular cells are damaged.

She returned to the clinic 4 weeks later for review and was found to be biochemically hypothyroid (raised TSH, low FT4). No treatment with thyroxine was required as the hypothyroidism is usually transient in this disorder.

Subclinical hyperthyroidism (FT4 and FT3 normal; TSH low)

Thyroid disease presents as a spectrum of clinical and biochemical features of varying severity. The clinical diagnosis of mild thyroid disorders is often difficult because the patient may have few if any clinical features and the only biochemical abnormality may be abnormal plasma TSH concentration. The combination of a persistent abnormality in TSH, together with normal thyroid hormone concentrations, is known as 'subclinical thyroid disease'. This description is unsatisfactory, since it rests solely on the results of biochemical investigations.

Many clinically euthyroid patients with multinodular goitre or with exophthalmic Graves' disease have 'subclinical hyperthyroidism', that is, TSH below 0.01 mU/L and FT4 and FT3 in the upper part of their respective reference ranges. Before assigning this diagnosis, however, other causes of a low TSH should be excluded, including NTI, pregnancy and drugs that suppress TSH (dopaminergic drugs, high dose glucocorticoids). The tests should be repeated 1–2 months later and if the abnormalities persist the patient should be referred to an endocrinologist to establish the diagnosis and give optimal treatment (Figure 8.5).

Secondary hyperthyroidism – TSH-secreting tumour (TSHoma)

Very rarely is hyperthyroidism caused by a TSH-secreting tumour. Persistent hyperthyroid symptoms associated with elevated FT4 and FT3 and raised or normal TSH are consistent with this diagnosis, once the common problems of assay interference or NTI have been eliminated.

The concentration of the α-subunit in the circulation is often increased in these patients.

Management of hyperthyroidism

Hyperthyroidism should be managed by an endocrinologist. Treatment depends on the cause of the hyperthyroidism. Thyroiditis may require no treatment; multinodular goiter is usually treated with radioiodine. The initial treatment for Graves' disease varies between countries. Radioiodine may be the treatment of choice in some countries but in others, including the UK, thionamide drugs such as carbimazole may be given for a period of around 18 months followed by radioiodine to those patients who relapse when thionomide medication is withdrawn. After radioactive iodine treatment many patients will develop hypothyroidism. Some patients may be treated by subtotal thyroidectomy; such patients may have temporary disturbances of thyroid function tests in the early post-operative

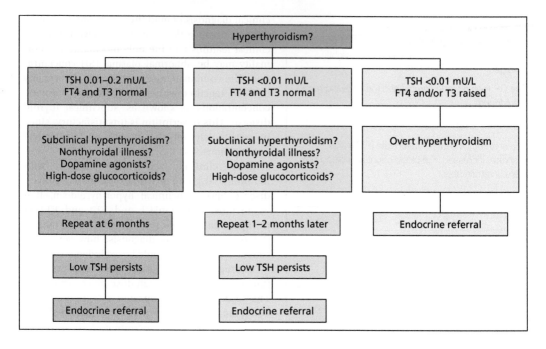

Figure 8.5 Interpretation of thyroid function tests in suspected hyperthyroidism.

period but in the long term are more likely to remain euthyroid than are patients treated with radioactive iodine. Annual follow-up of all patients is required.

Measurement of TSH is not a reliable guide of thyroid status during the first 4–6 months of treatment for hyperthyroidism, because TSH may still be suppressed even when plasma thyroid hormone concentrations have become abnormally low. Measurement of TSH concentration can be used to determine the adequacy of treatment after normal thyrotroph responsiveness has returned. The role of thyroid function testing in hyperthyroidism is summarised in Table 8.5.

Comment on the acceptability of these results. If they are not acceptable, what would you do?

Comments: Plasma TSH measurements are not a reliable indicator of thyroid status in the early months of treating hyperthyroid patients, as the responsiveness of the thyrotrophs lags behind the fall in plasma FT4 and FT3 for several weeks. During these early months, plasma free thyroid hormone measurements provide the most reliable indication of thyroid status. In this patient, the results for plasma FT4 and FT3 clearly indicated the need to reduce the dosage of carbimazole immediately.

 CASE 8.3

A 35-year-old secretary attended for follow-up review of her treatment for Graves' disease. Carbimazole administration (15 mg three times/day) had been started 1 month before. The results for thyroid function tests were as follows:

Serum	Result	Reference range
TSH	<0.01	0.2–4.5 mU/L
FT4	<5	9–21 pmol/L
FT3	2.5	2.6–6.2 pmol/L

Hypothyroidism

Overt primary hypothyroidism (FT4 low; TSH high)

TSH is often increased to more than 20 mU/L, as feedback inhibition of the pituitary (Figures 8.4 and 8.6) is diminished by the low FT4. Measurement of FT3 is unhelpful because normal concentrations are often observed.

The primary causes of hypothyroidism are listed in Table 8.6. Monitoring of thyroid function tests is essential to distinguish the transient from the permanent causes of hypothyroidism, as the former often require no specific treatment. The presence of a goitre

Table 8.5 Thyroid function testing when treating hyperthyroidism.

- Objective is to maintain FT4 in the upper half of the reference range
- FT4 provides the best indicator of thyroid status in the early months of treatment
- TSH may give an unreliable guide of thyroid status during the first 4–6 months of treatment
- Monitor every 4–6 weeks with TSH, FT4, FT3 until a stable euthyroid state is achieved
- Monitor every 3-6 months if long-term thionomides are being prescribed
- After radioactive iodine treatment many patients will develop hypothyroidism
- Annual follow-up of all patients is essential
- Patients with subclinical hyperthyroidism who are not treated should be monitored every 6–12 months

will distinguish Hashimoto's thyroiditis from atrophic thyroiditis, although the practical utility of separating these groups is limited as both will usually require lifelong replacement of T4. Congenital hypothyroidism will be detected in most countries by neonatal bloodspot screening programs (see Chapter 22).

Subclinical primary hypothyroidism (FT4 normal; TSH high)

Many cases of subclinical hypothyroidism are transient. It is essential to confirm that abnormalities in TSH are persistent or progressive. Studies suggest that the average patient will not get any clinical benefit from T4 therapy until TSH rises above approximately 10 mU/L. If a profile consistent with subclinical hypothyroidism is found, the tests should be repeated at 3 months to exclude a transient rise in TSH. Measurement of anti-thyroid peroxidase antibodies (TPOAbs) can help to determine if an autoimmune process is present and help predict risk of progression to overt hypothyroidism.

Secondary (central) hypothyroidism

Plasma TSH is normal in about half of patients with central (pituitary) hypothyroidism, but FT4 is usually low. Circulating TSH has been shown to have reduced bioactivity in hypopituitarism. It should be stressed that the most common cause of a normal TSH with low FT4 and FT3 is NTI, but it is essential to consider hypopituitarism in all patients with this combination of results. In patients with secondary hypothyroidism, the objective of replacement therapy is to maintain FT4 in the upper third of the reference range.

Table 8.6 The main causes of hypothyroidism.

Cause of hypothyroidism	Pathogenesis
Hashimoto's thyroiditis	Autoimmune destruction of thyroid gland
Atrophic thyroiditis	Autoimmune destruction of thyroid gland
Iatrogenic	
• Thyroidectomy	Used in the treatment of hyperthyroidism/thyroid malignancy
• Radioactive iodine	
• Anti-thyroid drugs	
• Other medication (Table 8.7)	
Transient	
• Viral thyroiditis (de Quervain's)	Inflammatory damage to thyroid gland (temporary)
• Post-partum thyroiditis	Autoimmune damage to thyroid gland (temporary)
Congenital	
• Thyroid aplasia	Structural abnormalities/absence of thyroid gland
• Dyshormonogenesis	Defects in enzyme synthesis of thyroid hormone
Iodine deficiency	Impaired hormone synthesis in susceptible geographical locations
Secondary hypothyroidism	
• Hypopituitarism	Deficiency of TSH/TRH
• Hypothalamic dysfunction	

CASE 8.4

A 38-year-old factory worker attended her GP because she was always tired and had a feeling of discomfort in her neck. She had been gaining weight. On clinical examination, she was found to have a goitre. The following results were reported for thyroid function tests:

Serum	Result	Reference range
TSH	18	0.2–4.5 mU/L
FT4	10	9–21 pmol/L
FT3	4.2	2.6–6.2 pmol/L

TPOAbs were present in the patient's serum in very high concentration.

What is the diagnosis and how should she be treated?

Comments: The patient has subclinical hypothyroidism. The very high concentration of TPOAbs in this patient's serum indicates that she had hypothyroidism due to Hashimoto's thyroiditis. Repeat thyroid function tests confirmed that she had subclinical hypothyroidism. Given that her TSH was >10 mU/L and she was symptomatic, she was treated with thyroxine.

Management of hypothyroidism

T4 replacement therapy

Aims

- To make the patient feel well and restore TSH and free T4 to within reference range.
- In some patients free T4 may have to be above the reference range to achieve a 'normal' TSH.
- Some patients report they 'feel better' only when T4 is given at a dose that produces a low or undetectable TSH. There are reports of decreased bone mineral density in post-menopausal women on T4 who have a TSH <0.1 mU/L; as a consequence many endocrinologists will attempt to fine-tune the T4 dose to allow the patient to feel well with a TSH that lies within the reference range. Therapeutic targets are different for pregnancy (Chapter 11: T4 replacement and pregnancy).

Monitoring

- When a patient is stabilised on T4, an annual check is required.
- If a change in dose is required, a period of around 6–8 weeks should elapse before re-testing.

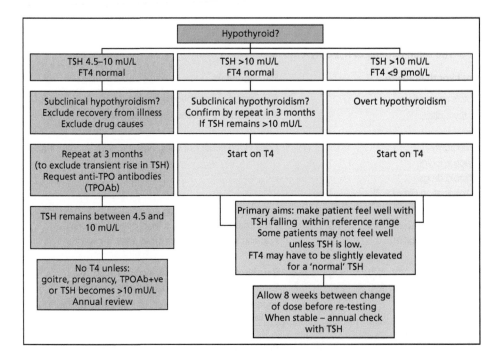

Figure 8.6 Interpretation of thyroid function tests in suspected hypothyroidism.

T4 replacement in subclinical hypothyroidism

The value of treating patients with subclinical hypothyroidism is controversial, but, in general, it is believed that only patients with a TSH greater than 10 mU/L will derive any benefit from therapy. If the TSH lies between 4.5 and 10 mU/L then T4 therapy is often withheld unless the patient has clear features of hypothyroidism; annual monitoring must be done and treatment initiated when TSH rises above 10 mU/L. Some endocrinologists may treat all patients with subclinical hypothyroidism who have positive anti-TPOAbs (Figure 8.6). This is because such patients have a high risk of developing overt disease and thus therapy is initiated with a view to preventing them from developing debilitating symptoms.

T4 therapy in central hypothyroidism (hypopituitarism)

TSH measurements are of no value in monitoring these patients. An endocrinologist should guide treatment and follow-up with the aim of maintaining FT4 in the upper third of the reference range.

Drugs and T4 therapy

Some over-the-counter medications can impair T4 absorption. These include: proton pump inhibitors, H_2 antagonists, calcium carbonate, soy protein, aluminium hydroxide and ferrous sulphate. Patients should not take their T4 within 4 hours of taking any other medications.

The requirement for T4 is likely to increase in hypothyroid patients who become pregnant or who are commenced on anti-convulsants or oestrogen-containing oral contraceptives (see Table 8.8).

CASE 8.5

A 65-year-old widow had been receiving treatment for primary hypothyroidism with thyroxine (150 mg/day) for the previous 12 months. She felt well and was clinically euthyroid; her weight had been steady. Results of thyroid function tests performed at a routine follow-up outpatient attendance were:

Serum	Result	Reference range
TSH	0.15	0.2–4.5 mU/L
FT4	28	9–21 pmol/L
FT3	6.0	2.6–6.2 pmol/L

Are these results indicative of satisfactory therapeutic control, or would you want to adjust the patient's dosage of thyroxine?

Comments: The aim of thyroxine replacement treatment for primary hypothyroidism is to keep the patient clinically euthyroid and to render plasma TSH normal (it would have been much increased before thyroxine treatment was started). In some of these patients, it is necessary to give sufficient thyroxine to increase the plasma FT4 to above the upper reference value in order to normalise plasma TSH. In this patient, although she was clinically euthyroid, the plasma FT4 was above normal and TSH was below normal, but not so suppressed as to be undetectable (i.e. it was not <0.01 mU/L). It was decided not to reduce the thyroxine dosage, and to reassess the patient 3 months later.

Situations in which thyroid function test results may be misleading

Nonthyroidal illness (NTI) and the sick euthyroid syndrome

Patients attending or admitted to a hospital suffering from any of a wide range of chronic or acute NTIs often have abnormalities in thyroid function tests. The abnormalities depend on the severity of the illness (Figure 8.7). A low T3 may often be found even though the patients are clinically euthyroid; this has been termed the *sick euthyroid syndrome*.

Several mechanisms are involved, including:

- induction of a central hypothyroidism – due to low hypothalamic TRH;
- suppression of TSH release by increased concentrations of cytokines, dopamine, cortisol and somatostatin;
- changes in the affinity and in the concentration of the thyroid hormone-binding proteins; these changes give rise to alterations (increase or decrease) in the concentrations of both the free and total thyroid hormones;
- impaired uptake of thyroid hormones by the tissues;

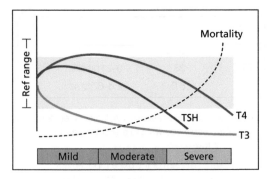

Figure 8.7 The effects of illness on the concentration of thyroid hormones and thyrotrophin. The shaded area represents the reference range.

Table 8.7 **Thyroid function testing in patients with nonthyroidal illness (NTI).**

- Abnormal thyroid function tests are commonly found in patients with NTI
- Thyroid testing should be performed only if thyroid disease is a possible contributor to the illness
- A low T3 is a very common finding
- A low TSH is twice as likely to be due to NTI as to hyperthyroidism
- NTI patients with low TSH usually have a TSH which is >0.01 mU/L
- Hyperthyroid patients usually have a TSH which is <0.01 mU/L
- A raised TSH is as likely to be due to recovery from illness as to hypothyroidism
- There is no persuasive evidence for the use of T4/T3 therapy

- decreased production of T3 from T4 in the peripheral tissues;
- changes in the T3 occupancy and function of the T3 receptors.

The contribution of each of the above mechanisms may vary with the severity and stage of the illness, and thus the pattern of thyroid function tests may be extremely variable and may mimic the profile seen in primary or secondary thyroid disease. Interpretation of thyroid function tests is complicated further by the effects of drugs and methodological problems associated with free hormone measurements.

Recovery from illness

When a patient recovers from illness, abnormalities in TSH, T4 and T3 eventually resolve. In some patients, TSH concentrations may rise transiently above the reference range in this recovery phase. In hospitalised patients, an elevated TSH is as likely to be due to recovery from nonthyroidal illness as primary hypothyroidism. It is essential that clinicians understand this in order to avoid misdiagnosis that could lead to inappropriate lifelong T4 replacement therapy. Table 8.7 summarises good practice points relating to thyroid function testing in patients with NTI.

Paediatrics and the neonate

Plasma TSH is widely used to screen for congenital hypothyroidism in the neonate. Marked changes in thyroid function occur in the early days of life, with an initial surge in TSH and thyroid hormone after delivery, followed by a marked decline in hormone levels over the next few days. Hormone levels then show a slow decline until adult values are reached at about

the age of 10. It is essential to apply appropriate age-related reference ranges, which should be provided by the local laboratory.

Pregnancy

Marked changes in thyroid hormone concentration and TSH occur throughout pregnancy, and it is essential to use trimester-related reference ranges. The diagnosis and management of thyroid disease in pregnancy is not straightforward, and close liaison between GP, endocrinologist, obstetrician and community midwife is essential. Thyroid disease and pregnancy is covered in Chapter 11.

Drug treatment

Drugs may interfere with TSH secretion or the production, secretion, transport and metabolism of thyroid hormones (Table 8.8). Some drugs modify thyroid status while others produce abnormal thyroid function test results in otherwise euthyroid subjects. Certain agents impair the absorption of thyroxine from the gut, and patients on thyroxine therapy should be advised to take their thyroxine at least 4 h apart from these medications. Patients taking thyroxine are likely to require an increase in replacement dose if drugs such as phenytoin or carbamazepine, proton pump inhibitors or H_2 antagonists are prescribed that increase hepatic metabolism of T4. Phenytoin, carbamazepine, furosemide and salicylate compete with thyroid hormone binding to serum-binding proteins and may increase FT4. However, it is important to note that the influence of

Table 8.8 Examples of drugs that alter thyroid hormone synthesis, secretion and metabolism.

Mechanism	Example of drug
Decrease in TSH secretion	Dopamine, glucocorticoids, octreotide, cytokines
Decrease in thyroid hormone secretion*	Lithium, amiodarone, iodide
Induce hyperthyroidism	Lithium, amiodarone, iodide
Decrease in thyroidal synthesis*	Carbimazole, methimazole, propylthiouracil, lithium
Increase in TBG	Oestrogens, tamoxifen, heroin, methadone
Decrease in TBG	Androgens, glucocorticoids, anabolic steroids
Displacement of thyroid hormones from plasma proteins	Furosemide, fenclofenac, salicylates, NSAIDs, mefenamic acid, carbamazepine
Increased hepatic metabolism	Proton pump inhibitors, H_2 antagonists, phenytoin, carbamazepine, rifampicin, barbiturates
Impaired T4 and T3 conversion	β-Antagonists, amiodarone*, radiocontrast dyes
Impaired absorption of thyroxine[†]	Colestyramine, aluminium hydroxide, ferrous sulphate, calcium, soya protein
Altered immunity[‡]	Interleukin-1, interferons, TNF-α
Modified thyroid hormone action	Amiodarone

* Cause a decrease in thyroid hormone synthesis or secretion and alter thyroid status.
[†] Interfere with absorption from the GI tract. Patients on T4 therapy should be advised to take their T4 at least 4 h apart from these medications.
[‡] These cytokines can cause transient hypothyroidism or thyrotoxicosis. The mechanism is unclear. Other drugs listed produce abnormal thyroid function tests but patients remain euthyroid. Amiodarone, lithium and iodine are exceptions (see text).

drugs on modifying free thyroid hormone concentrations may be method specific. For example, depending on the method, FT4 may be measured as normal, high or low in patients given heparin or taking phenytoin or carbamazepine.

Amiodarone, lithium and interferon can induce thyroid dysfunction. The anti-arrhythmic drug amiodarone is an iodine-containing drug that has complex effects on thyroid metabolism. These include inhibition of T4 to T3 conversion, inhibition of thyroidal iodine uptake and inhibition of T4 entry into cells. The drug may also induce a destructive thyroiditis. Patients may have an altered thyroid hormone profile without thyroid dysfunction, but 14–18% of patients taking amiodarone may develop clinically significant hypothyroidism or amiodarone-induced thyrotoxicosis.

It is important to evaluate patients before they commence therapy with amiodarone. This should include clinical examination and a basal measurement of TSH, FT4, FT3 and TPOAbs. After starting treatment, these tests should be repeated at 6 months and thereafter every 6 months including the year after the drug is stopped. Lithium can cause hypothyroidism or less commonly hyperthyroidism. Patients taking lithium should have their thyroid function tests measured at 6–12-month intervals.

 CASE 8.6

A 15-year-old schoolgirl presented to her GP complaining that she felt continually anxious and had palpitations. On examination she had a small goiter and a sinus tachycardia (98 beats per minute). She had a history of learning difficulties and anxiety attacks.

The GP took a blood sample and the following results were found:

Serum	Result	Reference range
TSH	4.2	0.2–4.5 mU/L
FT4	28	10–21 pmol/L
FT3	8.1	2.6–6.2 pmol/L

The laboratory could find no evidence of assay interference.

What might be the diagnosis and what further tests should be performed?

Comment: The patient may have either thyroid hormone resistance or a TSHoma. An MRI of the pituitary demonstrated no abnormality and the concentrations of α-subunit and other pituitary hormones were within normal limits. Blood was sent for genotyping, which identified a mutation in the carboxy terminal region of the TRβ gene consistent with a diagnosis of thyroid hormone resistance. No treatment will fully and specifically correct the defect. It is important not to intervene with the sole purpose of normalising the thyroid hormone levels. Sinus tachycardia can be controlled with the β-adrenoceptor blocking agent, atenolol. If goitre size is a problem this can be treated with supraphysiological doses of L-T$_3$, given as a single dose every other day.

Assay interference from endogenous antibodies

Some individuals have antibodies in their plasma that react with a range of animal immunoglobulins (heterophilic antibodies). These antibodies interfere with a wide range of immunoassays that are used to measure hormones. For example, a normal or elevated TSH result may be found in some thyrotoxic patients due to this type of assay interference.

Patients with anti-T4, anti-T3 and anti-TSH antibodies have also been described and these antibodies can interfere with the corresponding assays.

Thyroid hormone resistance (THR)

This is a rare disorder (1:40000 births) in which there is diminished end-organ sensitivity to thyroid hormone due to mutations in the beta form of the nuclear T3 receptor. The mutant TRβ receptors have either reduced affinity for T$_3$ or abnormal interaction with one of the cofactors involved in thyroid hormone action.

Patients usually have elevated FT4 and FT3 with normal or slightly raised TSH. THR has been classified into three categories but distinguishing between them is often difficult. The most common features are goitre, hyperkinetic behaviour and tachycardia.

Generalised thyroid hormone resistance The patient is clinically euthyroid as a consequence of the compensatory increase in thyroid hormone concentrations.

Pituitary thyroid hormone resistance The pituitary is particularly affected and is insensitive to feedback inhibition of TSH release by thyroid hormone. The inappropriately high TSH secretion leads to overproduction of T4 and T3 which may act on peripheral tissue to give rise to features of mild hyperthyroidism.

Peripheral thyroid hormone resistance The patient may present with clinical hypothyroidism because the sensitivity of peripheral tissues to thyroid hormones is decreased relative to that of the pituitary.

Recently, patients with mutations in the alpha form of the nuclear T3 receptor have been described. Thyroid function tests appear essentially normal; however patients display a clinical phenotype consistent with hypothyroidism, delayed growth and constipation.

Diagnosis

It is important to eliminate assay interference as a cause of any unusual thyroid function test profile. When this has been done, the important differential diagnosis is between TSHoma and THR. Family history, pituitary imaging, T3 suppression and TRH tests may help in the diagnosis. TSH secretion from a TSHoma is often unresponsive to T3 suppression and TRH stimulation whereas responses are seen in THR. The family history of a similarly affected first degree relative is virtually diagnostic of THR, as the disorder is familial in 80–90% of cases. Co-secretion of other pituitary hormones and measurement of free α-subunits may also help in the diagnosis of TSHoma. Serum α-subunit is increased, often markedly, in patients with thyrotroph adenomas, whereas normal concentrations are found in THR. Genotyping to identify a mutant allele may also be performed to confirm THR.

Causes of abnormal results for thyroid hormone measurements in euthyroid subjects

1 *Abnormal plasma TBG concentrations* occur frequently, leading to parallel changes in total thyroid hormone concentrations. The affinity and binding capacity of TBG for thyroid hormones may be diminished by NTI and by drugs (e.g. salicylates),

leading in turn to decreases in total T3 and total T4. Thyroid hormone concentrations may be increased in pregnancy or by oestrogen-containing medication that increases TBG concentration. Genetic causes of low and high TBG also exist.

Free hormone concentrations are unrelated to changes in the concentration of these proteins, but, in practice, some methods for free hormone measurement are unreliable and produce results that are influenced by changes in the concentration and binding capacity of albumin.

2 *Genetic variants of both albumin and pre-albumin* have been described which have a high affinity for T4. These variants give rise to increased total T4 but other tests are usually normal and the patient is clinically euthyroid.

Thyroid cancer

Patients with thyroid cancer (papillary and follicular) usually present with a thyroid swelling or nodule. A biopsy using a fine needle aspirate is required to make the diagnosis. Most patients are clinically euthyroid at presentation with normal TSH, FT4 and FT3. Treatment usually involves total thyroidectomy followed by an ablative dose of radioiodine to destroy any residual thyroid tissue and metastases. Lifelong therapy with sufficient thyroxine to suppress TSH to undetectable levels is required in order to prevent metastases from proliferating (see Chapter 17).

Miscellaneous tests and thyroid disease

TRH test

The only indication for the TRH test is in distinguishing secondary hyperthyroidism (due to a TSH-secreting tumour) from thyroid hormone resistance. In normal subjects, after IV TRH, serum TSH increases by more than 2 mU/L above the basal level at 20 min and returns towards the basal value at 60 min. Patients with T3 receptor defects also show a TSH response in a TRH test, but the TSH response is absent in patients with TSH-secreting tumours. There is no increase in the TSH response to TRH in patients with primary hyperthyroidism, and an absent response may also occur in hypopituitarism. In hypothyroidism, the response is exaggerated.

There may be problems in obtaining TRH for clinical use in some countries.

Anti-thyroid peroxidase antibodies (TPOAbs)

These are present in the serum of patients with a wide range of immunologically mediated thyroid disorders (e.g. Hashimoto's thyroiditis, Graves' disease). They may also be found in a small proportion of apparently healthy individuals, but the appearance of TPOAbs often precedes the development of overt thyroid disorders. The measurement of TPOAbs is of clinical use (1) in the diagnosis and risk stratification of autoimmune thyroid disorders and (2) as a risk factor for thyroid dysfunction during treatment with interferon, interleukin-2, lithium or amiodarone.

The highest titres of these antibodies are found in the serum of patients with Hashimoto's thyroiditis, and are present in ~90% of these patients.

Thyrotrophin receptor antibodies (TRAbs)

TSH receptor antibodies (TRAbs) are IgG antibodies directed against the TSH receptors in the thyroid. TRAbs are implicated in the pathogenesis of Graves' disease by inducing a direct stimulatory action on TSH receptors, leading to diffuse thyroid hypertrophy and increased thyroid hormone production. In addition, TRAbs appear to stimulate differentiation of retro-orbital fibroblasts within the eye, causing inflammation and the characteristic exophthalmic appearance associated with Graves' disease.

TRAbs are usually measured by assessing the ability of a patient's serum to inhibit the binding of labelled TSH to a suspension of TSH receptors. Very occasionally, TRAbs antagonise rather than stimulate the TSH receptor, and thus in rare circumstances are a cause of hypothyroidism.

TRAb measurements are of value in:

- the differential diagnosis of hyperthyroidism where the clinical picture is not obvious;
- predicting relapse in treated hyperthyroid patients who are to have their anti-thyroid medication withdrawn. If TRAbs are still strongly positive, then the patient has a high risk of immediate relapse;

Table 8.9 **Tests affected by changes in thyroid status**

Hyperthyroidism	Hypothyroidism
Hyperglycaemia/impaired glucose tolerance	Hyponatraemia
Hypocholesterolaemia	Hypercholesterolaemia
Abnormal liver function tests	Hyperprolactinaemia
Hypercalcaemia	Increased CK
Increased SHBG	Decreased SHBG

- predicting neonatal hyperthyroidism in babies born to mothers with high TRAbs after 20 weeks of pregnancy (TRAbs cross the placenta and stimulate the foetal thyroid);
- distinguishing between post-partum thyroiditis and Graves' disease; undetectable TRAbs are found in thyroiditis, while TRAbs are positive in 97% of patients with Graves' disease;
- investigation of suspected euthyroid Graves' ophthalmopathy.

Tests affected by thyroid dysfunction

Several laboratory tests may be affected by changes in thyroid status; these are listed in Table 8.9. It is particularly important to exclude abnormalities in thyroid function in patients with newly diagnosed diabetes, and also those with hypercholesterolaemia. Changes in sex hormone-binding globulin (SHBG) concentration can lead to marked changes in the free hormone concentration of testosterone; this is discussed further in Chapter 10.

9

Disorders of the adrenal cortex and medulla

Learning objectives

To understand:

✔ the mechanisms that regulate the hypothalamic–pituitary–adrenal axis;

✔ the biosynthetic pathways involved in adrenal steroidogenesis;

✔ the enzyme defects that are involved in the pathogenesis of congenital adrenal hyperplasia and how this can present in adulthood as well as in paediatrics (see also Chapter 22);

✔ the investigations that should be performed in suspected adrenocortical dysfunction;

✔ when and how to investigate suspected secondary hypertension;

✔ what investigations should be carried out to investigate suspected phaeochromocytoma.

Introduction

The adrenal gland consists of two distinct tissues of different embryological origin: the outer cortex and the inner medulla. The cortex secretes glucocorticoid, mineralocorticoid and sex steroid hormones which are synthesised from cholesterol obtained from both high-density lipoprotein (HDL) and low-density lipoprotein (LDL) in plasma. The medulla secretes catecholamines, principally adrenaline. Disorders of the adrenals are uncommon, but they are important to diagnose as they can be readily treated. The need for specific and sensitive screening tests is therefore important; additional tests can then be used to confirm or refute the results of screening tests.

After a brief review of the control of steroid hormone secretion from the adrenal cortex and the action of the different steroid hormones, the investigation of adrenocortical hyperfunction and hypofunction will be discussed. Finally, the investigation of catecholamine hypersecretion from an adrenomedullary tumour (phaeochromocytoma) is discussed.

Regulation of adrenal steroid hormone synthesis and secretion

Three anatomical zones can be recognised in the adrenal cortex (Figure 9.1). The outermost zona glomerulosa is the site of synthesis of aldosterone, the principal mineralocorticoid. The deeper layers of the cortex, the zona fasciculata and zona reticularis,

---

Clinical Biochemistry Lecture Notes, Tenth Edition. Peter Rae, Mike Crane and Rebecca Pattenden.
© 2018 John Wiley & Sons Ltd. Published 2018 by John Wiley & Sons Ltd.
Companion website: www.lecturenoteseries.com/clinicalbiochemistry

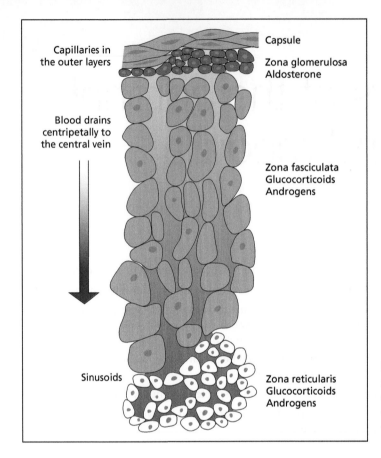

Capillaries in the outer layers

Blood drains centripetally to the central vein

Sinusoids

Capsule

Zona glomerulosa
Aldosterone

Zona fasciculata
Glucocorticoids
Androgens

Zona reticularis
Glucocorticoids
Androgens

Figure 9.1 The morphological zonation of the adrenal cortex, showing the three types of cells alongside their structural arrangement and hormone producing capability.

synthesise glucocorticoids, of which cortisol is the most important in man. Sex steroid production also occurs in the adrenal cortex, mainly in the zona reticularis and to some extent in the zona fasciculata.

Glucocorticoid secretion

Glucocorticoids have widespread effects on carbohydrate, fat and protein metabolism. In the liver, cortisol stimulates gluconeogenesis, amino acid uptake and degradation, and ketogenesis. Lipolysis is increased in adipose tissue, and proteolysis and amino acid release promoted in muscle. Glucocorticoids are also involved to some extent in regulating sodium and water homeostasis and the inflammatory and stress responses. In the circulation, glucocorticoids are mainly protein bound (~90%), chiefly to CBG (cortisol-binding globulin or transcortin). Plasma CBG is increased in pregnancy and with oestrogen treatment (e.g. oral contraceptives). It is decreased in hypoproteinaemic states (e.g. nephrotic syndrome). Changes in plasma cortisol concentration occur in parallel to

changes in CBG. The biologically active fraction of cortisol in plasma is the free (unbound) component, though usually the total (i.e. bound plus free) concentration of cortisol is measured for diagnostic purposes.

ACTH is the main stimulus to cortisol secretion. Three factors regulate ACTH (and therefore cortisol) secretion:

1 *Negative feedback control:* ACTH release from the anterior pituitary is stimulated by hypothalamic secretion of CRH. Increased plasma cortisol or synthetic glucocorticoids suppress secretion of CRH and ACTH (Figure 9.2).

2 *Stress* (e.g. major surgery, emotional stress) leads to a sudden large increase in CRH (and ACTH) secretion; the negative feedback control mechanism is temporarily over-ridden.

3 *The diurnal rhythm of plasma cortisol:* This control mechanism is related to the rhythm of an individual's sleeping–waking cycle (Figure 9.3). Cortisol levels are highest at the start of the working day, falling to the lowest levels in late evening with the onset of sleep.

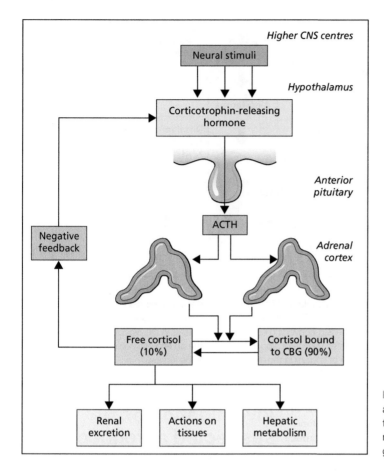

Figure 9.2 The hypothalamic–anterior pituitary–adrenal axis and the fate of cortisol following its release. CBG = cortisol-binding globulin.

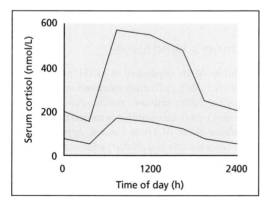

Figure 9.3 The diurnal rhythm of cortisol secretion; the shaded area represents values that lie within the reference range. There is a similar rhythm for the secretion of ACTH by the anterior pituitary. Patients with Cushing's syndrome lose this diurnal variation.

Aldosterone secretion

The principal physiological function of aldosterone is to conserve Na^+, mainly by facilitating Na^+ reabsorption and reciprocal K^+ or H^+ secretion in the distal renal tubule and in other epithelial cells. Although its rate of production is less than 1% of the rate of cortisol production, aldosterone is a major regulator of water and electrolyte balance, as well as blood pressure.

The renin–angiotensin system is the most important system controlling aldosterone secretion (Figure 9.4). *Renin* is a proteolytic enzyme produced by the juxtaglomerular apparatus of the kidney and released into the circulation in response to a fall in circulating blood volume or renal perfusion pressure, and by loss of Na^+. Renin then acts on angiotensinogen (a 485 amino acid peptide produced by the liver) in plasma to produce angiotensin I (AI), a decapeptide which is then converted by ACE in the lung to the octapeptide angiotensin II (AII). AI and particularly AII stimulate aldosterone

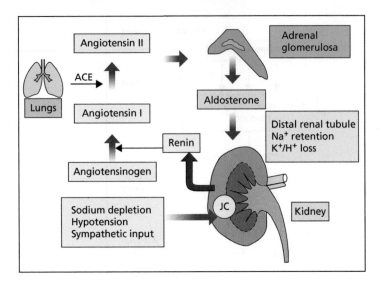

Figure 9.4 The renin–angiotensin system. Renin is released from the renal juxtaglomerular cells (JC) in response to hypotension, low blood volume or sodium depletion. Renin catalyses the conversion of angiotensinogen to angiotensin I. During passage through the lung, angiotensin-converting enzyme (ACE) catalyses the production of angiotensin II from angiotensin I. The angiotensin II stimulates release of aldosterone from the adrenal glomerulosa and the mineralocorticoid then promotes reabsorption of sodium in the distal tubules of the kidney.

production in the adrenal glomerulosa. Measurements of both aldosterone and renin are often helpful to establish whether aldosterone production is autonomous. Under normal circumstances, plasma aldosterone varies with posture, and measurement of aldosterone in the supine and erect position is sometimes helpful in elucidating the cause of hyperaldosteronism (Chapter 9: Investigation of suspected primary hyperaldosteronism). An increase in plasma K^+ also stimulates aldosterone, while ACTH is relatively unimportant, except possibly in stress conditions and in congenital adrenal hyperplasia (CAH) due to 21-hydroxylase deficiency (Chapter 22: 21-Hydroxylase deficiency). No specific aldosterone-binding protein has been demonstrated.

Androgen secretion

The zona reticularis and to some extent the zona fasciculata produce the androgens androstenedione, dehydroepiandrosterone (DHEA) and dehydroepiandrosterone sulphate (DHEAS). The measurements of these androgens are important in the investigation of hirsutism, virilisation (Chapter 10: Hirsutism and virilism) and CAH (Chapter 22: Congenital adrenal hyperplasia).

The pathways for the production of the various adrenal steroids are shown in Figure 9.5.

Investigation of suspected adrenocortical hyperfunction

Hyperfunction of the adrenal cortex can lead to overproduction of cortisol (Cushing's syndrome) or aldosterone (Conn's syndrome).

Cushing's syndrome

This can be ACTH dependent or ACTH independent (Figure 9.6; Table 9.1). If iatrogenic causes are excluded (e.g. use of hydrocortisone, prednisolone or dexamethasone), then the condition is caused by tumours that release either ACTH or cortisol. Approximately 70% of cases are due to a pituitary adenoma secreting ACTH (this is known as Cushing's disease). Ectopic ACTH secretion (often from a small-cell carcinoma of the bronchus or a carcinoid tumour) is the cause of approximately 10% of the cases. Glucocorticoid-secreting adrenal adenoma or carcinoma are each responsible for about 10% of the cases. Most ACTH-dependent forms of Cushing's syndrome lead to diffuse bilateral adrenocortical hyperplasia, but about 10–15% of patients with ACTH-driven Cushing's syndrome demonstrate a macronodular hyperplasia.

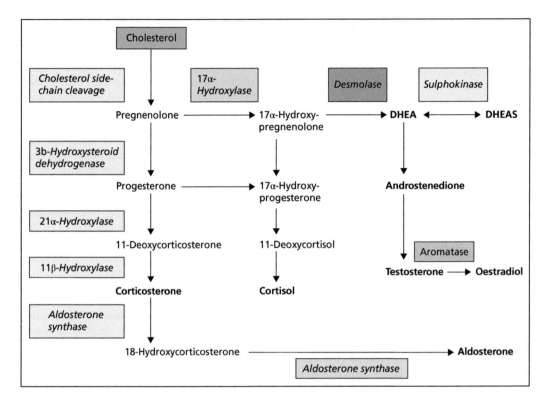

Figure 9.5 Steroid biosynthetic pathways in the adrenal cortex. Enzymes are shown in the boxes, and major steroid products are shown in bold. The conversion of corticosterone to aldosterone is restricted to the zona glomerulosa.

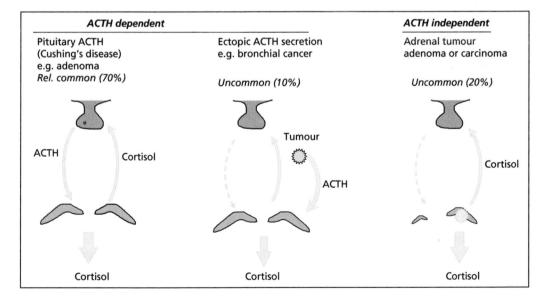

Figure 9.6 Pathological causes of Cushing's syndrome. Cushing's disease is caused by a pituitary adenoma autonomously secreting ACTH. The production of ACTH from the pituitary is suppressed (dotted arrow) when Cushing's syndrome is caused by an ectopic ACTH-secreting tumour or an adrenal adenoma autonomously secreting cortisol.

Table 9.1 Causes of glucocorticoid excess.

ACTH dependent
- Pituitary (Cushing's disease)
- Ectopic
- Ectopic CRH or related peptides
- ACTH therapy

ACTH independent
- Adrenal adenoma
- Adrenal carcinoma
- Glucocorticoid therapy
- Micronodular hyperplasia (partially ACTH dependent)

While Cushing's syndrome is uncommon, many of the clinical features of the disease such as hypertension, obesity, menstrual irregularities, depression, glucose intolerance or diabetes are commonly seen in general practice. It is therefore essential that patients with suspected Cushing's syndrome should be investigated according to a logical scheme that involves the use of simple screening tests to establish a likely diagnosis of Cushing's syndrome before the more involved investigations are carried out to establish the cause.

Some patients have 'cyclical Cushing's syndrome' in which there is intermittent and cyclical abnormal secretion of ACTH. This may be reflected by a history of variable and intermittent depression with anxiety, or variability in the severity of the symptoms and signs characteristic of Cushing's syndrome. Such patients may require tests to be performed on a number of occasions to make the diagnosis; salivary cortisol measurements can provide a convenient means of providing this long-term assessment.

A suggested plan of investigation is shown in Figure 9.7. Table 9.2 gives a summary of the commonly observed (but not invariable) findings in these hormonal tests.

Tests used to establish if a clinical diagnosis of Cushing's syndrome is likely

Initial screening tests

Low-dose dexamethasone suppression test

The best initial screening test for adrenocortical hyperfunction is to perform, as an outpatient, a low-dose overnight dexamethasone suppression test. Under normal circumstances, dexamethasone sup-

presses the secretion of CRH (negative feedback – Figure 9.2) and thus ACTH. As a consequence, cortisol levels fall below 50 nmol/L.

In the *overnight suppression test*, the patient takes dexamethasone (1 mg) at 11–12 pm the night before attending the clinic. Serum cortisol is measured on a blood specimen taken the following morning at 8–9 am. A cortisol concentration of less than 50 nmol/L in this morning sample effectively excludes Cushing's syndrome. This test performed using a 1 mg dose of dexamethasone has a false-positive rate of around 12% with a false-negative rate of less than 2%.

The *48-h suppression test* is superior, but less convenient than the overnight test. Dexamethasone (0.5 mg) is taken every 6 h, beginning at 9 am on the first day, and serum cortisol is measured 48 h later (interpretation as for the overnight test). The true-positive rate is reported to be better than 97%, with a false-negative rate of less than 1% for the 48-h test.

Drugs that affect hepatic microsomal enzymes (e.g. phenytoin, phenobarbitone, fluoxetine) can affect the metabolism of dexamethasone, leading to either false-positive or false-negative results. False positives can also occur in women taking exogenous oestrogens (e.g. contraceptive pill), and in patients with poorly controlled diabetes.

Urinary free cortisol (UFC)

Cortisol undergoes hepatic metabolism with the production of a number of metabolically inactive compounds that are excreted in the urine mainly as conjugated metabolites (e.g. glucuronides). A small amount of cortisol is excreted unchanged in the urine. Urinary cortisol excretion is related to the biologically active plasma free cortisol during the period of urine collection.

The measurement of UFC excretion in a 24-h collection is an acceptable screening test, but it suffers from the disadvantage that an incomplete collection of urine may lead to a false-negative result. Cushing's syndrome is generally excluded if the cortisol excretion is less than 250 nmol/24h. Even if a complete urine collection is obtained, the test has a false-negative rate of 8–15%.

Late night salivary cortisol

This test has emerged as a useful screening and monitoring test for patients with Cushing's syndrome. Salivary cortisol reflects free (unbound) cortisol, and its measurement carries the advantage of allowing for home collection, where the stress effects of the hospital environment can be minimised. Sampling should be performed between 11 pm and midnight on two

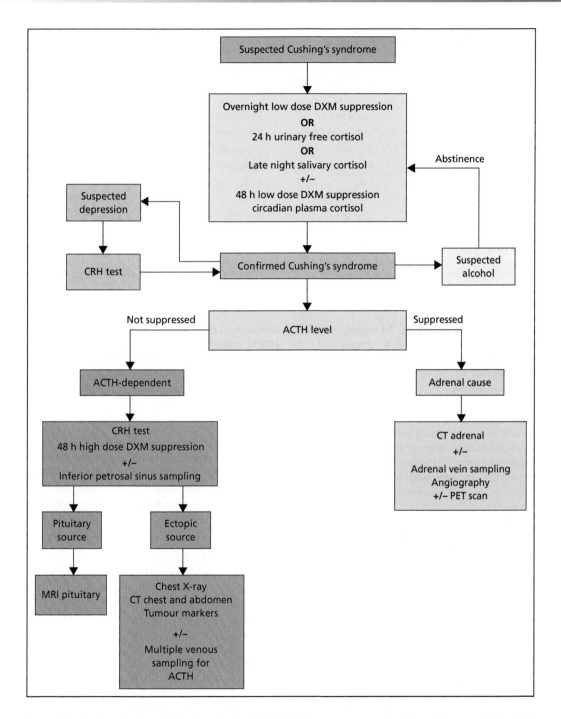

Figure 9.7 Algorithm for the investigation of suspected Cushing's syndrome and elucidation of its cause. CRH = corticotrophin-releasing hormone; CT = computed tomography; DXM = dexamethasone.

separate occasions. Studies report an overall test sensitivity and specificity between 92 and 100%.

False-positive results can occur with contamination from steroid-containing lotion or oral gels, and higher values have also been reported in elderly patients, smokers and individuals with hypertension or diabetes. The test should also be avoided in shift workers or patients with variable bedtimes, which can

Table 9.2 **Results of hormonal tests in patients with adrenal hyperfunction.**

Test	Cushing's disease	Adrenal tumour	Ectopic ACTH-secreting tumour
Tests to confirm the diagnosis			
• Midnight serum cortisol	Increased	Increased	Increased
• Dexamethasone, low-dose test	Not suppressed	Not suppressed	Not suppressed
• Urinary free cortisol*	Increased	Increased	Increased
• Late night salivary cortisol	Increased	Increased	Increased
• Diurnal rhythm	Lost	Lost	Lost
Tests to differentiate cause			
• Plasma ACTH	Normal or increased	Not detectable	Often much increased
• Dexamethasone, high-dose	Suppressed	Not suppressed	Not suppressed
• CRH test	Increased response	No response	No response

*This test may be performed on a 24-h collection of urine or on an early morning specimen when the results are expressed as the urinary cortisol : creatinine ratio.

lead to falsely elevated results. An important advantage of salivary cortisol is that it appears useful in detecting mild cases of Cushing's syndrome, and is useful not only for diagnosis but also in monitoring response to treatment.

Interpretation of screening tests

The screening tests usually serve to distinguish simple nonendocrine obesity from obesity due to Cushing's syndrome. Abnormal results may, however, be obtained in depressed or extremely anxious patients, in the presence of severe intercurrent illness or in alcoholism (pseudo-Cushing syndrome). Further tests (as an inpatient) may be required to rule out pseudo-Cushing syndrome and help determine the specific cause of the adrenocortical hyperfunction (Figure 9.7).

Confirmatory tests

In normal subjects, plasma cortisol is highest in the morning and lowest around midnight (Figure 9.3). Patients with Cushing's syndrome lose this rhythm such that in most patients the 8 am plasma cortisol is normal but midnight plasma cortisol is raised. Patients need to be hospitalised for at least 48 h prior to stress-free venepuncture (e.g. in-dwelling catheter) to obtain meaningful results. It is also convenient to collect a series of 24-h urine samples for urine free cortisol measurement.

Patients with pseudo-Cushing syndrome may also show abnormal diurnal variation in cortisol; however, such patients can usually be distinguished from patients with true Cushing's by their ACTH response to CRH (see Chapter 9: CRH stimulation test). In

alcoholism, other clues (e.g. raised mean cell volume (MCV), abnormal liver function tests) may be helpful; abstinence will lead to normalisation of the HPA axis.

Determining the cause of Cushing's syndrome

Once the diagnosis is established, other investigations may help to determine the cause (Table 9.2); difficulties sometimes arise in distinguishing between ectopic ACTH production and Cushing's disease. Biochemical results need to be considered together with the findings from other methods of investigation, particularly radiological, including MRI and CT scanning.

Plasma ACTH

ACTH is unstable and samples must be collected into EDTA preservative, with the plasma ideally being separated and frozen within 30 min of collection. Temporary, often large, increases in ACTH may be observed as a response to emotional stress. Plasma ACTH should be measured on blood specimens collected both in the morning and in the evening (e.g. at 8 am and 10 pm). If ACTH is undetectable, this is diagnostic of a functional adrenal tumour and should be confirmed by an abdominal CT or MRI scan to detect an adrenal mass. Rare types of nodular adrenocortical disease (also ACTH independent) are also described.

If the patient has Cushing's disease (pituitary-dependent Cushing's syndrome), ACTH will be present in plasma in normal or increased concentration, particularly in the evening specimen. Results for plasma ACTH overlap considerably for patients with Cushing's disease and ectopic ACTH secretion.

However, a very high plasma ACTH often points to an ectopic ('non-endocrine') origin.

The following additional tests are used to distinguish Cushing's disease from ectopic ACTH secretion.

High-dose dexamethasone suppression test

This uses 2 mg of dexamethasone 6-hourly for 48 h in an attempt to suppress cortisol secretion. Basal (pre-dexamethasone) serum cortisol or 24-h urine free cortisol is compared with values obtained at the end of the 48-h period. Suppression is defined as a fall to less than 50% of the basal value. An overnight suppression test using a single dose of 8 mg of dexamethasone is reported to achieve similar diagnostic accuracy to the standard 48-h high-dose test.

About 90% of patients with pituitary-dependent Cushing's show suppression of cortisol output. In contrast, only 10% of patients with ectopic ACTH production show suppression.

CRH stimulation test

This test measures ACTH and cortisol concentration prior to and at 15, 30, 45, 60, 90 and 120 min after injection of 100 µg of CRH. Normal individuals (and depressed patients without Cushing's syndrome) demonstrate an ACTH peak less than 120 ng/L, and a variable increase in cortisol, with a mean peak of approx 700 nmol/L. Little or no response to CRH is found in patients with ectopic ACTH production or an adrenal tumour. Most patients with pituitary Cushing's show exaggerated ACTH and cortisol responses to human CRH (Figure 9.8). In distinguishing between Cushing's disease and ectopic ACTH production, the CRH test has a specificity of about 95%. Together, the high-dose dexamethasone suppression test and the CRH test provide almost 100% specificity and sensitivity in the diagnosis of Cushing's disease.

Other biochemical tests

1 *Potassium:* Hypokalaemic alkalosis may be a prominent feature of ectopic ACTH production, possibly due to the increased output of mineralocorticoids or high cortisol concentration (with renal loss of K^+ and H^+ in the urine). Patients with Cushing's syndrome are often treated with diuretics (for hypertension and oedema), and this treatment may itself lower the plasma K^+ concentration.

2 *Selective venous sampling:* Blood specimens can be collected from selected sites for measurement of plasma ACTH, to help identify the source of the ACTH (e.g. inferior petrosal sinus: peripheral vein ACTH ratio, which, if it increases following CRH injection, supports a pituitary source for the ACTH). In patients with an ectopic ACTH syndrome, there is no ACTH gradient between the inferior petrosal sinus samples and the samples drawn from peripheral veins.

3 *Pituitary function tests* (Chapter 7) may be abnormal in Cushing's syndrome due to the suppressive effect of cortisol on the hypothalamus and pituitary. The LH and TSH responses to GnRH and TRH respectively are often impaired, and the increase in plasma GH in response to hypoglycaemia is reduced.

4 *Tumour markers:* As many as 70% of patients with ectopic ACTH secretion also secrete one or more marker peptides (e.g. carcinoembryonic antigen, gastrin, somatostatin and calcitonin); a peptide tumour marker screen may assist in difficult cases.

5 *Glucose tolerance test:* Patients with adrenocortical hyperfunction may develop steroid-induced diabetes and have a diabetic response to an OGTT (Chapter 6: Oral glucose tolerance test).

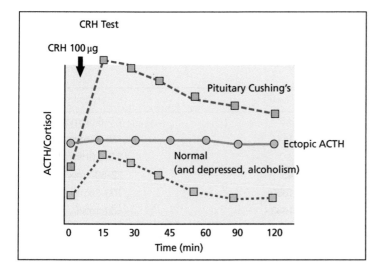

Figure 9.8 The cortisol and ACTH response in the CRH test. An exaggerated response is seen in Cushing's disease (pituitary adenoma), while a flat response is seen in ectopic ACTH production and adrenal adenoma. The test is usually not required for confirmation of adrenal adenoma as in such patients the diagnosis is made on the basis of an undetectable ACTH concentration.

Treatment

Surgery is the mainstay of treatment for Cushing's syndrome, although patients may benefit from medical therapy with ketoconazole or metyrapone to control steroid hormone excess prior to surgery. Adrenal adenomas are treated by unilateral adrenalectomy. After surgery it may be many months or even years before the suppressed adrenal recovers, and treatment with glucocorticoids may be required as a temporary measure. Pituitary-dependent Cushing's disease is treated by selective removal of the pituitary microadenoma by trans-sphenoidal surgery. Again glucocorticoid cover may be required until the HPA axis recovers from suppression. A nonsuppressible serum cortisol post-operatively suggests that the patient has not been cured, even if basal cortisol secretion has fallen to normal.

Treatment of ectopic ACTH syndrome involves removal of the tumour or occasionally bilateral adrenalectomy if the source of ACTH cannot be found.

 CASE 9.1

A 34-year-old housewife was admitted to hospital with a provisional diagnosis of Cushing's syndrome. As an outpatient, her serum cortisol had not been suppressed when an overnight dexamethasone suppression test (1 mg of dexamethasone) was performed. She was obese (weight 74 kg, height 1.7 m), hypertensive (blood pressure, 165/105 mmHg) and had wasting of the proximal limb muscles. The following results were obtained for adrenal function tests:

Test		Result		Usual response
Diurnal rhythm of serum cortisol nmol/L		400 (8 am) 380 (10 pm)		Reference range 100–565 nmol/L Reference range up to 200 nmol/L
Dexamethasone suppression test	Basal	After 48 h 0.5 mg qid	After 48 h 2 mg qid	
Serum cortisol nmol/L	420	410	500	Cortisol should suppress to <50 nmol/L
Plasma ACTH ng/L	<2			Reference range 7–51 ng/L

How would you interpret these results?

Comments: These results are consistent with a diagnosis of Cushing's syndrome due to an adrenal adenoma (low basal ACTH, no cortisol suppression with high dose dexamethasone). These tumours account for 5–10% of all cases of Cushing's syndrome. Ultrasound examination and imaging confirmed the presence of a tumour in the right adrenal, and the patient was treated successfully by right adrenalectomy.

 CASE 9.2

A 58-year-old man was admitted to a hospital with weight loss and respiratory distress. He was pigmented and his blood pressure was 140/80. Urea electrolytes, a random cortisol and an overnight (1 mg) dexamethasone test gave the following results:

Serum	Result	Reference range
Urea	8.6	2.5–6.6 mmol/L
Sodium	144	135–145 mmol/L
Potassium	2.0	3.6–5.0 mmol/L
Total CO_2	45	22–30 mmol/L
Cortisol (random)	1650	100–565 nmol/L
Post-overnight dexamethasone	1530	<50 nmol/L

Further investigation revealed the following:

Test		Result		Usual response
Dexamethasone suppression test	Basal	After 48h, 0.5mg qid	After 48h, 2.0mg qid	
Serum cortisol nmol/L	1350	1420	1100	Suppression to <50nmol/L
Plasma ACTH ng/L		750	723	Suppression to <2ng/L

A CRH test showed a flat response for cortisol and ACTH.

How would you interpret these results?

Comments: The very high cortisol and ACTH that are not suppressed by dexamethasone (overnight, low-dose and high-dose dexamethasone test) together with the marked hypokalaemic alkalosis strongly suggest that the patient has Cushing's syndrome caused by ectopic ACTH production. The flat response to the high-dose dexamethasone suppression test supports this diagnosis. Imaging demonstrated that the patient had carcinoma of the bronchus.

 CASE 9.3

A 68-year-old retired woman with long-standing type 2 diabetes presented with continued problems of obesity and poorly controlled hypertension. The GP noticed that she had plethoric moon facies and a blood pressure of 210/115mmHg. An overnight dexamethasone (1mg of dexamethasone) suppression test failed to suppress her cortisol below 50nmol/L and ACTH below 40ng/L. Urea, sodium, potassium and total CO_2 were all within the reference range but her glucose was 22.0mmol/L. Further tests performed as an outpatient at the endocrine clinic gave the following results for adrenal function tests:

Test	Result		
Dexamethasone	Basal	After 48h, 0.5mg qid	After 48h, 2.0mg qid
Serum cortisol 9am	520	230	110

A CRH test gave the following results:

Time (min)	Cortisol (nmol/L)	Time (min)	Cortisol (nmol/L)
0	590	60	1220
15	710	90	890
30	1300	120	735
45	1660		

What is the likely diagnosis? What further investigations should be performed?

Comments: These results are consistent with a diagnosis of Cushing's syndrome due to a pituitary adenoma secreting ACTH (Cushing's disease). Approximately 90% of patients with Cushing's disease suppress cortisol to less than half of the basal values when given high-dose dexamethasone. Most patients with Cushing's disease show an exaggerated cortisol response (>600nmol/L) following CRH injection. In this patient MRI showed bilateral adrenocortical hyperplasia and a microadenoma (~5mm in diameter) in the anterior pituitary. If imaging had failed to demonstrate an adenoma then petrosal sinus sampling for ACTH may have been required to detect the source of the ACTH. She was treated surgically by trans-sphenoidal removal of the microadenoma. Cure is likely if the patient develops hypocortisolism in the first few days to weeks after surgery. During this post-operative period, glucocorticoid replacement therapy is required.

Investigation of suspected adrenocortical insufficiency

Adrenocortical insufficiency may be primary (e.g. destruction of the gland by autoimmune disease or infection) or secondary (e.g. hypothalamic or pituitary disease leading to ACTH deficiency or after long-term steroid therapy). The causes are listed in Table 9.3.

In primary adrenal failure, patients present with lethargy, weakness, nausea and weight loss. They are typically hypotensive, with characteristic hyperpigmentation affecting the buccal mucosa, scars and skin creases. The condition may present itself when a patient suffers from trauma or infection, or undergoes surgery. Patients with primary adrenal failure usually have deficiencies of both glucocorticoids and mineralocorticoids. Often there is hypoglycaemia with hyponatraemia, hyperkalaemia, raised serum urea levels and acid–base disturbance. The condition is life threatening, and requires urgent investigation if suspected.

The hypotension and electrolyte abnormalities are generally less severe in secondary adrenal insufficiency, with preservation of aldosterone secretion; the patient is typically pale. Where hypothalamic or pituitary disease is the cause, associated deficiency of other pituitary hormones may be found (Chapter 7). An enlarging pituitary tumour often first affects gonadotrophin secretion (with loss of libido and secondary sexual characteristics), followed by loss of growth hormone, thyrotrophin and ACTH.

The diagnosis of adrenocortical hypofunction is relatively straightforward, once the suspicion of the condition arises. Patients should be immediately referred to a hospital, and blood should be collected for basal measurements of serum urea, electrolytes, glucose, cortisol and plasma ACTH concentrations *before* the patient is given cortisol. Definitive tests for the diagnosis of this condition should be carried out later, after the crisis. A suggested plan of investigation is shown in Figure 9.9.

Table 9.3 Causes of adrenocortical insufficiency.

Primary adrenocortical insufficiency (Addison's disease)
1 Autoimmune adrenalitis
2 Infective (e.g. tuberculosis (TB), cytomegalovirus, histoplasmosis, meningococcal)
3 Secondary tumour deposits
4 Infiltrative lesions (e.g. amyloidosis, haemochromatosis)
5 CAH or hypoplasia
6 Adrenoleukodystrophy (X-linked)
7 Drugs (e.g. etomidate)

Secondary to pituitary disease
1 Congenital deficiency (isolated or with GH deficiency)
2 Pituitary tumours (functional or non-functional)
3 Infections (e.g. TB, syphilis)
4 Secondary tumour deposits
5 Vascular lesions (e.g. post-partum haemorrhage)
6 Trauma
7 Iatrogenic (e.g. surgery or radiotherapy)
8 Secondary to hypothalamic disease
9 Others

Diagnosis of primary adrenal insufficiency (Addison's disease)

Cortisol and ACTH measurements

A normal serum cortisol at 8 am (or normal 24-h UFC) does *not* exclude Addison's disease; patients may be able to maintain a normal basal output but be unable to secrete adequate amounts of cortisol in response to stress. Nevertheless, a serum cortisol below 50 nmol/L at 8 am is strong presumptive evidence for Addison's disease, while a value (at 8 am) of 400 nmol/L or more (in the absence of steroid therapy) makes the diagnosis unlikely. Simultaneous measurement of cortisol and ACTH improves diagnostic accuracy such that a low serum cortisol (<100 nmol/L) and a raised ACTH (>200 ng/L) are diagnostic of adrenal failure.

Short tetracosactrin (Synacthen) test

Stimulation of the adrenal cortex with synthetic ACTH (tetracosactide, Synacthen, comprising the first 24 amino acids of ACTH) allows confirmation of the diagnosis of Addison's disease and an assessment of adrenocortical reserve. For patients with equivocal results, it allows a firm diagnosis to be made or dismissed. Basal cortisol is measured and a further measurement is taken 30 min after an IM injection of 250 μg tetracosactrin. In some centres, a lower dose (1 μg) Synacthen test has been adopted, for the reason that 250 μg dose is supraphysiological and may be falsely reassuring in patients with mild or partial deficiency.

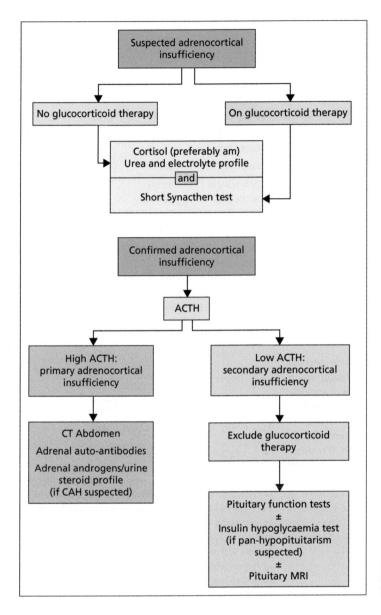

Figure 9.9 Suggested plan of investigation of adrenocortical insufficiency.

A normal response is defined as a rise in serum cortisol to at least 450 nmol/L, although the absolute value will depend on the local laboratory method. A normal response excludes primary adrenocortical insufficiency. Conversely, failure of cortisol to respond to Synacthen, together with elevated plasma ACTH, confirms primary adrenocortical insufficiency. Adrenocortical insufficiency secondary to hypothalamic or pituitary disease is also extremely unlikely if the response is normal, because, in the prolonged absence of ACTH, the cells of the adrenal cortex become atrophic and unresponsive.

Severe emotional stress, treatment with glucocorticoids within 12 h prior to the tetracosactrin injection, and the taking of oestrogen-containing oral contraceptives may invalidate the test. Where a patient with suspected Addison's disease is receiving glucocorticoid therapy, an agent that does not cross-react in the cortisol assay should be prescribed (e.g. dexamethasone rather than prednisolone) unless it is possible to stop glucocorticoid therapy for 24 h prior to the tests. With this proviso, adrenal reserve in patients on glucocorticoid therapy can also be assessed using this test.

Further testing in confirmed adrenocortical insufficiency

Patients with detectable adrenal auto-antibodies and primary adrenal insufficiency have autoimmune Addison's disease; however many patients with autoimmune Addison's fail to demonstrate a detectable antibody titre. Abdominal imaging may help to confirm the presence of enlarged or calcified adrenal glands that point to an alternative diagnosis.

In congenital adrenal hyperplasia (CAH), adrenal insufficiency is caused by an inherited enzyme deficiency that results in abnormal steroid secretion; most patients present as neonates or in early infancy, but in some cases the clinical symptoms may not manifest until adult life. Testing for CAH is discussed in more detail in Chapter 22.

Patients who receive prolonged glucocorticoid therapy are at risk of adrenal insufficiency on withdrawal of glucocorticoid treatment; the short Synacthen test can be useful to assess adrenal reserve in such patients.

The finding of a frankly low serum cortisol accompanied by a *low* plasma ACTH supports a diagnosis of adrenocortical insufficiency secondary to hypothalamic or pituitary disease. Baseline pituitary functions will almost certainly be abnormal by the time hypopituitarism is severe enough to produce adrenocortical hypofunction. It is usual in these patients, therefore, to measure basal concentrations of FT4 and TSH, prolactin, testosterone (male), oestradiol (female), LH and FSH and to investigate dynamic growth hormone responses in addition to the cortisol response (Chapter 7: Dynamic function tests – insulin hypoglycaemia test).

 CASE 9.4

A 25-year-old woman presented to her GP complaining of tiredness, loss of appetite and some weight loss. She also complained of feeling dizzy when she stood up and generally feeling very depressed. She appeared pigmented, which she attributed to sunbathing, but on closer examination her buccal mucosa were also pigmented. Her blood pressure (supine) was 110/70 and she was hyponatraemic with serum sodium of 128 mmol/L. Further investigations gave the following results:

Serum	Result	Reference range
Urea	8.0	2.5–6.6 mmol/L
Sodium	130	135–145 mmol/L
Potassium	5.2	3.6–5.0 mmol/L
Basal cortisol	160	100–565 nmol/L
Cortisol 30 min post-Synacthen	190	>450 nmol/L
Basal ACTH	450	7–50 ng/L
Anti-adrenal antibodies	Strong positive	

How would you interpret these results?

Comments: The high basal ACTH, borderline low basal serum cortisol and lack of cortisol response to the short Synacthen test confirmed a diagnosis of primary adrenal failure. The presence of anti-adrenal antibodies suggests that she has autoimmune primary adrenal failure. She was given glucocorticoid and mineralocorticoid replacement therapy.

Biochemical tests in the investigation of hypertension

Hypertension is common and in most patients no underlying cause is apparent, that is, they have 'essential hypertension'. Laboratory tests are usually aimed at assessing end-organ damage and cardiovascular risk. In a few cases biochemical investigations are performed to determine if there are secondary causes of hypertension such as renal disease, hypercalcaemia, Cushing's syndrome, hyperaldosteronism and phaeochromocytoma (Table 9.4).

Secondary hypertension

This is most often due to renal disease or adrenal disorders. Adrenal causes are given in Table 9.5.

Patients with hypertension who have a clinical history or features suggestive of a renal or adrenal lesion require further investigation, that is:

- hypertension with spontaneous or low-dose diuretic-induced hypokalaemia;
- severe hypertension (>160/100 mm), or drug-resistant hypertension (defined as sub-optimal control under a three-drug antihypertensive program);

Table 9.4 **Laboratory tests and the investigation of hypertension.**

All patients

Assessing end-organ damage and cardiovascular risk

- Triglycerides, cholesterol, LDL and HDL
- Creatinine, electrolytes, eGFR
- Glucose
- Urine protein and blood (dipstick)

Patients with suspected secondary hypertension

Tests will be steered by history and clinical features

- Aldosterone : renin ratio
- Calcium and, if raised, PTH
- Urine/plasma metadrenalines
- Overnight dexamethasone test and/or 24-h urine cortisol
- IGF-1
- Renal ultrasound

Table 9.5 **Biochemical investigations in suspected adrenal hypertension.**

Adrenal disorder	Biochemical tests
Cushing's syndrome	Cortisol >50 nmol/L after dexamethasone suppression test Raised 24-h urine free cortisol
Primary aldosteronism (Conn's syndrome) and bilateral adrenal hyperplasia	Hypokalaemia, hypernatraemia, increased aldosterone : renin ratio
Phaeochromocytoma	Increased urinary or plasma metadrenalines

- strong family history of early hypertension or stroke;
- documented adrenal tumour or incidentaloma;
- hypokalaemia with hyponatraemia (may suggest secondary hyperaldosteronism).

Noncompliance with medication, excessive sodium intake and white coat hypertension should be excluded before further investigations are initiated.

Primary hyperaldosteronism (low-renin hyperaldosteronism)

Primary hyperaldosteronism is a rare but potentially reversible cause of hypertension, responsible for

approximately 5–10% of cases of hypertension. The commonest causes are:

- Idiopathic or bilateral adrenal hyperplasia (~60–70% of cases).
- A unilateral single small aldosterone-producing adenoma, as originally described by Conn (Conn's syndrome; ~30–40% of cases).
- Rare causes include:
  - glucocorticoid-suppressible hyperaldosteronism (GSH), an autosomal dominant inherited disorder produced by a hybrid gene (11β-hydroxylase + aldosterone synthase), which allows aldosterone to be produced by the fasciculata under the control of ACTH; in GSH, aldosterone production can be suppressed by giving glucocorticoids;
  - primary adrenal hyperplasia (unilateral);
  - aldosterone-producing carcinoma (rare).

Establishing the cause is important to guide appropriate treatment; for example, Conn's adenoma is potentially cured by surgery, and GSH has the potential for remission with specific treatment using a synthetic glucocorticoid such as dexamethasone to suppress ACTH secretion. Standard protocols to establish the differential diagnosis involve demonstrating suppression of plasma renin activity and investigating responsiveness of plasma aldosterone concentrations to variations in angiotensin II (e.g. in response to change in posture, ACE inhibition, or diuretics) and ACTH (e.g. diurnal variation). Adrenal imaging is reserved for those with biochemically proven adrenal disease. These tests are disrupted by anti-hypertensive medication and are both complex to perform and interpret.

Symptoms are usually absent or nonspecific, and include tiredness, muscle weakness, thirst and polyuria. The condition may be suspected in a hypertensive patient with low plasma K+ (<3.5 mmol/L) or in a patient where plasma K+ concentration falls below 3 nmol/L during therapy with a thiazide diuretic; however, up to 50% of patients are normokalaemic. Common causes of hypertension with a reduced plasma K+ need to be considered in the differential diagnosis (e.g. essential hypertension with diuretic therapy). If hypokalaemia is found in patients taking diuretics and primary hyperaldosteronism is suspected, then the diuretic should be withdrawn, potassium stores replenished and plasma K+ measured 2 weeks later.

Investigation of suspected primary hyperaldosteronism

Screening

A ratio of plasma aldosterone : renin is often used as a screening test. If possible, the patient should be off anti-hypertensive medication before the test is performed. Cut-offs depend on the assay used for measurement of plasma renin, and therefore local protocols and reference ranges for the investigation of suspected primary hyperaldosteronism should always be followed. Samples should be taken after the patient has been seated for 30 min. An increase in both the aldosterone : renin ratio *and* an absolute increase in plasma aldosterone concentration is usually required for the diagnosis of primary hyperaldosteronism; typically aldosterone is > 400 pmol/L.

Confirmation testing

Defined protocols are required and involve the patient being admitted as a day case to study. There are often local preferences that determine which further investigations are performed; currently accepted confirmatory tests include the oral salt-loading test, saline infusion test, captopril challenge or fludrocortisone suppression test. Each protocol is designed to suppress the endogenous secretion of aldosterone; a lack of suppression of aldosterone secretion under the different stimuli confirms the presence of primary hyperaldosteronism. Currently, there is little evidence to determine which of these is the most reliable.

Subtype classification

In patients with confirmed primary hyperaldosteronism, further testing is required to distinguish idiopathic hyperplasia from Conn's adenoma. Adrenal CT imaging is used to detect the presence of adrenal tumours, and adrenal vein sampling (with the measurement of aldosterone) can confirm if lateralization is present in cases where surgery is being considered.

The posture stimulation test can be used to distinguish adrenal hyperplasia from adenoma. This test typically involves taking measurements of aldosterone and renin at 8 am (supine), followed by an upright sample at noon after 4 h of ambulation. Patients with adrenal hyperplasia have a characteristic rise in aldosterone concentration in response to the standing position, whereas those with adrenal adenoma do not, in view of autonomous secretion. Patients with adenomas also tend to be more responsive to ACTH stimulation, and demonstrate higher aldosterone excretion on the early morning sample.

The measurement of urine 18-hydroxycortisol (18-OHF) may also be of help in the differential diagnosis of primary hyperaldosteronism; 18-OHF is a hybrid steroid, secreted by the adrenal cortex from the action of aldosterone synthase on cortisol, rather than on its usual substrate corticosterone. Patients with Conn's adenoma or GSH excrete more of the steroid than patients with adrenal hyperplasia. In Conn's adenoma, abnormal expression of steroidogenic enzymes in the tumour may explain over-production of 18-OHF.

Patients presenting with a strong family history of primary hyperaldosteronism should prompt genetic testing of the *CYP11B2* gene to exclude GSH.

Treatment

Adrenal tumours are removed. Patients with bilateral adrenal hyperplasia are treated with spironolactone, a diuretic that antagonises the action of aldosterone. GSH is treated with dexamethasone.

Secondary hyperaldosteronism (high-renin hyperaldosteronism)

This is much more common, and is only sometimes associated with hypertension. It is due to conditions that stimulate the secretion of renin, often as a result of reduced renal Na^+ filtration (e.g. congestive heart failure, cirrhosis, Na^+ deprivation). Diagnosis of these conditions is usually straightforward and further investigation of the renin–angiotensin–aldosterone system is not necessary. The most common cause of secondary hyperaldosteronism is diuretic therapy.

 CASE 9.5

A 50-year-old lady was referred to the hypertension clinic with uncontrolled blood pressure for the past year despite using multiple combinations of anti-hypertensive drugs. Hypertension had first been diagnosed 20 years previously. Her blood pressure was 160/110 mm Hg with a resting pulse of 74. She had been put on potassium supplements because of previous intermittent hypokalaemia which she had developed despite not being on potassium wasting diuretics.

Her hypokalaemia was corrected with further potassium supplements and her anti-hypertensive medication was withdrawn for a week prior to further blood tests being performed with the sample taken sitting at 9 am.

	Result	Reference range
Aldosterone	850	70–570 pmol/L (sitting)
Renin	4	5–45 miU/L (sitting)
Aldosterone : renin ratio	212	<35

How would you interpret these results?

Comments: The aldosterone : renin ratio is high and the aldosterone is >400 pmol/L, results which are highly suggestive of primary hyperaldosteronism. The clinical presentation and the hypokalaemia that the patient had developed previously are also consistent with the diagnosis. A saline suppression test was subsequently performed, that is, saline was infused (2 L of normal saline infused over 4 h) and the response in plasma aldosterone was measured. This patient failed to suppress aldosterone during this test which is consistent with hyperaldosteronism. MRI of the adrenals revealed a 2.5 cm left adrenal tumour, consistent with a diagnosis of primary hyperaldosteronism due to a left adrenal adenoma (Conn's syndrome). The patient was successfully treated by a left adrenalectomy. NB hypokalaemia must be corrected prior to investigation because hypokalaemia can suppress aldosterone levels and lead to a false-negative result.

Phaeochromocytoma

These tumours arise from chromaffin cells (90% are in the adrenal medulla; the rest can occur anywhere from the base of the brain to the testes). About 5% of tumours are bilateral and about 10% malignant. They secrete excessive amounts of the catecholamines noradrenaline and adrenaline, and the metabolites normetadrenaline, metadrenaline and 4-hydroxy-3-methoxymandelic acid (HMMA – also known as vanillylmandelic acid or VMA). The catecholamines and their metabolites can be further metabolised in various tissues, especially the liver, to produce sulphated and glucuronide derivatives that are then excreted in urine (Figure 9.10).

Phaeochromocytoma is a rare cause of hypertension, accounting for less than 0.2% of cases. Characteristically, the hypertension is episodic. Even when present all the time, symptoms (e.g. headache, pallor, palpitations, sweating, panic attacks, abdominal pain) can be paroxysmal. The episodic nature is important when selecting the time for collecting specimens for laboratory investigations.

Phaeochromocytoma sometimes occurs as a familial condition, in association with the MEN IIa and IIb syndromes (see Chapter 17).

Catecholamines and their metabolites are also secreted by neuroblastomas; these are rare rapidly growing tumours that occur in infants and young children.

Diagnosis

The diagnosis of phaeochromocytoma depends crucially on demonstrating excessive production of catecholamines or their metabolites in plasma or urine. The measurements of plasma-free metadrenalines or urinary fractioned metadrenalines are the most sensitive tests, having sensitivities of 96–100%. The measurement of plasma or urine catecholamines (sensitivity 84–86%), urinary total metadrenalines (sensitivity 77%) or urinary VMA (sensitivity 64%) is much less reliable for detecting phaeochromocytoma. However, the measurement of urinary catecholamines, VMA and dopamine metabolites does form the mainstay for the diagnosis of neuroblastoma in children (Chapter 22).

The measurement of plasma or urine metadrenalines for the diagnosis of phaeochromocytoma is more reliable because tumours produce metadrenalines continuously while the release of catecholamines is usually episodic. Furthermore, stimulation of the adrenal via the sympathetic nervous system causes a large increase in the release of catecholamines but, under such circumstances, plasma free metadrenalines remain relatively unaffected.

The choice of urine versus plasma metadrenaline measurement will depend on the local availability of assays and the clinical circumstance. In an outpatient setting 24-h urine collections are usually first choice of test, due to the greater specificity of urine testing and greater stability of metabolites in urine. Conversely, plasma measurements are particularly beneficial in monitoring patients with a high risk of phaeochromocytoma (e.g. those with a family history or a previously resected tumour), on account of greater sensitivity. Measurement of plasma metadrenalines is also useful in a paediatric population where the collection of an accurate 24-h urine sample can be problematic.

Several drugs are known to interfere with the analysis of catecholamines and metadrenalines in plasma and urine; these are listed in Table 9.6. Interference

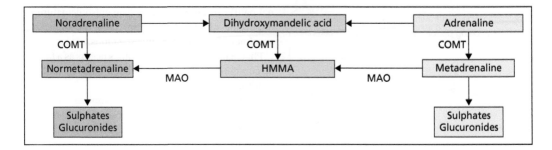

Figure 9.10 Pathways for the metabolism of catecholamines. COMT = catechol-O-methyltransferase; MAO = monoamine oxidase; HMMA = 4-hydroxy-3-methoxymandelic acid.

Table 9.6 **Medications that can interfere with the analysis of plasma/urine catecholamines and metadrenalines.**

Analytical interference

- Paracetamol
- Anti-adrenergic agents: labetalol, sotalol, α-methyl dopa
- Anxiolytics: buspirone
- Sulfasalazine
- Levodopa*

Pharmacodynamic interference

- Tricyclic antidepressants
- Monoamine oxidase inhibitors
- Phenoxybenzamine
- Sympathomimetics
- Cocaine

*Levodopa may also cause pharmacodynamic interference if dopamine metabolites are measured.

---

may be either analytical or pharmacodynamic, and may be specific to both the sample type and the analysis method involved. The local laboratory should provide a list of medications to avoid; occasionally re-testing may be necessary to avoid interference from a particular agent. Interference from dietary constituents should also be considered; in particular the measurement of some catecholamine metabolites including VMA requires the patient to be placed on a vanilla-free diet. Caution should also be exercised in patients who have undergone testing under extreme illness, where physiological stress can lead to marked elevations in catecholamine secretion.

In the case of paroxysmal attacks, patients should ideally collect a baseline 24-h urine sample alongside a second urine collection when the next attack occurs.

A single collection is usually sufficient in patients with persistent hypertension. When the clinical index of suspicion is low (e.g. a middle-aged or elderly patient who is hypertensive but without paroxysmal symptoms), there is little justification for requesting these investigations, which should be restricted to those with appropriate symptoms or young patients with hypertension.

Further testing

Due to the low prevalence of phaeochromocytoma, false positives are common. Both the extent of the abnormality and the nature of increased results (e.g. if both metadrenaline and normetadrenaline are increased) should guide follow-up testing. Imaging with abdominal CT is usually used to locate any tumour mass. In borderline cases, clonidine suppression testing can be used to biochemically confirm elevated catecholamine secretion. Clonidine is an α2-adrenergic receptor agonist that prevents noradrenaline release in patients without phaeochromocytoma, but not in patients with autonomous tumoural secretion of noradrenaline; measurement of plasma normetadrenaline before and after infusion of clonidine can reportedly distinguish true from false positives with a sensitivity of 96–100%.

In those with confirmed phaeochromocytoma, genetic testing should be considered. Current testing strategies can identify mutations in up to one-third of patients.

Treatment

Laparoscopic adrenalectomy is performed in patients with adrenal phaeochromocytomas. Prior to surgery, patients should be rendered stable with α-adrenergic blockade to prevent hypertensive crisis. Calcium channel and β-adrenergic blockers can also be used as adjunctive agents.

10

Investigation of gonadal function infertility, menstrual irregularities and hirsutism

---

Learning objectives

To understand:

✔ the mechanisms that regulate the hypothalamic–pituitary–gonadal axis in males and females;

✔ the endocrine investigations that should be performed in males for erectile dysfunction, low libido, infertility and gynaecomastia;

✔ the endocrine investigations that should be performed in women for infertility, menstrual irregularities, hirsutism, suspected polycystic ovarian syndrome and suspected menopause and premature ovarian failure;

✔ how to interpret the results of the endocrine tests performed for the investigation of the clinical problems listed above in males and females.

Introduction

Infertility in women and menstrual irregularities are relatively common clinical problems. They often have an endocrine cause and result from abnormal ovarian, thyroid, hypothalamic, pituitary or adrenal function. The laboratory can help with the diagnosis of these endocrine abnormalities. Biochemical tests are also useful in screening hirsute women for the presence of occult ovarian or adrenal tumours and in determining if polycystic ovarian syndrome is a likely cause of their presenting complaints. Although endocrine causes of male infertility and erectile dysfunction are rare, mild hypogonadism associated with an ageing male population is becoming an increasingly recognised finding. Biochemical tests play an important role in assessing such patients.

This chapter outlines the function of the hypothalamic–pituitary–gonadal axis, and describes the biochemical tests that are required for the investigation of the disorders listed above. Guidance on interpretation of the test employed is also provided.

Clinical Biochemistry Lecture Notes, Tenth Edition. Peter Rae, Mike Crane and Rebecca Pattenden.
© 2018 John Wiley & Sons Ltd. Published 2018 by John Wiley & Sons Ltd.
Companion website: www.lecturenoteseries.com/clinicalbiochemistry

Male gonadal function

Spermatogenesis and its control

Spermatogenesis takes place in the seminiferous tubules, and requires normal function of both the Leydig and the Sertoli cells.

Leydig cells produce testosterone, the principal androgen, under the control of LH. Sertoli cells provide other testicular cells with nutrients, and also produce several regulatory proteins, of which inhibin, activin, anti-Mullerian hormone (AMH) and androgen-binding protein (ABP) are the best characterised. Sertoli cell function is regulated by FSH. Testosterone has crucial paracrine actions in the testes which are required for normal spermatogenesis and fertility.

The entire hypothalamic–pituitary–testicular axis (Figure 10.1) must function normally for spermatogenesis. GnRH from the hypothalamus stimulates the release of LH and FSH; its effect on LH release is more marked than that on FSH release. The secretion of GnRH, and thus of LH, occurs in pulses; the secretion of FSH is less markedly pulsatile. The amplitude and frequency of the pulses of LH release appear to be important in exerting effects on testosterone production.

The secretion of LH is under negative feedback control from testosterone, and the release of FSH is inhibited by inhibin and stimulated by activin, both released by Sertoli cells. A high testicular testosterone concentration is ensured by the anatomical proximity of Leydig, Sertoli and spermatogenic cells, and by the local release of ABP. Inhibin is a dimeric glycopeptide, comprising a 20 kDa α-subunit and a 15 kDa β-subunit. Two forms of β-subunit occur, thus two forms of inhibin (inhibin A and inhibin B) occur, although in males inhibin B is the most important form in plasma. Both FSH and testosterone are necessary for inhibin production in normal men. Activin is a dimer of inhibin β-subunits and has a stimulatory action on FSH

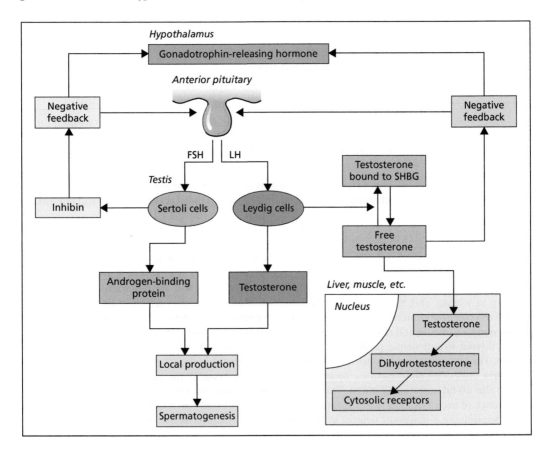

Figure 10.1 The hypothalamic–pituitary–testicular axis. SHBG = sex hormone-binding globulin. Activin from Sertoli cells stimulates FSH release.

release. AMH causes regression of the Mullerian ducts, and in the absence of AMH and testosterone the ducts differentiate into female internal genitalia.

Transport, metabolism and actions of testosterone

In the circulation in males, about 60% of testosterone is strongly bound to sex hormone-binding globulin (SHBG), 38% is weakly bound to albumin and approximately 2% is unbound (free). A large proportion of testosterone is bound to SHBG in both males and females, thus the factors that alter the concentration or affinity of SHBG will have a significant effect on the circulating total testosterone concentration. Factors that modify the concentration of SHBG are shown in Table 10.1. There is continued debate concerning which components of circulating testosterone are capable of exerting bioactivity on target tissues. Classically androgens have been considered to exert their effect through interactions with a cytosolic receptor that then translocates to the nucleus and interacts with androgen-responsive genes. As such it was believed that only the small unbound 'free' fraction could enter cells and exert a biological effect. However, some consider that both the 'free' and 'albumin-bound fraction' of testosterone may be able to enter cells and thus be the 'bioavailable testosterone' fraction. Few laboratories measure the 'free' testosterone concentration or 'bioavailable testosterone'. Most laboratories will offer a 'free androgen index' (FAI) which requires the measurement of SHBG and total testosterone and applying these in the formula:

$$FAI = \frac{total\ testosterone}{SHBG} \times 100.$$

This effectively corrects for changes in SHBG but it does not take into account changes in the albumin-bound fraction. The FAI is unreliable in males and tends to overestimate the free testosterone concentration; its use should be confined to females. More complicated mathematical formulae based on the law of mass action have been produced that can calculate free testosterone and estimate bioavailable testosterone from measured total testosterone, albumin and SHBG. These formulae do not take into account changes in the affinity of SHBG and albumin but appear to work well for most male subjects.

Androgens are thought to exert their action in target tissues through high-affinity cytosolic receptors that transport the androgens into the cell nucleus. In the nucleus, the androgens then interact with androgen receptors, which in turn modify the expression of androgen-responsive genes. In many tissues, testosterone is converted to the more biologically active compound 5α-dihydrotestosterone (5α-DHT) by 5α-reductase. It would seem that some actions of testosterone might be mediated through oestrogen receptors after local conversion of testosterone to oestrogen by the enzyme 'aromatase'. It has thus become apparent that many of the actions of testosterone may be regulated in target tissues by both 5α-reductase and aromatase. In addition, because oestradiol and testosterone bind to SHBG with differing affinities, changes in the concentration of SHBG may modify the relative clearance rates of testosterone and oestradiol and thus alter the ratio of these hormones in plasma; this may in turn have a biological consequence.

Investigation of infertility and male hypogonadism

Endocrine causes of subfertility are rare in men. Most infertile males are eugonadal, with oligospermia due to failure of the seminiferous tubules. In a eugonadal male with a normal sperm count, endocrine investigations are not required. Causes of male hypogonadism are given in Table 10.2.

If on two occasions the sperm count is less than 15×10^6/mL and/or motility is poor in more than 50% of the sperm, measurements of serum LH, FSH and testosterone should be made to determine whether hypogonadism is caused by a primary defect in the testes or in the hypothalamic–pituitary region. Both forms lead to infertility (Figure 10.2). Azoospermia with a raised FSH suggests severe seminiferous tubular damage, while azoospermia with normal FSH and normal testicular volume indicates bilateral genital tract obstruction. Plasma

---

Table 10.1 **Causes of abnormal SHBG in males and females.**

Increased SHBG	Decreased SHBG
Anorexia nervosa	Obesity
Hyperthyroidism	Hypothyroidism
Androgen deficiency (males)	Polycystic ovarian syndrome
Liver disease	Glucocorticoid (high dose)
Anti-convulsants	Androgens
Oestrogens	Insulin resistance
Excess alcohol	Hyperprolactinaemia

Table 10.2 **Causes of hypogonadism in the male.**

Primary hypogonadism (low testosterone, high LH, FSH)

- Klinefelter's syndrome
- Androgen resistance*
- Androgen synthesis defects
- Anorchia or cryptorchidism
- Epididymo-orchitis (e.g. mumps)

- Testicular torsion
- Trauma
- Iron overload
- Drugs including alcohol

Secondary hypogonadism (low testosterone, LH, FSH low or normal)

- Kallmann's syndrome
- Hypothalamic–pituitary disease
- Isolated GnRH deficiency
- Panhypopituitarism
- Destructive pituitary tumour
- Cushing's syndrome
- Hyperprolactinaemia

- Opiates, cocaine, 'anabolic' steroids
- Excessive exercise
- Stress
- Weight loss
- Moderate illness (acute or chronic)
- Iron overload
- Oestrogen-secreting tumours

* Testosterone appears high against female reference range.

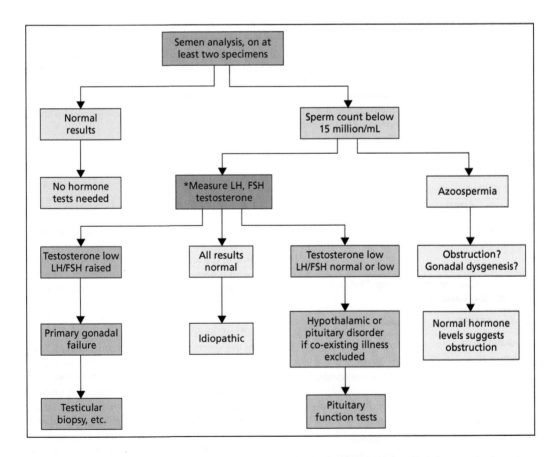

Figure 10.2 The investigation of male infertility. *Prolactin should also be measured to exclude hyperprolactinaemia.

prolactin should also be determined (Chapter 7: Hyperprolactinaemia and its investigation), as hyperprolactinaemia can lead to diminished libido, hypogonadism and impotence.

Misleadingly high values for LH and FSH might be observed because of pulsatile release. Serum total testosterone results are affected by changes in serum SHBG. The calculated free testosterone should be derived for all males who have abnormalities in serum SHBG concentration or a low total testosterone. The calculation of the FAI provides an unreliable and often misleading estimate of free testosterone in male patients, and its use should be avoided.

CASE 10.1

During investigations for infertility, a 27-year-old man was found to have azoospermia. On examination he had bilateral gynaecomastia and firm but small testes. He also complained of fatigue and low libido. Results of blood tests were as follows:

Serum	Result	Reference range
Prolactin	300	<500 mU/L
LH	36	1.0–9.0 U/L
FSH	21	1.0–10.0 U/L
Testosterone	5	10–30 nmol/L
Oestradiol	280	<160 pmol/L
FT4	15	9–21 pmol/L
TSH	2.0	0.2–4.5 mU/L
Cortisol	400	100–565 nmol/L

What do these results suggest as regards the cause of the patient's infertility?

Comments: The low testosterone with markedly raised LH and FSH suggest that the patient has primary gonadal failure (hypergonadotrophic hypogonadism). The most common cause is Klinefelter syndrome. Chromosomal analysis in this patient showed he had karyotype 47XXY, confirming the diagnosis of Klinefelter syndrome. The disorder affects 1 in 500 men across all ethnic groups, but the diagnosis is often delayed because of substantial variation in clinical presentation. This patient was treated with regular injections of testosterone (200 mg of testosterone enanthate IM) which gave improvements in fatigue and libido. The couple were referred to an infertility clinic for artificial insemination with donor sperm.

Hypergonadotrophic and hypogonadotrophic hypogonadism

Causes of hypogonadism are listed in Table 10.2.

Primary gonadal failure: hypergonadotrophic hypogonadism

The primary abnormality is in the testes, and serum testosterone is reduced while gonadotrophins are increased. This group of conditions includes congenital defects such as Klinefelter syndrome (usually 47XXY) and acquired lesions due to drugs, viruses or systemic diseases that affect testicular function. In some cases of abnormal spermatogenesis, FSH may be raised but LH and testosterone may remain normal.

Hypothalamic–pituitary disease: hypogonadotrophic hypogonadism

The primary abnormality is in the hypothalamus or the pituitary; the deficiency may be part of a generalised failure of pituitary hormone production. Serum gonadotrophins and testosterone are often both reduced, but in many cases gonadotrophins remain

CASE 10.2

A 17-year-old boy was investigated for delayed onset of puberty. There was nothing of note in his medical history, and he had not been receiving any medication; his 14-year-old brother was already more advanced developmentally. The patient was on the 25th centile for height, and had poorly developed secondary sexual characteristics. There were no signs of endocrine disturbances. However, it was noticed that the patient had a poor sense of smell. Hormone investigations on blood samples gave the following results:

Serum	Result	Reference range
LH	1.2	1.0–9.0 U/L
FSH	<0.5	1.0–10.0 U/L
TSH	1.3	0.2–4.5 mU/L
FT4	17	9–21 pmol/L
Prolactin	200	<500 mU/L
Testosterone	2	10–30 nmol/L
Cortisol (8 am)	500	100–565 nmol/L

How would you interpret these results in light of the patient's history and clinical findings?

Comments: The findings suggest that the patient had hypogonadotrophic hypogonadism as the sole endocrine abnormality, but a combined test of pituitary functional reserve (Chapter 7: Anterior pituitary disease and its investigation) would be worth considering; it would provide information about growth hormone. The lack of a sense of smell is typical of Kallmann's syndrome, in which there is an isolated deficiency of GnRH. Stimulation with exogenous GnRH can be used both diagnostically and as treatment, but usually puberty is induced in these patients with sex steroids.

within the reference range. Low testosterone is a common finding in those who have moderate to severe chronic or acute illnesses.

Disorders of male sex differentiation

Many conditions have been described, all rare. In some, the gonads degenerate; in others, there is a defect affecting enzymatic steroid synthesis or action at the receptor level (termed 'androgen insensitivity syndrome', or AIS). In many of the conditions, testosterone is low, both in childhood and in adult life. In AIS, however, a mutation in the gene coding for the androgen receptor results in genetic (XY) males developing female secondary sexual characteristics; serum testosterone is often abnormally high for age and LH is also often elevated. Depending on the severity of the mutation, patients may appear as a phenotypically normal female (complete AIS) or can demonstrate both male and female sexual organs (partial AIS). Patients with complete AIS are often only diagnosed at puberty following investigation into primary amenorrhoea.

Most patients with a disorder of sexual differentiation (DSD) are diagnosed shortly after birth, when the appearance of atypical genitalia becomes apparent. The results of biochemical tests, alongside karyotyping, genetic investigations and imaging studies, are required to generate an accurate diagnosis. The use of biochemical tests for the diagnosis of congenital adrenal hyperplasia is further discussed in Chapter 22.

Erectile dysfunction (impotence) and late-onset hypogonadism (andropause)

Erectile dysfunction (ED) is most commonly caused by diabetes, neurological disorders, cardiovascular

disease, medication such as β-blockers, alcohol abuse, thyroid disease, liver and renal disease and psychological problems. Androgen deficiency and hyperprolactinaemia are uncommon causes of erectile dysfunction and such patients often complain of loss of libido in addition to their ED.

Androgen deficiency may also present with a variety of clinical features (Table 10.3) and its potential involvement in a range of common pathologies including osteoporosis, Alzheimer's disease, type 2 diabetes, ischemic heart disease, hypercholesterolaemia and hypertension has been prominent in both the medical and lay press. Whereas classical androgen deficiency (such as that caused by inherited disorders, pituitary tumours and testicular abnormalities) is an unequivocal indication for testosterone replacement, a growing number of older men are being identified with borderline testosterone deficiency with no clear underlying cause; this is known as 'late-onset male hypogonadism'. The evidence supporting replacement therapy in these patients is conflicting.

Testosterone concentrations decline with age and borderline testosterone deficiency may be a normal consequence of ageing. However current guidelines recommend that age related reference ranges are not used. Similarly a large proportion of obese men, and those with type 2 diabetes mellitus, will have low testosterone levels of uncertain clinical significance. Sleep disturbances may also cause low testosterone. The limited evidence available suggests that in unequivocal testosterone deficiency, sexual symptoms may be ameliorated by replacement therapy; the response to therapy is less predictable when borderline androgen deficiency is found. No clear benefits upon morbidity or mortality have been observed and replacement may be harmful in some elderly individuals.

Who to test

Male patients with symptoms of hypogonadism, particularly those with low libido, loss of early morning erections and erectile dysfunction or other features of well-developed hypogonadism should be tested (see Table 10.3). Patients referred to a hospital clinic because of isolated infertility, gynaecomastia or osteoporosis, as a principal problem, should have testosterone measured at consultation.

Investigation

Investigation should follow a protocol similar to that shown in Figure 10.3.

Table 10.3 Symptoms and signs associated with male hypogonadism.

Physical	Psychological	Sexual
Decreased muscle mass and strength	Depression	Decreased sex drive (libido)
Decreased bone mineral density or osteoporosis	Lack of energy	Decreased sexual thoughts
Gynaecomastia	Fatigue	Erectile dysfunction
Reduced body hair		Infertility
Hot flush		
Sweating		

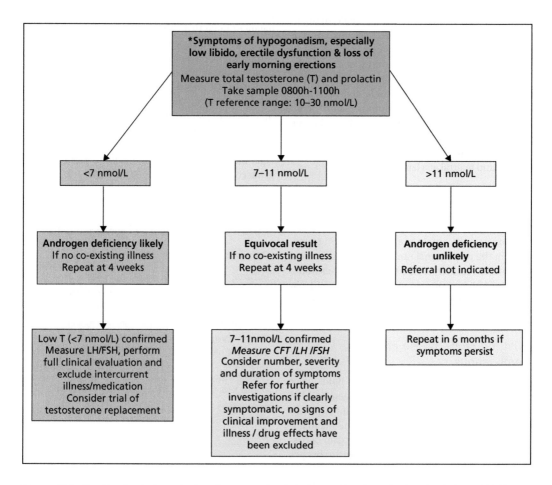

Figure 10.3 Algorithm for the investigation of suspected male hypogonadism. Investigation should be avoided in patients with acute illness and those with only vague symptoms.

Serum total testosterone is the initial laboratory investigation, and if sexual dysfunction is the main presenting complaint, prolactin should also be measured. There is a diurnal rhythm in testosterone, and samples must be taken before 11.00 am when testosterone concentrations are at their highest.

If testosterone remains low or equivocal on repeat testing, LH and FSH should be measured in the sample to help to identify possible endocrine causes of the androgen deficiency. In patients with equivocal testosterone a calculated free testosterone (CFT) may help to determine if replacement therapy is required.

Effects of illness, lifestyles and drugs on testosterone

Significant illness and certain drugs (particularly drugs of abuse, anabolic steroids, anti-convulsants and drugs that cause hyperprolactinaemia) and life-style factors (e.g. excessive alcohol, stress, excessive exercising, poor sleep patterns and obesity) can all contribute to hypogonadal symptoms and diminish total testosterone. These factors should be considered prior to testing. Co-existing illness can be the cause of features overlapping with those of hypogonadism, especially nonspecific features such as fatigue, weight loss and muscle wasting, but also erectile dysfunc-tion, low libido and diminishing testosterone. For many illnesses such effects may begin within a day of onset and correlate with the severity of the illness. These features may lag behind disease recovery. It is recommended that important treatment decisions are not based on assessments during or shortly after acute/subacute illness or during an escalation in drug treatment. These effects are often temporary/reversi-ble and thus may influence the need for subsequent retesting and referral at a later date.

Treatment and monitoring

Patients have a choice of intramuscular injections or topical gels containing testosterone. For those on tes-tosterone gels, the aim is to achieve a serum testos-terone in the mid-normal range. For those receiving injections the aim should be to achieve levels in the lower third of the normal range (11–17 nmol/L) just prior to an injection or levels in the mid-normal range around 6 weeks after an injection.

Monitoring for adverse effects/complications

It is advisable to do full blood count, lipids, liver function tests and prostate specific antigen (PSA) at baseline, 3 and 6 months thereafter annually if no problems occur. Testosterone may elevate haemato-crit and PSA, and if concomitant weight gain occurs there may occasionally be associated adverse changes to the lipid profile. Although any such changes are usually modest, if haematocrit rises to >0.5 and/or Hb >180 g/L or PSA >3 µg/L (>5 µg/L in those >70 years) then consideration should be given to reducing the dose or stopping treatment. If change persists, an appropriate specialist referral is indicated.

Gynaecomastia in males

Gynaecomastia is a benign enlargement of the male breast resulting from a proliferation of the glandular component of the breast. Although the condition is usually bilateral, it can be unilateral. Care must be taken to differentiate gynaecomastia from breast cancer, the latter being much less common. The causes of gynaecomastia in males can be of either physiological or pathological origin. About 25% of cases of gynaecomastia occur in puberty and around 25% are idiopathic. Most cases of pubertal gynaecomastia resolve spontaneously within 1–2 years of onset, although occasionally it persists into early adulthood.

The principal endocrine causes of gynaecomastia are conditions that affect the oestrogen–androgen balance (Table 10.4). These include decreased andro-gen activity in hypogonadism and increased oestro-gen production resulting from a variety of endocrine tumours; these tumours may synthesise oestrogens or secrete hCG, which then act as a stimulus of oestro-gen production. Thyrotoxicosis, hyperprolactinae-mia, renal failure, liver failure and androgen resistance are other pathological causes that lead to an imbalance of oestrogens and androgens. The prin-cipal biochemical investigations to be performed in gynaecomastia are shown in Table 10.5.

Table 10.4 **Some causes of gynaecomastia.**

Common	Uncommon
Pubertal gynaecomastia	Hyperthyroidism
Hypogonadism (primary or secondary)	Haemochromatosis
	Chronic renal failure
Hyperprolactinaemia	Tumours – including testicular, adrenal, bronchial, hepatic, haematological, etc.
Drugs – including cannabis, methadone, cimetidine, phenothiazines, oestrogens	
Malnutrition and liver disease	
Idiopathic	

Table 10.5 **Routine laboratory investigations in gynaecomastia.**

- Testosterone
- Oestradiol
- LH & FSH
- Prolactin and full drug history
- TSH and FT4

- hCG and AFP (to exclude germ cell tumours)
- Liver function tests
- Creatinine

Drugs account for about 25% of cases of gynaeco-mastia, and over 300 drugs have been reported as having the potential for producing the condition. Most drugs cause gynaecomastia by modifying the androgen : oestrogen ratio by direct or indirect mechanisms. In the elderly, mild gynaecomastia may commonly occur as a result of a decline in testosterone production. Pseudogynaecomastia, a condition that occurs in obese men where there is only fat deposition in the subareolar area, should be excluded prior to further investigation

Female gonadal function

Menstrual disorders and infertility

The changes that occur in normal menstrual cycles depend on cyclical variations in the output of FSH and LH, influenced by the output of GnRH (Figure 10.4). The effects of GnRH on LH and FSH release, in terms of the amounts secreted at different stages of the menstrual cycle, are strongly influenced by negative feedback control effects exerted by oestradiol and progesterone.

The developing Graafian follicles in the ovaries respond to the cyclical stimulus of gonadotrophins by secreting two oestrogens, oestradiol and oestrone; these are metabolised to a third oestrogen, oestriol. After ovulation, the corpus luteum secretes progesterone as well as oestrogens. The changes in the uterus are determined by the ovarian steroid output at each stage. These changes are modified if pregnancy occurs.

Changes in plasma concentrations of FSH, LH and the principal gonadal steroids in the normal menstrual cycle (i.e. a cycle unmodified by oral contraceptives) are shown diagrammatically in Figure 10.5. Reference ranges for these hormones are given in Table 10.6, but these may vary slightly between laboratories.

Oestrogens act on several target tissues, including the uterus, vagina and breast; progesterone mainly acts on the uterus, and is essential for the maintenance of early pregnancy. Both oestrogens and progesterone are important in the control of the hypothalamic–pituitary–ovarian axis. Oestradiol may stimulate or inhibit the secretion of gonadotrophins, depending on its concentration in plasma; the stimulating effect of oestradiol can be prevented by high plasma progesterone. Inhibins and activins also play a role in regulating ovarian function and they change during the cycle; however, their measurement is not performed as part of routine investigation. Inhibin B originates from developing follicles whereas inhibin A is derived from the dominant follicle and corpus luteum.

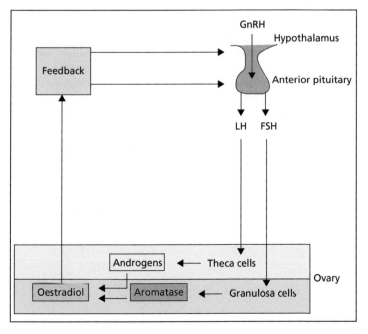

Figure 10.4 The hypothalamic–pituitary–ovarian axis. Activins, inhibins and progesterone also have a role in regulating the cycle.

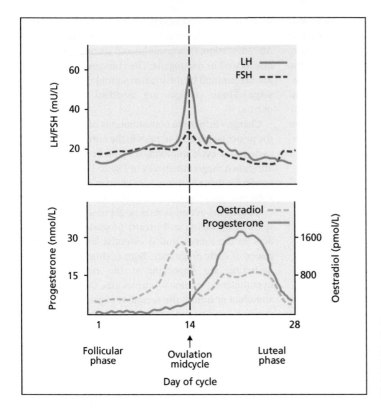

Figure 10.5 Cyclical changes in the plasma concentrations of the pituitary gonadotrophins and the principal ovarian steroid sex hormones in a normal 28-day menstrual cycle.

Ovarian dysfunction and its investigation

The complex relationships between the hypothalamus, pituitary, ovary and uterus in controlling gonadal function mean that abnormality in any of these organs may cause abnormal menstruation and infertility. Other endocrine diseases (e.g. Cushing's syndrome, thyroid disease) and general ill-health or stress can also have these effects. The patient history may provide important clues as to the cause of the problem. The regularity of the cycle is an important determinant of the rate of conception. Oligomenorrhoea, defined as an interval between periods of more than 6 weeks but less than 6 months, is often due to polycystic ovarian syndrome (PCOS; see Chapter 10: Polycystic ovarian syndrome). Amenorrhoea (no periods for >6 months) has many causes (see Table 10.7). Details of general health and weight fluctuations are also important because weight loss is a common cause of amenorrhoea, while a large increase in body weight may precipitate PCOS. Presentation of amenorrhoea with galactorrhoea may

Table 10.6 Typical reference ranges in men and women for the plasma concentrations of the pituitary gonadotrophins and of the principal sex hormones.

Hormone	Males	Menstruating female			Post-menopausal
		Early follicular	Mid-cycle	Luteal	
FSH (IU/L)	1.5–9.0	2.0–10.0	<15	1.5–10.0	30–115
LH (IU/L)	1.5–9.0	2.0–9.0	<80	1.5–9.0	30–115
Oestradiol (pmol/L)	<160	75–140	550–1650	370–700	<150
Testosterone (nmol/L)	10–30	0.4–2.0			

suggest hyperprolactinaemia, although hyperprolactinaemia can occur without galactorrhoea. Menstrual disturbance with features of hyperandrogenism (hirsutism, acne, etc.) is often due to PCOS.

Oligomenorrhoea and amenorrhoea

Women with oligomenorrhoea or amenorrhoea may present because of concerns they have regarding their bleeding pattern, infertility, hirsutism, virilism or a combination of these.

Physiological causes of amenorrhoea (pregnancy, lactation) and anatomical abnormalities should first be excluded as the possible cause. Amenorrhoea may be primary, that is, the patient has never menstruated, in which case abnormal development is a likely cause, or secondary to various causes (Table 10.7). Investigation of primary amenorrhoea is required if the patient has reached the age of 16 and has undergone normal secondary sexual development or at the age of 14 if the patient has no breast development.

Measurements of plasma concentrations of prolactin, FSH, LH, oestradiol, TSH and FT4 are required. In addition, plasma testosterone should be measured if PCOS is suspected; other androgens such as androstenedione and DHEAS concentrations may

need to be measured if there is hirsutism or virilisation. Figure 10.6 summarises one scheme for interpreting the investigations commonly performed in patients with menstrual abnormalities or hirsutism or who are infertile.

Infertility

Table 10.7 summarises the endocrine causes of infertility that may have to be considered, particularly if there are also menstrual abnormalities. Approximately one third of female factor infertility can be attributed to an endocrine cause; the remaining causes are primarily related to endometriosis, pelvic adhesions and fallopian tube abnormalities. Once it has been established that known endocrine diseases (e.g. diabetes mellitus, hypothyroidism) are not the cause of the infertility, investigation should proceed according to the schemes outlined in Figures 10.6 and 10.7, depending on whether or not the patient has regular cycles.

FSH and fertility

FSH is often measured in the early follicular phase (days 1–5 of the cycle) in patients undergoing assisted conception, because an elevated FSH even in the presence of normal menstruation indicates diminished fertility.

Table 10.7 Endocrine causes of amenorrhoea and infertility.

Site of lesion	Examples
Hypothalamus	Anorexia nervosa Severe weight loss Stress (psychological and/or physical) GnRH deficiency (Kallmann's syndrome) Tumours (e.g. craniopharyngioma, acromegaly)
Anterior pituitary	Hyperprolactinaemia Hypopituitarism Functional tumours (e.g. Cushing's disease) Isolated deficiency of FSH or LH
Ovarian	PCOS Ovarian failure* Ovarian dysgenesis – Turner's syndrome Ovarian tumours
Receptor defect	Androgen insensitivity syndrome
Other endocrine diseases	Diabetes mellitus Thyrotoxicosis Adrenal dysfunction (e.g. late-onset CAH)

*Ovarian failure may be autoimmune, chromosomal, iatrogenic (e.g. after cancer therapy) or idiopathic.

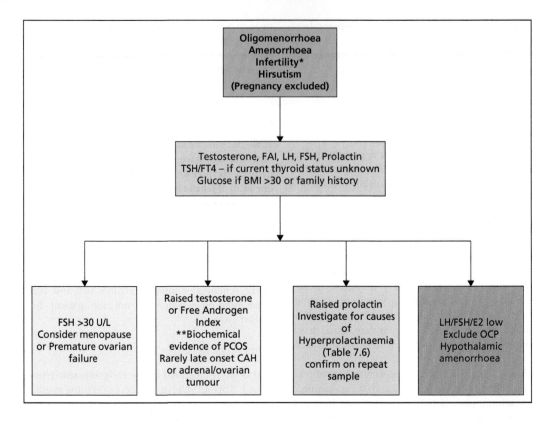

Figure 10.6 The investigation of oligomenorrhoea, amenorrhoea and hirsutism. It is assumed that other endocrine causes of these conditions (e.g. pregnancy, thyroid disease) have been excluded. *If infertility is being investigated progesterone should also be measured (see Chapter 10: Menstrual disorders and infertility). **It is unusual for PCOS to present with a testosterone of >5 nmol/L: in such patients the test should be repeated and further testing carried out to exclude other causes of hyperandrogenism (e.g. tumour, Cushing's etc).

Anti-Müllerian hormone (AMH) and fertility

AMH is a dimeric glycoprotein that is produced exclusively in the gonads and is involved in the regulation of follicular growth and development. In the ovary AMH is produced by the granulosa cells of early developing follicles and seems to be able to inhibit the initiation of primordial follicle growth and FSH-induced follicle growth. AMH values in women are low until the onset of puberty, thereafter rising rapidly during puberty before declining from the middle of the third decade until menopause. There is good evidence to suggest that serum levels of AMH may represent both the quantity and quality of the ovarian follicle pool and as such may be a very useful predictor of fertility, particularly in older women. AMH values are also elevated in PCOS, although the usefulness of measurement for this purpose is contentious. Analysis of AMH can, however, be useful in the assessment

of patients undergoing assisted conception to predict ovarian responsiveness to therapy and help prevent the risk of ovarian hyperstimulation.

Hirsutism and virilism

Hirsutism is a fairly common complaint among women. Most hirsute women have normal menstruation and no evidence of virilism. By itself, hirsutism rarely signifies an important disease, but it still requires investigation because patients with ovarian or adrenal tumours have been described with normal menstrual cycles. Patients who have menstrual disorders in addition to hirsutism are more likely to have endocrine dysfunction. The main causes of hirsutism are PCOS (60–75%), idiopathic hyperandrogenism (25%), and idiopathic hirsutism without biochemical hyperandrogenism (10%). Congenital adrenal hyperplasia (3–5%), androgen-secreting tumours (0.2%), glucocorticoid excess, hyperprolactinaemia, acromegaly, thyroid dysfunction and drugs (including exogenous androgens, glucocorticoids and sodium valproate) constitute rare but important causes.

 CASE 10.3

A 22-year-old secretary presented to her doctor complaining of a white, milk-like discharge from the nipple of each breast. She had had these symptoms intermittently for the previous month. On questioning, it was found that she had also been experiencing menstrual irregularities over the previous year, and had not had a period for at least 6 months. She was a nonsmoker, and was not taking any medication.

Plasma prolactin was found to be elevated at 1846 mU/L (reference range 60–500), and a second sample taken 2 weeks later showed a similar elevation at 1240 mU/L. Macroprolactin was not detected.

She was referred to an endocrinologist. The patient was clinically euthyroid, not pigmented and had normal secondary sexual characteristics. Visual fields were normal.

The following hormones were measured in blood:

Serum	Result	Reference range
Prolactin	1400	<500 mU/L
LH	1.6	2.0–9.0 U/L
FSH	3.5	2.0-10.0 U/L
TSH	2.2	0.2–4.5 mU/L
FT4	15	9–21 pmol/L

How would you interpret these results in light of the history and clinical findings? What further investigations should be performed?

Comments: The high prolactin level, accompanied by galactorrhoea and amenorrhoea, suggests the presence of a prolactinoma. In patients with a prolactin level >700 mU/L, stress, hypothyroidism and pharmacological causes of a raised prolactin level should be excluded, and the test should be repeated to confirm an elevated level. An MRI scan of the pituitary should be performed in patients with unexplained hyperprolactinaemia. In this patient, an MRI scan demonstrated a microadenoma in the anterior pituitary. The patient was treated successfully with dopamine agonists.

Clinical evaluation

Clinical evaluation of a patient with hirsutism should look for features of underlying hyperandrogenism such as oligo/amenorrhoea, infertility, central obesity, acanthosis nigricans, clitoromegaly or presence of risk factors for type 2 diabetes.

When taking a history the following information is useful:

- Has it been present since puberty?
- Rapid onset – hirsutism of sudden onset or of rapid progression should raise suspicion of an androgen-secreting tumour.
- Associated with any changes in body weight, presence of acne or alopecia, use of oral contraceptives or other medications.

Preliminary investigations and interpretation

This should follow that shown in Figure 10.6.

If serum testosterone is >4 nmol/L or virilization is found, 17α-hydroxyprogesterone (17-OHP), DHEAS and androstenedione should be measured to exclude late-onset CAH or ovarian or adrenal androgen-secreting tumours. If the underlying cause is thought to be *late-onset CAH*, due to partial deficiency of 21-hydroxylase (Chapter 22: 21-Hydroxylase deficiency), this can be confirmed by injecting Synacthen, (250 mg IM) and measuring serum 17-OHP 1 h later. In a patient with CAH, the increase in serum 17-OHP is typically more than 2–3-fold the upper reference value.

Treatment

If PCOS is thought to be the cause of hirsutism, oral contraceptives are effective in greater than 60% of cases. Specific formulations that contain cyproterone acetate (an anti-androgen) and ethinyloestradiol are often first-line treatment as they suppress secretion of gonadotrophins, thereby reducing the secretion of ovarian androgens, but also act peripherally with anti-androgen actions. Cosmetic treatments or more permanent treatment such as electrolysis or laser photoepilation may also be used.

Polycystic ovarian syndrome (PCOS)

PCOS is very common, with a prevalence of 5–10% in women of child-bearing age. There is no single diagnostic criterion to confirm the clinical diagnosis.

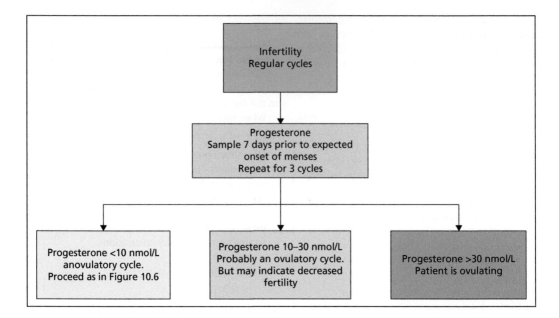

Figure 10.7 The investigation of female infertility in patients with regular menstrual cycles. Note that samples must be taken 7 days prior to the expected onset of next menses. If patients have irregular long cycles, samples should be taken at weekly intervals from day 21 until the onset of next menstrual period. If patients have irregular short cycles, samples should be taken at weekly intervals from day 14 until the onset of next menstrual period. Monitor the response in three cycles.

Clinical manifestations include infrequent or absent menses, anovulatory infertility and signs of androgen excess (hirsutism, acne or seborrhoea). Although the classical profile of PCOS is that of hypersecretion of LH and androgens with normal concentrations of FSH, a wide spectrum of findings are seen and abnormalities in LH are not always present.

In addition to establishing the diagnosis, it is also important to exclude disorders with similar presenting features such as CAH, Cushing's syndrome and androgen-secreting tumours.

Many women with PCOS have an increased risk of insulin resistance which, with the high prevalence of obesity, is a powerful risk factor for progression to type 2 diabetes. They also have an increased long-term risk of endometrial hyperplasia/cancer. Investigation of glucose tolerance (initially by a random glucose) should be considered in women with PCOS with relevant *additional* risk factors such as obesity and a family history.

Definition

An international consensus definition of PCOS has defined patients with PCOS as having at least two of the following three criteria:

- Oligomenorrhoea or amenorrhoea.
- Clinical and/or biochemical signs of excessive androgen secretion, i.e. hirsutism, acne, raised total testosterone and/or a raised free androgen index.
- Presence of at least 12 follicles measuring 2–9 mm in diameter, an ovarian volume >10 mL, or both. Only one ovary needs to meet this criterion. An ultrasound scan is therefore not essential to make the diagnosis.

Gonadotrophins and PCOS

Although increases in LH and the LH/FSH ratio occur in many women with PCOS, such abnormalities are not required for the diagnosis. LH is often normal in PCOS, and a raised LH and LH/FSH ratio is commonly found in women who do not have the syndrome, reflecting the pulsatile nature of LH secretion (or blood sampling shortly before ovulation). However, measurement of LH (and FSH) can be useful in identifying *other* causes of amenorrhoea, for example the low gonadotrophins and oestradiol found in 'hypothalamic' amenorrhoea associated with weight loss, stress and excess exercise (Figure 10.6).

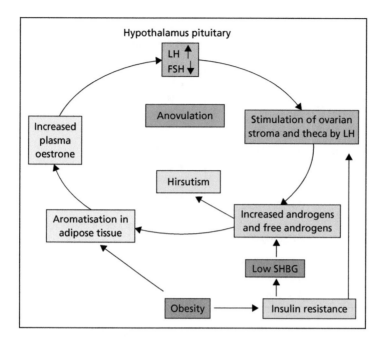

Figure 10.8 Biochemical, metabolic and endocrine changes in PCOS. Treatment is aimed at breaking the cycle (see text).

Androgens and PCOS

Most patients with PCOS have evidence of androgen excess but the measurement of total testosterone may not be as sensitive at detecting an abnormality as a measure of free testosterone such as the FAI. This is because in PCOS the concentration of SHBG often decreases, which in turn tends to decrease total testosterone but increase free testosterone. Androstenedione and DHEAS may also be increased in some patients with PCOS.

The cause of PCOS is unclear, but abnormalities in the adrenal, ovary and pituitary gland have been suggested. The high prevalence of PCOS suggests that it may not be a single disease. Approximately 50% of women with PCOS have insulin resistance, and the ensuing hyperinsulinaemia can give rise to increased ovarian synthesis of testosterone and androstenedione. The high insulin also gives rise to reduced synthesis of SHBG and thus an increase in free testosterone. Impaired conversion of androgens to oestrogens in the ovary also leads to increased release of ovarian androgens. These androgens are then converted in adipose tissue by aromatase to oestrone that in turn inhibits the release of FSH and stimulates secretion of LH. These effects on the gonadotrophins tend to produce persistent anovulation and the excess LH also tends to stimulate androgen production from

the theca cells, thus perpetuating the abnormalities. Figure 10.8 summarises how a cycle may be set up that tends to perpetuate the clinical problems. Clearly obesity is a risk factor because it may produce insulin resistance, and excess adipose tissue will increase oestrone production from androgens. Treatment of PCOS is directed towards interrupting the cycle by lowering LH levels with oral contraceptives, weight reduction in obese patients or enhancement of FSH production with clomiphene, etc. Table 10.8 outlines the investigations that should be performed if PCOS is suspected on clinical grounds.

 CASE 10.4

A 17-year-old girl consulted her doctor because she was embarrassed about the amount of dark hair that was growing on her face. She told the doctor that her menstrual periods had never been regular (menarche age 13) and that she had not had a period for over 4 months. She was not pregnant. On examination, the doctor found that the patient was slightly overweight and had an extensive growth of dark hair on her lower abdomen (an escutcheon), as well as much dark hair on her upper lip, arms and legs. The patient was referred to an endocrinologist. After it was confirmed that the patient was not pregnant, the following hormones were measured in blood (reference ranges are for the early follicular phase, where relevant):

Serum	Result	Reference range
Prolactin	550	<500 mU/L
LH	14	2.0–9.0 U/L
FSH	2.0	2.0–10.0 U/L
Oestradiol	135	75–140 pmol/L
Testosterone	3.1	0.8–2.0 nmol/L
SHBG	27	30–120 nmol/L
Free androgen index	11	<5
Androstenedione	13	0.6–8.8 nmol/L
DHEAS	11	1.8–11.7 µmol/L
TSH	0.4	0.2–4.5 mU/L
FT4	18	9–21 pmol/L

What do you think is the most likely diagnosis? What is your differential diagnosis?

Comments: This girl had the clinical and biochemical features of PCOS. The gonadotrophin pattern excludes hypogonadotrophic hypogonadism and ovarian failure as the cause of amenorrhoea (pregnancy had already been excluded). The testosterone concentration was high and the patient had a low SHBG giving a significantly elevated free androgen index. The androgens were not sufficiently high, however, to indicate that the patient had an androgen-secreting tumour. Late-onset CAH can present with all the features of PCOS, and could be excluded by measuring the 17-hydroxyprogesterone response to Synacthen stimulation.

Ovarian failure

Perimenopause and menopause

The menopausal transition, or perimenopause, is defined as the time from the start of irregular menstrual cycles until at least 1 year after periods have ceased. This menopausal transition takes 2–8 years, with the menopause occurring at an average age of about 51 years. The menopause can only be defined retrospectively when 12 months have elapsed since the last period. During the perimenopause, hormone levels in serum fluctuate erratically such that a single blood sample may not show biochemical evidence of the perimenopause. A raised serum FSH (often >30 U/L) is the most consistent finding in the peri-

Table 10.8 Biochemical investigations in suspected PCOS.

Sample timing
- Unless the patient is amenorrhoeic, the sample should be taken on days 1–5 of the menstrual cycle
- (Misleading increases in testosterone, FSH and LH may occur later in the cycle)

First-line tests
- LH, FSH, testosterone/free androgen index and prolactin
- Thyroid function tests – if current thyroid status unknown
- Random glucose if BMI is >30 or family history of diabetes

Additional tests
- Ultrasound
- Oestradiol: if menses are erratic and a raised testosterone is found, an oestradiol measurement may help to establish if sampling is within the (preferred) early follicular phase
- If testosterone is >4 nmol/L: measure androstenedione, DHEAS, 17-hydroxyprogesterone

Interpretation
- This should follow that shown in Figure 10.6

menopause but FSH is not invariably raised. Also women with raised FSH may continue to have further ovulatory cycles. Samples for FSH measurement should be collected if possible during the early follicular stage of the cycle. It is only later in the menopausal transition that oestradiol levels may become low. In most women, the perimenopause can be diagnosed clinically. In women over the age of 45 years with oligomenorrhoea or amenorrhoea, biochemical investigations will add little to the diagnosis of the perimenopause. Younger women with menstrual disturbances should be investigated as described in Figure 10.6. See also Table 10.9.

 CASE 10.5

A 45-year-old shop assistant presented to her GP complaining of fatigue, weight gain, trouble sleeping, anxiety and hot flushes. Her periods were regular.

Her hormone profile was as follows, with the sample being taken at day 3 of her menstrual cycle.

Serum	Result	Reference range
Prolactin	500	<500 mU/L
LH	9.0	2.0–9.0 U/L
FSH	25	2.0–10.0 U/L
Oestradiol	120	75/140 pmol/L
TSH	6.5	0.2–4.5 mU/L
FT4	12	9–21 pmol/L

How would you interpret these results in light of the history and clinical findings?

Comments: The high FSH would be consistent with perimenopause, which would also explain her symptoms. The thyroid function tests are consistent with subclinical hypothyroidism, but with such a modest elevation in TSH it is unlikely that this mild thyroid disorder is contributing to her clinical problems. The thyroid function tests should be repeated in 3 months time to exclude transient elevation of TSH. If the raised TSH were confirmed, the patient should have T4 therapy commenced if TSH became greater than 10 mU/L. For management of the menopause see Figure 10.9.

Table 10.9 Practice points for investigation of menopause.

Who to test

- Women aged <45 who are not on OCP and have amenorrhoea or menstrual irregularity should be investigated as outlined in Figure 10.6
- Measurement of FSH is rarely necessary in women who clearly have menopausal symptoms and are within the age range expected for menopause

Testing

- If testing is indicated, and the woman is having periods, take sample on days 1–5 of the cycle

Interpretation

- FSH >20 U/L on days 1–5 of the cycle is suggestive of perimenopause or ovarian failure
- Random FSH >30 U/L is highly suggestive of ovarian failure or perimenopause but exclude mid-cycle peak as a cause especially if the LH concentration is greater than that of FSH
- Ovarian failure and perimenopause cannot be excluded by normal FSH levels

Use of FSH to assess need for continued contraception during menopause

In women of menopausal age who are on oral contraceptives with amenorrhoea, the protocols shown in Figures 10.9 and 10.10 should be followed.

Premature ovarian failure or 'premature menopause'

This refers to the occurrence of menopause before the age of 40 and may manifest itself in 1–3% of women. It may be due to genetic factors, autoimmune disorders, viral agents, chemotherapy, radiation therapy, surgery or exposure to toxic substances, or it may be idiopathic. Although a normal menopause is an irreversible condition, about 50% of women with premature ovarian failure may have intermittent ovarian function and sometimes ovulate despite the presence of high gonadotrophin levels. The diagnosis of premature ovarian failure is made by finding persistently elevated serum FSH (>30 mU/L) on two or three occasions with samples taken 3–4 weeks apart. If premature ovarian failure occurs at a young age, a karyotype is often performed to investigate chromosome abnormalities (Turner's syndrome). There is a high prevalence of autoimmune disorders in premature ovarian failure, and additional tests may be advisable to rule out autoimmune disorders of the adrenal, parathyroid, thyroid, pancreas and GI tract. Annual follow-up to exclude these autoimmune disorders is also desirable. Risks associated with early menopause include osteoporosis and cardiovascular disease. Some also advocate that androgen replacement should also be considered in women who are receiving hormone replacement therapy (HRT) but who continue to experience fatigue and low libido.

Hysterectomy

After hysterectomy, women are at risk of undergoing early menopause. Such patients should have FSH measured annually or earlier if symptoms develop.

Hormone replacement therapy

In HRT, natural oestrogens are often used in combination with a progestogen (oestrogen-only replacement is usually avoided due to risk of endometrial cancer). There is little place for the measurement of reproductive hormones in patients taking HRT because often such therapy does not suppress gonadotrophins to pre-menopausal levels and many of the natural

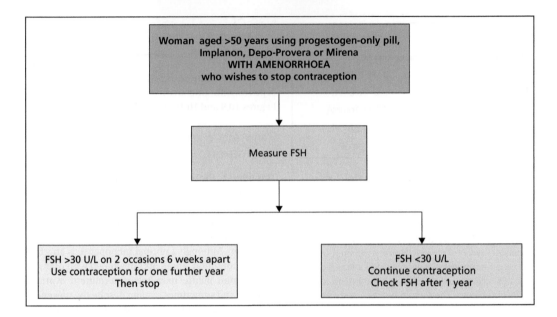

Figure 10.9 The use of FSH to assess the need for continued contraception in women over the age of 50 years who are taking the progesterone only or combined oral contraceptive.

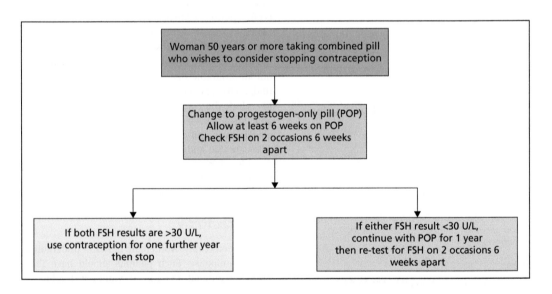

Figure 10.10 The use of FSH to assess the need for continued contraception in women over the age of 50 years who are taking the combined oral contraceptive.

oestrogens used are not detected by the specific assay used in the laboratory to measure oestradiol. The exception is perhaps the use of oestradiol measurements to check whether an implant containing oestradiol needs replacing; a serum oestradiol above 400 pmol/L suggests that the implant is still function-

ing. Oestradiol implants are more potent than natural oestrogens at decreasing gonadotrophin levels and may suppress LH and FSH into the pre-menopausal ranges. The effect on plasma lipids and other biochemistry and risk to the patient will depend on the particular preparation used and also on whether the hormones are given orally or as a dermal patch or gel. The safety and efficacy of 'bio-identical hormones', custom-made hormone regimens designed to be identical to their human hormone equivalents, are not currently advocated, and the use of biochemical tests to monitor such regimens is controversial.

Steroid contraceptives

Combined oral contraceptives (COCs)

Ethinyl oestradiol in COCs can suppress LH and FSH to less than 15 U/L; thus primary ovarian failure cannot be excluded by the usual method of FSH testing. Patients aged over 50 years who have amenorrhoea who wish to stop contraception should be advised to change to a progestogen-only pill (POP) and FSH checked after 6 weeks. The protocol shown in Figure 10.10 should then be followed.

Progestogen-only pill (POP)

Women aged over 50 years taking the POP or who use a synthetic progesterone implant with amenorrhoea who wish to stop contraception should have their FSH measured. If FSH is less than 30 mU/L, the POP should be continued for a further 12 months and FSH re-checked. If FSH is >30 U/L on two occasions 6 weeks apart, contraception should continue for one further year then can be stopped (Figure 10.9).

Young women who remain amenorrhoeic when they stop taking oral contraceptives may have premature menopause and should be investigated accordingly. Progesterone-only medications do not suppress FSH and LH to pre-menopausal levels; thus an FSH of less than 15 U/L makes primary ovarian failure unlikely in women who become amenorrhoeic when taking these medications.

Steroid contraceptives, principally those containing synthetic oestrogens, may cause diverse metabolic effects. For example, increases in plasma hormone-binding proteins and lipids may occur. Contraceptives that only contain progestogens are largely free from these effects. Progestogens largely oppose the effects of oestrogens; thus, in preparations containing combinations of oestrogen and progestogens, the net effect on the lipid profile and hormone binding proteins, etc. will depend on the balance of these hormones in the individual preparations.

11

Pregnancy and antenatal screening

Learning objectives

To understand:

✔ how the physiological changes in pregnancy may affect biochemical reference ranges;

✔ the use of biochemical investigations in monitoring complications of pregnancy;

✔ antenatal screening strategies for trisomies 13, 18 and 21.

Introduction

Pregnancy is associated with many hormonal, physiological and metabolic changes. This chapter considers how the results of biochemical tests may be affected, how they may help in the diagnosis and management of some complications of pregnancy, and how biochemical tests are applied in antenatal screening programmes for the identification of pregnancies at risk of trisomies 13, 18 and 21.

The foetoplacental unit

The placenta produces several proteins, including human chorionic gonadotrophin (hCG) and (human) placental lactogen. It also produces large amounts of steroid hormones and is the main source of progesterone during pregnancy.

Human chorionic gonadotrophin

There are several pregnancy-specific proteins, all of which normally originate in the trophoblast. The most commonly measured is hCG. Following synthesis, hCG is secreted into the maternal circulation. There is a surge in maternal hCG in early pregnancy, peak blood levels being reached at 12 weeks; thereafter, production of hCG rapidly declines. hCG becomes detectable in urine about 10 days after conception, and this forms the basis of readily available pregnancy tests.

Trophoblastic tumours also secrete hCG. These tumours can occur in males and females, and they include hydatidiform mole and choriocarcinoma, both of which may secrete hCG in very large amounts. A female who is found to be excreting hCG and who is not pregnant most frequently has a tumour of the trophoblast; in males, testicular teratoma is the most common source (Chapter 17: Malignancy and tumour markers).

Clinical Biochemistry Lecture Notes, Tenth Edition. Peter Rae, Mike Crane and Rebecca Pattenden.
© 2018 John Wiley & Sons Ltd. Published 2018 by John Wiley & Sons Ltd.
Companion website: www.lecturenoteseries.com/clinicalbiochemistry

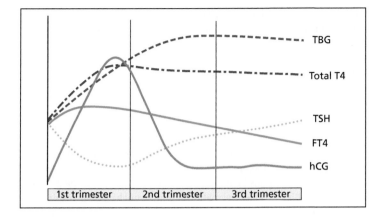

Figure 11.1 Changes in TSH, thyroid hormones, hCG and TBG in normal pregnancy. For TSH and thyroid hormones it is important to use gestational or trimester-related reference ranges. In some pregnancies TSH may fall to <0.1 mU/L in the first trimester. Total T3 and FT3 follow the same pattern as total T4 and FT4, respectively.

Steroids in pregnancy

Oestrogens and progesterone are secreted by the corpus luteum during the first 6 weeks of pregnancy, but after this the placenta is the most important source of these steroids. Oestriol is the oestrogen produced in the greatest amounts, but oestradiol-17β and oestrone are also produced in large amounts. The placenta cannot synthesise oestriol *de novo*, but it can produce oestriol from C-19 adrenal steroids that are supplied by the foetal adrenal in the form of DHEAS. The oestriol produced in this way is secreted into the maternal and foetal circulation. Oestriol production thus requires the involvement of both the placenta and the foetus, and recognition of this interdependence led to the concept of the foetoplacental unit.

Effect of pregnancy on biochemical tests

Reproductive hormones

Serum prolactin, oestrogens and testosterone show a steady increase in pregnancy, as does the concentration of SHBG. The concentrations of growth hormone and the pituitary gonadotrophins are decreased. Historically, some less specific methods for the measurement of LH have shown cross-reactivity with hCG, leading to apparently high LH levels.

Cortisol

There are large increases in serum cortisol due to increased serum CBG, but the diurnal rhythm is retained. However, increased free and total cortisol levels in pregnancy may also be related to resetting of

the sensitivity of the HPA axis and not merely to raised levels of CBG, progesterone or CRH. There is also an increase in serum free cortisol and in the 24-h urinary excretion of cortisol. This may be related to a resetting of the HPA axis and also the production of an ACTH-like substance by the placenta that is not completely suppressible by low- or high-dose glucocorticoids such as dexamethasone. This may help to explain why pregnant women often show intolerance of glucose and occasionally develop Cushingoid features. These changes make the diagnosis of Cushing's syndrome difficult in pregnancy, and several variations in the work-up, when compared with nonpregnant women, may be required. An absence of diurnal variation is a useful clue to the diagnosis.

Thyroid function tests

In normal pregnancy there is an increase in the pool size of extra-thyroidal T4 and an increase in the deiodination of thyroid hormones from the developing placenta. As a consequence there is a marked increase in the requirement for iodine (approximately 200 μg/day) and for T4 production. Women with hypothyroidism taking T4 replacement thus need an increase in the dose of T4 during pregnancy.

In early pregnancy, free T4 and free T3 concentrations may initially show a small rise, thought to be due to the weak thyroid-stimulating action of hCG, present in very high concentration in early pregnancy. This increase in free hormone suppresses TSH, sometimes to undetectable concentrations. It is important that these changes in early pregnancy are not construed as suggesting that the patient has thyrotoxicosis requiring treatment. As pregnancy progresses, the concentrations of free thyroid hormones fall and TSH begins to rise, although rarely increasing above the reference range seen in nonpregnant subjects.

The magnitude of the changes in free hormones is method dependent. It is important that trimester-related reference ranges are used for both TSH and free thyroid hormones, and for the free thyroid hormones the ranges should be those derived for the specific method used by the laboratory. TBG concentrations rise in pregnancy leading to an increase in total T4 and total T3 (Figure 11.1).

Plasma volume and renal function

During pregnancy, the plasma volume and GFR increase, sometimes by as much as 50%. This is accompanied by decreases in, for example, serum sodium, urea and creatinine.

Serum lipids and proteins

Serum triglyceride may increase as much as 3-fold in pregnancy; serum cholesterol, LDL and HDL increase to a lesser extent. Serum albumin and pre-albumin fall because of the increase in plasma volume. Plasma fibrinogen and ceruloplasmin increase.

Liver function tests

In pregnancy, the placental isoenzyme of ALP is released, and total ALP activity in serum may rise to as much as three times nonpregnant levels. In contrast, the expansion of the extracellular fluid leads to a fall (~20%) in the activities of the transaminases and γ-glutamyltransferase (GGT) and in the concentration of bilirubin.

Iron and ferritin

During pregnancy, increased maternal red cell synthesis and transfer of iron to the developing foetus cause a greater demand for iron. Unless iron supplements are given, iron stores generally fall, with accompanying falls in serum ferritin and serum iron, and rises in serum transferrin and total iron binding capacity (TIBC).

Complications in pregnancy

Ectopic pregnancy

In ectopic pregnancy, serum hCG fails to rise at the normal rate (approximately doubling every 2–3 days).

If levels have failed to rise by 63% in 2 days, there is an increased chance of an abnormal pregnancy. In practice, the diagnosis is made on a high index of clinical suspicion, qualitative pregnancy tests, ultrasound and, if indicated, laparoscopy.

Diabetes mellitus

Women with type 1 diabetes are at greater risk from both diabetic and obstetric complications during pregnancy. Rates of foetal and neonatal complications including late intrauterine death, foetal distress, congenital malformation, hypoglycaemia, respiratory distress syndrome and jaundice are also increased. To minimise these risks, it is essential that maternal glucose control and HbA_{1c} are optimised prior to conception and that tight control is maintained throughout pregnancy. Particular emphasis is placed on the need for careful home glucose monitoring (4–6 times a day) and intensive insulin regimens. Women should aim to maintain blood glucose and HbA_{1c} concentrations as near to the nondiabetic range as possible without excessive risk of hypoglycaemia. Although less common, the prevalence of type 2 diabetes during the reproductive years is increasing; management during pregnancy should follow the same intensive pattern.

Gestational diabetes mellitus

'Gestational diabetes mellitus' (GDM) is the term used to describe the abnormal glucose tolerance or diabetes mellitus that may develop during pregnancy. Controversy remains over the most appropriate strategies for screening and diagnosis. Risk factors for gestational diabetes include a BMI >30 kg/m², a previous macrosomic baby, previous gestational diabetes, a family history of diabetes (first degree relative) or a minority ethnic family origin with a high prevalence of diabetes. It is particularly important to identify women with previously undiagnosed type 1 or type 2 diabetes mellitus as urgent action is required to normalise metabolism.

At the first gestational visit, it has been recommended that all women with risk factors should be offered screening for GDM; furthermore, all women with risk factors but not already showing overt or gestational diabetes should have a 75 g oral glucose tolerance test at 24–28 weeks. A fasting plasma glucose at 24–28 weeks is recommended for women at low risk.

Post-natal care

Women with gestational diabetes are at increased risk of developing type 2 diabetes in the future. If diabetes is not immediately apparent post-partum, all women should be reassessed not less than 6 weeks after delivery with fasting plasma glucose. A 75 g OGTT should also be performed if clinically indicated. Glycaemic control should then be assessed on an annual basis using fasting plasma glucose or HbA_{1c}.

Thyroid disorders

Screening for thyroid disorders in pregnancy

The following categories of patient should have TSH and FT4 measured, preferably prior to conception or, if not, at booking:

- current thyroid disease;
- previous history of thyroid disease;
- family history of thyroid disease;
- goitre or other features of thyroid disease;
- other autoimmune disease, e.g. coeliac disease;
- type 1 and type 2 diabetes, gestational diabetes.

Management of thyroid disease requires close liaison between the GP, endocrinologist, obstetrician and community midwife.

Hypothyroidism

The developing foetal brain requires optimal thyroxine levels from early in the first trimester of pregnancy. The foetus relies on maternal thyroxine until 12 weeks' gestation, when its own thyroid gland develops. Overt untreated hypothyroidism is associated with foetal loss, gestational hypertension, placental abruption, poor perinatal outcome and severe neurodevelopmental delay. The offspring of women whose free thyroxine levels are in the lowest 10% of the reference range in the first trimester of pregnancy have significant neurodevelopmental delays at the age of 2 years.

There is an increased requirement for T4 in pregnancy; it is thus very important to ensure adequate thyroxine replacement from as early as 5 weeks' gestation. It is recommended that patients with established hypothyroidism have the dose of T4 dose increased by 25 µg/day when a pregnancy is confirmed.

Assessing hypothyroidism in pregnancy

Ideally women with established hypothyroidism should be seen pre-pregnancy to ensure that they are euthyroid. They should also be encouraged to present as soon as they become pregnant in order that their thyroxine dose may be increased and TSH and FT4

monitored regularly. The ideal monitoring regimen is to assess TSH and FT4:

- before conception (if possible);
- at diagnosis of pregnancy or at antenatal booking;
- 2 weeks after the dose of T4 has been increased;
- at least once in each trimester;
- 2–6 weeks post-partum.

Patients with a history of Graves' disease who have been rendered euthyroid or hypothyroid through radioiodine treatment or surgery must also have TSH-receptor antibodies (TRAbs) measured early in pregnancy irrespective of the thyroid function test profile. *If TRAbs are undetectable* they do not need to be repeated. *If TRAbs are positive* the consultant obstetrician and consultant endocrinologist should be informed. Further TRAbs measurements and ultrasound scans are likely to be required, and possibly anti-thyroid medication may need to be given if the TRAbs concentration is very high.

T4 replacement and pregnancy

T4 requirements increase by up to 50% by 20 weeks and then plateau. Thus:

- When pregnancy is confirmed the daily T4 dose should be increased by 25 µg and rechecked after approximately 2 weeks. Further dose increases may be required to achieve a satisfactory FT4 level.
- Patients newly diagnosed with hypothyroidism while pregnant should have T4 treatment commenced immediately and be closely monitored to ensure an optimal FT4 and TSH is achieved.
- TSH and FT4 should be monitored as a minimum once in each trimester. If the thyroid function tests are unstable, the patient should be seen by a consultant obstetrician and consultant endocrinologist as early as possible as growth scans may need to be performed in the third trimester.
- Thyroid function should be assessed 2–6 weeks post-partum and reduced as required. TSH and T4 should be rechecked 6–8 weeks later.

Hyperthyroidism

All women with hyperthyroidism in pregnancy need to be seen by a consultant endocrinologist and a consultant obstetrician to ensure appropriate management.

Patients being treated with anti-thyroid drugs require careful monitoring during pregnancy because these drugs cross the placenta and can induce foetal hypothyroidism. Similarly, TRAbs in maternal blood also cross the placenta and may give rise to intrauterine and neonatal thyrotoxicosis if present in high concentration. For these reasons it is essential to identify new cases of Graves' disease in pregnancy and also to assess TRAb status pre-conception or at booking in patients with previous Graves' disease irrespective of their current thyroid status.

Managing hyperthyroidism in pregnancy

A scheme for the investigation of hyperthyroidism in pregnancy is shown in Figure 11.2. The aim is for good control of hyperthyroidism on the minimum dose of carbimazole/propylthiouracil possible.

If TRAbs are positive the endocrinologists and obstetricians should be informed. Such women should be advised to deliver in hospital. Further TRAb measurements and ultrasound scans will probably be required. Paediatricians should be informed on the woman's admission to the labour ward and FT4 and TSH measured in cord blood to assess the thyroid status of the baby.

Hyperemesis gravidarum – undetectable TSH

Patients with hyperemesis gravidarum and some 'normal' pregnancies are associated with a mild transient 'physiological' hyperthyroidism during the first trimester due to the stimulatory action of high hCG on the thyroid. In approximately 3% of pregnancies the TSH in the first trimester will be suppressed to <0.01 mU/L and FT4/FT3 may be slightly elevated. It is essential to exclude Graves' disease in such pregnancies, and TRAbs should be measured and an endocrine and/or obstetric opinion sought.

Post-partum thyroiditis

This occurs in 5% of women within 2–6 months of delivery or miscarriage. It presents with nonspecific symptoms such as tiredness, anxiety and depression. Typically the patient will initially have a hyperthyroid hormone profile, which will resolve or be followed by a transient hypothyroidism, neither of which usually requires treatment. Occasionally, thyroid function may not return to normal after post-partum thyroiditis, and persistent hypothyroidism may require treatment with T4.

Post-partum patients should have thyroid function tests checked at 8–12 weeks if they have symptoms of thyroid disease, goitre, previous history of post-partum thyroiditis or other autoimmune disease or positive TPOAbs.

If a hyperthyroid profile is found (i.e. TSH <0.01 mU/L; FT4/FT3 raised) an endocrine opinion is warranted to differentiate post-partum thyroiditis from other causes of hyperthyroidism such as Graves' disease; a TRAb measurement will be helpful for this.

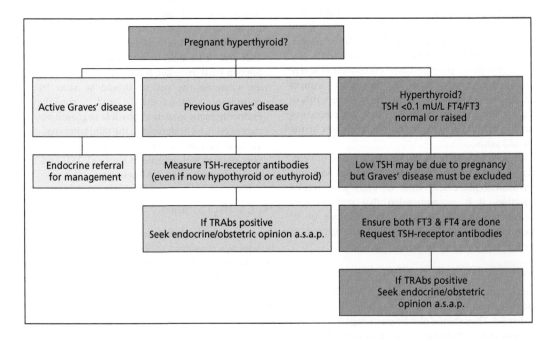

Figure 11.2 Scheme for the investigation of hyperthyroidism in pregnancy.

CASE 11.1

A 24-year-old housewife was 4 months pregnant when she consulted her doctor because she felt extremely uncomfortable in the current warm weather. She was concerned because, 20 years before, her mother had had similar symptoms and had been found to have Graves' disease. Furthermore, she had read an article in a medical column in a magazine concerning the potential hazards to the foetus if the mother had Graves' disease.

The patient showed no signs or symptoms of thyroid disease. However, the doctor decided to request the following thyroid function tests (reference ranges for TSH and free thyroid hormones relate to the second trimester of pregnancy):

Hormone	Result	Reference range
TSH	<0.01	0.06–3.4 mU/L
FT4	14	9–16 pmol/L
Total T4	190	70–150 nmol/L
FT3	4.5	3.2–6.2 pmol/L
Total T3	3.0	0.9–2.4 nmol/L
TRAbs	<1	<2.5 U/L

How would you interpret these results?

Comments: Serum TSH was below the limits of sensitivity of the assay. Undetectable TSH could be due to hyperthyroidism, but it could also be due to the mild thyrotrophic action of the high plasma hCG that is found in pregnancy.

Serum TBG increases in pregnancy. This causes increases in plasma total T4 and total T3 without, at the same time, causing raised levels of the free thyroid hormones. When interpreting results for serum FT4 and FT3 in pregnant women, it is important to use the appropriate trimester-related reference ranges. In this patient, the results for these analyses were both normal, and TRAbs were not detectable in the patient's serum; thus Graves' disease was not the cause of the low serum TSH.

It was concluded that the undetectable TSH was due to the effects of hCG and the patient was reassured that she had a normal pregnancy. A repeat blood test 1 month later showed that TSH had become detectable as the hCG levels fell.

Pre-eclampsia

Pre-eclampsia is a hypertensive syndrome that occurs after 20 weeks' gestation. It is a major cause of maternal and foetal morbidity and mortality, affecting approximately 4–6% of pregnancies worldwide. It usually develops during the third trimester, often after 32 weeks, and is strongly associated with primiparity. The biochemical and haematological abnormalities most commonly associated with pre-eclampsia are proteinuria, raised serum creatinine, abnormal liver function tests, raised serum urate, thrombocytopenia and a low platelet count.

At the antenatal clinic, urine specimens should be routinely tested for protein. Proteinuria, if detected, may be the first evidence of pre-eclampsia. Proteinuria may be detected using reagent strip testing (with or without automatic readers), measuring a protein : creatinine ratio (>30 mg/mmol is diagnostic) or protein estimation in a 24-h collection (>0.3 g protein/24 h is considered diagnostic). Patients with pre-eclampsia may develop impaired renal function with increasing serum creatinine and urea as the renal impairment worsens, or as a result of vomiting and dehydration. A serum urea of 7.0 mmol/L should be regarded as definitely abnormal, because plasma urea is normally reduced in pregnancy due to the increase in plasma volume.

Impaired renal function causes reduced tubular clearance of urate. Serum urate may be measured to assess the severity of pre-eclampsia and to provide an index of prognosis. A serum urate greater than 0.35 mmol/L before 32 weeks' gestation, or greater than 0.40 mmol/L after 32 weeks, is significantly raised.

Intravascular coagulation and hepatic ischaemia can result in the HELLP (haemolysis, elevated liver enzymes and low platelets) syndrome which is seen in 4–12% of women with pre-eclampsia. The platelet count is the main criterion used for classifying the severity of HELLP syndrome. Serum LDH may also increase as a result of haemolysis, and renal function tests may be abnormal.

Obstetric cholestasis

Obstetric cholestasis usually occurs in the third trimester of pregnancy and affects approximately 0.5% of all pregnancies in the UK. The prevalence varies between populations and it is thought to relate to a genetic predisposition resulting in increased susceptibility to environmental and hormonal factors, especially oestrogens. The foetus is at risk from intrauterine/perinatal death, foetal distress and spontaneous pre-term delivery.

Although a prominent clinical feature is generalised pruritus, itching is common in pregnancy and it is important to distinguish obstetric cholestasis from other forms of liver disease. The most sensitive and important biochemical test is the measurement of serum bile acids, which may be elevated by up to 100 times normal. However, there is no correlation between serum bile acid concentrations and foetal outcome. Most affected women will also have increased levels in at least one other liver function test. Although bilirubin is raised only infrequently (approximately 25% of cases), modest elevations in transaminase levels (2- to 3-fold) or GGT may also be observed. Because of the presence of the placental isoenzyme, the reference range for ALP is so wide in the third trimester of pregnancy that its measurement contributes little to the diagnosis. In patients with persistent unexplained pruritus, but no biochemical abnormalities, liver function tests should be performed every 1–2 weeks.

 CASE 11.2

A 32-year-old woman, in her second pregnancy, was seen during the 29th week of gestation. She complained of pruritus which had increased in severity over the past 2 weeks, particularly affecting her palms and the soles of her feet. She had experienced intermittent epigastric pain and complained of nausea and vomiting. Her blood pressure was 135/78. The following biochemistry results were obtained:

Serum	Result	Reference range
Urea	2.0	2.5–6.6 mmol/L
Creatinine	62	50–98 µmol/L
Bilirubin	10	3–21 µmol/L
ALT	131	10–50 U/L
GGT	79	5–35 U/L
Bile acids	178	<14 µmol/L

Comments: A provisional diagnosis of obstetric cholestasis was made in view of the elevations in serum bile acids and liver enzymes. This was confirmed following a negative liver ultrasound examination and after obtaining negative viral screens for hepatitis A, B and C, Epstein–Barr and cytomegalovirus, and negative liver autoimmune screens for chronic active hepatitis and primary biliary cirrhosis. The patient was treated with ursodeoxycholic acid and the pruritus and abnormal liver function tests resolved within 3 weeks. A healthy girl was born vaginally after induction at 38 weeks 2 days.

Pre-natal diagnosis of foetal abnormalities

Screening for trisomies 13, 18 and 21

Trisomy 21 (Down's syndrome) affects about 1 in every 1000 births, trisomy 13 (Patau's syndrome) about 2 in 10 000, and trisomy 18 (Edwards' syndrome) about 3 in 10 000. In all cases, affected pregnancies can be identified by chromosome analysis of cells obtained at amniocentesis in the second trimester. The incidence of trisomies 13, 18 and 21 varies greatly with maternal age, for example, a 37-year-old woman has a chance of 1 in 250 of carrying an affected Down's syndrome foetus at term, whereas for a woman aged 25 years this is reduced to approximately 1 in 1100.

Abnormalities in a number of maternal serum analytes are associated with Down's, Edwards' and Patau's syndrome pregnancies. These analytes include AFP, pregnancy-associated plasma protein A (PAPP-A), unconjugated oestriol, total hCG, free β-hCG and inhibin A. Each of these parameters shows overlap between affected pregnancies and the unaffected population. However, if the distributions of the concentrations of these analytes for affected and unaffected pregnancies are known, a likelihood ratio for the chance of a foetus with trisomy 13, 18 and 21 can be calculated. This is combined with the maternal age-related chance of trisomy 13, 18 and 21 in order to calculate the overall probability that the pregnancy may be affected. Women with a high probability of carrying an affected child may then be offered amniocentesis.

First trimester screening

Screening in the first trimester has now become an established part of obstetric practice. The chance of an affected pregnancy is calculated using the Combined Test which is based on maternal age, biochemical measurements (maternal serum free β-hCG and PAPP-A) and the ultrasonographic measurement of foetal nuchal translucency thickness, which is increased in trisomy 21 pregnancies. This protocol can yield detection rates approaching 90% for a screen positive rate of approximately 2% for trisomy 21.

Additional parameters which may be incorporated into the risk calculation include smoking status, ethnic origin and diabetic status.

Second trimester screening

The Quadruple Test is recommended for women who present too late for first trimester screening, or in whom a foetal nuchal translucency thickness measurement is not available. This involves the measurement of maternal serum AFP, either serum total hCG or free β-hCG, unconjugated oestriol and inhibin A. For trisomy 21 second trimester testing can achieve a detection rate of 80% for a screen positive rate approximately 3–4%, but screening performance is inferior to that of first trimester programmes.

Noninvasive prenatal testing (NIPT)

NIPT detects foetal DNA fragments in a blood sample taken from the mother. Although it is thought to be more accurate than the combined test, it remains a screening test rather than a diagnostic test and therefore is not proposed to replace current diagnostic testing.

Its improved accuracy means that fewer women will go on to have invasive diagnostic testing therefore avoiding the miscarriage risk associated with confirmatory tests.

NIPT is currently not routinely available in the UK.

Neural tube defects

The foetal liver begins to produce α-foetoprotein (AFP) from the sixth week of gestation, and the highest concentration of AFP in foetal serum occurs in the second trimester, after which it falls progressively until term. If the foetus has an open NTD, abnormal amounts of AFP are present in both amniotic fluid and maternal serum. Although the measurement of maternal serum AFP has previously been the basis of second trimester screening programmes for neural tube defects, this has now been superseded by the widespread introduction of 18-week foetal anomaly scanning.

 CASE 11.3

First trimester antenatal screening for trisomy 21 was performed on a 33-year-old school teacher who was seen by the community midwives. The results were as follows:

Patient details provided		Laboratory data	
Maternal weight	68 kg	Maternal age at EDD	33.3 years
? current smoker	Yes	Gestation at sample date	13 wks 2 days
Family origin	Caucasian	Age-related chance	1 in 593
Nuchal translucency	1.7 mm	Free β-hCG MOM*	2.11
		PAPP-A MOM*	0.34
		Nuchal translucency MOM*	1.55

Combined chance of trisomy 21 at term: 1 in 27

*Results expressed as multiples of the median (MOM).

Comments: Free β-hCG, PAPP-A and nuchal translucency are expressed as MOMs for the appropriate gestational age, having made an adjustment for the effect of family origin and smoking on the screening markers. In pregnancies affected by trisomy 21, the free β-hCG and nuchal translucency MOMs tend to be elevated and the PAPP-A MOM reduced. This pattern was observed in the current pregnancy, but, because there are no clearly defined cut-offs between affected and unaffected pregnancies, the overall chance that the pregnancy may be affected is calculated by modifying the maternal age-related chance using the likelihood ratios for the overlapping free β-hCG, PAPP-A and nuchal translucency distributions. If the combined chance of an affected pregnancy is >1 in 150, amniocentesis and chromosomal analysis are offered.

In this woman the chance that the foetus was affected by trisomy 21 was increased at 1 in 27. She underwent amniocentesis and chromosomal analysis indicated that the pregnancy was affected by trisomy 21.

FURTHER READING

Fetal Anomaly Screening Programme (2015) FASP handbook, August 2015. Available at: www.gov.uk/government/publications/fetal-anomaly-screening-programme-handbook

National Institute for Health and Care Excellence (2015) NICE Guideline (NG)3 – Diabetes in pregnancy: management from preconception to the postnatal period 2015. Available at: https://www.nice.org.uk/guidance/NG3

Scottish Intercollegiate Guidelines Network (2010) SIGN 116 – Management of diabetes. Available at: http://www.sign.ac.uk/guidelines/fulltext/116/

Walker, J.J. and Morley, L. (2016) *BMJ Best Practice – Pre-eclampsia*. BMJ, London.

12

Cardiovascular disorders

Learning objectives

To understand:

✔ the biochemical tests used in the diagnosis of acute coronary syndromes and in disorders of skeletal muscle;

✔ cardiovascular risk factors, including lipids, and how these risk factors can be used to calculate an estimate of overall cardiovascular risk.

The diagnosis of myocardial infarction

Myocardial infarction (MI) can be defined pathologically as myocardial necrosis due to prolonged ischaemia and may be recognised clinically through some combination of clinical features, electrocardiographic (ECG) findings and elevated values of biochemical markers or by imaging. After the onset of myocardial ischaemia, histological cell death takes from possibly as little as 20 minutes up to 4 hours or longer, and the entire process leading to a healed infarction takes at least 5–6 weeks.

The diagnosis of MI has in past decades been based on WHO criteria, which comprise a typical history of chest pain, the presence of diagnostic ECG abnormalities, and a rise in biochemical markers. The presence of two or more of these three defined the diagnosis. This long-established definition has been overtaken by the advent of more sensitive biochemical markers, and in particular the troponins (see Chapter 12: Troponin). Many studies have shown that troponins are released in some patients without conventional ECG changes of infarction, in particular elevation of the ST segment and T wave inversion. These patients are found to be at increased risk of subsequent cardiac events. This has given rise to the concept of the 'acute coronary syndromes', which comprise unstable angina, non-ST segment elevation MI and ST segment elevation MI.

The use of troponin measurement thus potentially reveals biochemical changes that would not previously have been detected in patients with chest pain. This has major implications in the definition of MI, and of course for the patients (and their families, employers and insurers) who may now be given this diagnosis but who would formerly have been reassured that they had not had an infarct.

A task force drawn from a number of expert bodies has published a consensus 'Universal Definition of Myocardial Infarction' (see Chapter 12: Further reading). This places biomarkers central to the definition, requiring the detection of a rise and/or fall of a biomarker (preferably troponin). At least one troponin value should be above the 99th percentile of a 'normal' population. In addition there should be at least one of the following:

- symptoms of ischaemia;
- ECG changes indicative of new ischaemia;
- development of pathological Q waves in the ECG;
- imaging evidence of new loss of viable myocardium or new regional wall motion abnormality;
- identification of an intracoronary thrombus by angiography or autopsy.

The assay should have an analytical performance at the 99th percentile level defined by a coefficient of variation of less than 10%. This is a challenging analytical

---

Table 12.1 Types of MI, and biochemical marker criteria for diagnosis.

Type of MI	Cause	Multiples of cardiac marker rise required for diagnosis*
Type 1	Spontaneous MI: spontaneous rupture, ulceration or dissection of atherosclerotic plaque, with intraluminal thrombus occluding one or more of the coronary arteries	>1×
Type 2	MI secondary to ischaemic imbalance: imbalance between oxygen supply and demand in the absence of atherosclerotic plaque, e.g. due to coronary artery spasm, tachy- or brady-arrhythmias, severe anaemia, respiratory failure, hypotension, aortic dissection, severe aortic valve disease, etc.	>1×
Type 3	Sudden cardiac death: strongly suggestive clinical history, but antemortem blood samples may not be available	>10× or not defined
Type 4a	MI associated with PCI	>5×
Type 4b	MI associated with stent thrombosis	>1×
Type 4c	MI associated with stent restenosis	>1×
Type 5	MI associated with CABG	>10×

*Multiples of the 99th percentile of cardiac marker required for diagnosis; PCI = percutaneous coronary intervention; CABG = coronary artery bypass grafting.

standard that not all currently available assays meet. There are implications for the laboratory in this stringent analytical requirement and in potential increases in testing, and for cardiology services in the increase in patients receiving a diagnosis of MI.

MI can be classified according to cause. Some of these causes occur in the presence of procedures such as cardiac catheterisation or coronary artery bypass grafting, which might be expected in themselves to cause elevations of biochemical markers, so the thresholds vary according to the cause (Table 12.1).

Biochemical tests in myocardial infarction and ischaemia

After MI, a number of intracellular proteins are released from the damaged cells. The proteins of major diagnostic interest include:

- troponin I and troponin T;
- enzymes, such as creatine kinase (CK), CK-MB, aspartate aminotransferase (AST) and lactate dehydrogenase (LDH);
- myoglobin.

The troponins and CK will be considered in detail (Chapter 12: Troponin and Creatine kinase) because they are the most widely established biochemical indices of myocardial damage, although troponins

have essentially taken the place of the enzymes in recent years. CK is, however, still used in some countries, and retains a use in the investigation of muscle disorders. Myoglobin is also a sensitive index of myocardial damage, and it rises very rapidly after the event. However it is nonspecific because it is raised following any form of muscle damage. It is not in wide laboratory use, but has a role in point of care analysers in the emergency setting. A negative result on an appropriately timed sample can be used to rule out myocardial damage and thereby determine early patient management. A positive result requires further investigation.

Time-course of changes

After an MI, the time-course of plasma biochemical markers always follows the same general pattern (Figure 12.1). After an initial 'lag' phase, they rise rapidly to a peak between 18 and 36 h, and then return to normal at rates that depend on the half-life of each marker in plasma. The biphasic response of troponins with a rapid rise and prolonged elevation, and the rapid rise and fall of CK and CK-MB activity should be particularly noted. In patients treated by angioplasty or with thrombolytic agents, the general pattern of plasma marker changes shown in Figure 12.1 is slightly modified, with a 'washout' of markers from the infarcted area, causing levels to rise rapidly to reach an early peak at 10–18 h.

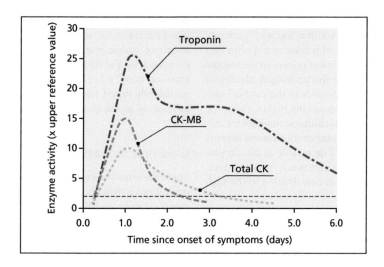

Figure 12.1 Patterns of biochemical markers in the first few days after an uncomplicated MI.

Optimal times for blood sampling

A sample taken on admission with an appropriate clinical history, if sufficiently elevated, will make the required diagnosis, but if not elevated will not rule out the diagnosis if insufficient time has elapsed for a significant rise in CK or troponin to have occurred (Table 12.2). Detection of a rise and/or fall in measurements is ideally required for the diagnosis of an acute MI, so testing should be repeated after 3–6 hours. It is likely that hospitals will have a local protocol for the initial diagnosis and management of patients suspected of MI, and this should be consulted.

Except for the occasional patient seen for the first time 2 days or more after the episode, in whom troponin measurements might still be useful, it is very rarely of any value to take samples for plasma markers after 48 h from the onset of symptoms that suggest a diagnosis of MI.

Troponin

The troponin complex is exclusively present in striated muscle fibres and regulates the calcium-mediated interactions of actin and myosin. It comprises equimolar quantities of the structurally unrelated proteins troponin T, troponin I and troponin C. Troponin T binds tropomyosin, troponin I is an inhibitory protein and troponin C is responsible for binding calcium. Three distinct isoforms of troponin T and I exist, one each in slow twitch and fast twitch fibres of skeletal muscle, and one in cardiac muscle. These cardiac-specific forms of troponin can be recognised and measured in the plasma. There are two isoforms of troponin C, one found in slow twitch and cardiac muscle, and one in fast twitch muscle, so there is not a troponin C species unique to myocardium.

In human heart the cardiac-specific troponin T and troponin I are largely insoluble, but 3–5% exists

Table 12.2 **Time-course of plasma biochemical marker elevation after MI.**

Enzyme	Abnormal activity detectable (h)	Peak value of abnormality (h)	Duration of abnormality (days)
Troponin T or I	4–6	12–24	3–10
CK-MB isoenzyme	3–10	12–24	1.5–3
Total CK	5–12	18–30	2–5
'Heart-specific' LDH	8–16	30–48	5–14

as a soluble cytoplasmic pool. Following cardiac myocyte necrosis, this soluble fraction probably accounts for the early rapid release of troponin into the circulation, and the slower release of the insoluble fraction accounts for the prolonged plateau of troponin release. The existence of the cardiac-specific isoforms of these troponins makes them the most specific of all the biochemical markers for cardiac damage. Under normal circumstances there is no cardiac troponin T or I detectable in the circulation by conventional troponin assays, so any detectable rise is of significance, contributing to the high sensitivity of these tests.

Highly sensitive troponin assays are coming into clinical use. These are sufficiently sensitive that they are able to detect troponin levels in most healthy control subjects. Some but not all studies suggest that age- and gender-specific reference ranges may be needed. The improved sensitivity of highly sensitive troponin assays is offset by reduced specificity,

because more patients are detected with myocardial injury not related to ischaemia (Table 12.3). A characteristic of cardiac marker release in acute ischaemic events is a rise and fall in concentration, thus, whereas most of these other conditions will demonstrate persistently raised results, the distinction can often be made by repeat measurements of troponin levels.

Creatine kinase

There are three principal CK isoenzymes, each comprising two polypeptide chains, either B or M; these give the dimers BB, MB and MM.

- Skeletal muscle has a very high total CK content; over 98% normally comprises CK-MM and less than 2% CK-MB. CK-MB may rise to 5–15% in some patients with muscle disease, and also in athletes in training.
- Cardiac muscle also has a high CK content. It comprises 70–80% CK-MM and 20–30% CK-MB. As a general rule, cardiac muscle is the only tissue with more than 5% CK-MB. Before troponin analyses were widely available, CK-MB measurement was useful in confirming the cardiac origin of a raised CK.
- Other organs, such as brain, contain less CK, often CK-BB. However, CK-BB rarely appears in plasma and is not of diagnostic importance. Plasma normally contains more than 95% of its CK as CK-MM.

CK is used in the diagnosis of some muscle diseases (see the following paragraphs). It used to be used in the diagnosis of MI, but this is no longer recommended because of its lack of specificity. Increases, sometimes large, may occur after trauma or surgical operations, IM injections, in comatose patients, in diabetic ketoacidosis, acute renal failure and

---

 CASE 12.1

A 66-year-old man had experienced central chest pain on exertion for some months, but in the afternoon of the day prior to admission he had had a particularly severe episode of the pain, which came on without any exertion and lasted for about an hour. On admission there were no abnormalities on examination and the ECG was normal. The troponin was clearly detectable.

Comment on these results. Has he suffered an MI?

Comments: He has an elevated troponin plus a typical history. This is sufficient to diagnose an MI by the most recent definition, even in the absence of ECG changes.

Table 12.3 Elevations of cardiac troponin due to myocardial injury but not due to MI.

Myocardial injury not related to myocardial ischaemia	Multifactorial or indeterminate myocardial injury
• Cardiac contusion, surgery, pacing, defibrillator shocks • Rhabdomyolysis with cardiac involvement • Myocarditis • Cardiotoxic agents	• Heart failure • Severe pulmonary embolism or pulmonary hypertension • Sepsis • Renal failure • Severe acute neurological disease, e.g. subarachnoid haemorrhage • Strenuous exercise

hypothyroidism, and after prolonged muscular exercise, especially in unfit individuals.

CK-MB isoenzyme

CK-MB is a more sensitive and specific test for myocardial damage than total CK. Its use has been largely overtaken by the widespread availability of troponin measurement. CK-MB (preferably by a mass measurement method) may be a more suitable alternative to troponin in less well-resourced settings and countries.

Creatine kinase and muscle disease

Plasma CK, AST, LDH and ALT activities may be increased in muscle disease. However, plasma total CK is usually the measurement of choice, irrespective of the aetiology of the disorder, since it is increased in the greatest number of cases and shows the largest changes.

- *Muscular dystrophy:* In Duchenne-type dystrophy, high plasma CK activity is present from birth, before the onset of clinical signs. During the early clinical stages of the disease, very high activities are usually present, but these tend to fall as the terminal stages of the disease are reached. Smaller CK increases are present in other forms of muscular dystrophy. About 75% of female carriers of the Duchenne dystrophy gene have small increases in plasma CK activity.
- *Malignant hyperpyrexia:* This is a rare but serious disorder, characterised by raised body temperature, convulsions and shock following general anaesthesia. Many of the patients show evidence of myopathy. Extremely high plasma CK activities are seen in the acute, post-anaesthetic stage, but smaller increases often persist and can also be detected in the relatives of affected patients. Pre-operative screening of plasma CK is not a reliable way of detecting patients liable to develop malignant hyperpyrexia, and should be limited to those patients with a family history of anaesthetic deaths or of malignant hyperpyrexia.
- *Miscellaneous muscle diseases:* CK is variably increased in various myopathies, including that due to a side effect of treatment with β-hydroxy β-methylglutaryl-coenzyme A (HMG-CoA) reductase inhibitor ('statin') cholesterol-lowering drugs. It is also raised in polymyositis.
- *Neurogenic muscle disease:* Plasma CK activity is usually normal in peripheral neuritis, poliomyelitis and motor neuron disease.

 CASE 12.2

A well-trained marathon runner collapsed as he was approaching the finishing line. An ECG was normal, but CK was elevated at 9500 U/L (male reference range 55–170 U/L), and the CK-MB was 14% of the total CK (normally <6%). Troponin was undetectable. Comment on these results.

Comments: The total CK is substantially elevated, and CK-MB >6% can usually be taken to mean that it is of myocardial origin. However, the normal ECG and troponin are both reassuring. In trained endurance athletes, the proportion of CK-MB in muscle increases from the normal low levels and may be as high as 10–15%. An elevated CK-MB in such individuals can no longer be taken to imply a cardiac origin for the raised CK. Extreme exercise, especially in unfit individuals, causes an elevated CK, potentially to very high levels.

The diagnosis of heart failure

Heart failure is a complex clinical condition in which the heart's ability to pump is compromised by one or more of a number of underlying conditions, commonly ischaemic heart disease, but also heart valve abnormalities. The prognosis is poor if untreated, with a 2-year survival rate of under 50%.

The diagnosis of heart failure can be difficult, especially because the usual presenting symptoms such as breathlessness or ankle swelling are common and can be due to many different conditions. Physical examination is neither sensitive nor specific for heart failure, even in expert hands, with incorrect diagnoses in up to 50% of patients. The definitive diagnosis is best made by echocardiography, but access to this may be limited or delayed. B-type natriuretic peptide (BNP) is a neurohormone secreted by cardiac myocytes in response to volume expansion and pressure overload, and plays a role in circulatory homeostasis. In heart failure the level of BNP increases, enabling differentiation of cardiac and pulmonary causes of breathlessness. It has an evolving role in the diagnosis of heart failure in both primary care and the emergency setting because it costs considerably less than echocardiography, and the result can be available much more rapidly.

Laboratory and point of care assays for BNP and for the inactive peptide N-terminal-proBNP (NT-proBNP) are available and provide qualitatively similar information.

Their accuracy is greatest in patients with more severe disease and poorest in those already receiving treatment. Levels rise with age, so age-related cut-offs should be used.

A number of other conditions can cause elevated BNP levels but, in a patient who is not on heart failure treatment, if levels are below the cut-off level then heart failure is highly unlikely and the patient should be investigated for other conditions. If the level is elevated the patient should proceed to further assessment, including echocardiography. The introduction of this strategy has the potential to speed up accurate diagnosis of heart failure, and to save money by restricting the use of echocardiography to those patients most likely to benefit from its use.

The diagnosis of thromboembolic disease

Laboratory investigations have a part to play in the investigation of possible thromboembolic disease. As the fibrinolytic system breaks down clots formed of cross-linked fibrin, degradation products are produced, including D-dimers. These are not detectable in the circulation under normal circumstances but are present in thromboembolic disease and in disseminated intravascular coagulation. Measurement of D-dimer levels is used in the diagnosis (or, more accurately, exclusion) of thromboembolic disease such as deep venous thrombosis (DVT) and pulmonary embolism (PE). In carefully selected patients at relatively low risk of DVT or PE, a normal result can effectively rule out these conditions, avoiding the need for more expensive and time-consuming imaging techniques. Careful clinical assessment is needed, because false-positive results are possible in nonthrombotic pathologies such as neoplasia, recent surgery, MI and trauma.

Both laboratory and point of care tests are available for D-dimers and can help in the immediate management of patients presenting with symptoms or signs suggestive of DVT or PE, because a negative result offers reassurance. A positive result will require further investigation.

Cardiovascular risk factors

Many factors are associated with or cause increased cardiovascular risk. These can pragmatically be divided into those which cannot be influenced and those which can be influenced and reduction of which has been demonstrated to reduce risk. Those that cannot be influenced include a family history of premature vascular disease, age and pre-existing vascular disease. Those whose modification has an established role include cigarette smoking and hypertension (not considered further here), diabetes (see Chapter 6) and the hyperlipidaemias, especially hypercholesterolaemia. Lipid metabolism and the hyperlipidaemias are covered in the following paragraphs, followed by a description of how cardiovascular risk is assessed and treated. Other novel biochemical markers of vascular risk are briefly described.

Lipids

Lipids act as energy stores (triglycerides) and as important structural components of cells (cholesterol and phospholipids). They also have specialised functions (e.g. as adrenal and sex hormones). The main lipids, being insoluble in water, are transported in plasma as particulate complexes with proteins, the lipoproteins.

From the clinical viewpoint, it is the strong relationship between plasma lipid levels and the incidence of ischaemic vascular disease, particularly of the coronary arteries, that is of major importance. In the following section, we outline:

- the biochemistry of the main body lipids;
- the mechanisms for lipid transport in plasma;
- the importance of lipids, and other factors, in the pathogenesis of arterial disease;
- the role of plasma lipid measurements in the management of hyperlipidaemia and in cardiovascular risk assessment.

Cholesterol

This is a steroid that is present in the diet, but it is mainly synthesised in the liver and small intestine, the rate-limiting step being catalysed by HMG-CoA reductase. HMG-CoA reductase inhibitors, commonly referred to as statins, are effective cholesterol-lowering drugs. Cholesterol is a major component of cell membranes, and acts as the substrate for steroid hormone formation in the adrenals and the gonads. It is present in plasma mainly esterified with fatty acids. The body cannot break down the sterol nucleus, so cholesterol is either excreted unchanged in bile or converted to bile acids and then excreted. Cholesterol and bile acids both undergo an enterohepatic circulation.

Triglycerides

These are fatty acid esters of glycerol, and are the main lipids in the diet. They are broken down in the small intestine to a mixture of monoglycerides, fatty acids and glycerol. These products are absorbed, and triglycerides are resynthesised from them in the mucosal cell. Most of these exogenous triglycerides pass into plasma as chylomicrons (see Chapter 12: Chylomicron metabolism).

Endogenous triglyceride synthesis occurs in the liver from fatty acids and glycerol. The triglycerides synthesised in this way are transported as VLDL (see Chapter 12: VLDL and IDL metabolism).

Fatty acids

These are mostly straight-chain monocarboxylic acids. They are mainly derived from dietary or tissue triglyceride, but the body can also synthesise most of them, apart from certain polyunsaturated (essential) fatty acids. Fatty acids act as an alternative or additional energy source to glucose.

Phospholipids

These have a structure similar to triglycerides, but a polar group (e.g. phosphorylcholine) replaces one of the three fatty acid components. The presence of both polar and nonpolar (fatty acid) groups gives the phospholipids their characteristic detergent properties. Phospholipids are mainly synthesised in the liver and small intestine; they are important constituents of cell membranes.

Lipoproteins

Cholesterol and its esters, triglycerides and phospholipids are all transported in plasma as lipoprotein (Table 12.4) particles. Fatty acids are transported bound to albumin.

Lipoprotein particles comprise a peripheral envelope, consisting mainly of phospholipids and free cholesterol (which each have both water-soluble polar and lipid-soluble nonpolar groups) with some apolipoproteins, and a central nonpolar core (mostly triglyceride and esterified cholesterol). The molecules in the envelope are distributed in a single layer in such a way that the polar groups face out towards the surrounding plasma, while the nonpolar groups face inwards towards the lipid core in which the insoluble lipids are carried. Most lipoproteins are assembled in the liver or small intestine. Five main types of lipoprotein particle can be recognised:

- Chylomicrons are the principal form in which dietary triglycerides are carried to the tissues.
- VLDLs are triglyceride-rich particles that form the major route whereby endogenous triglycerides are carried to the tissues from the liver and, to a lesser extent, from the small intestine.
- Intermediate-density lipoproteins (IDLs or 'VLDL remnants') are particles formed by the removal of triglycerides from VLDLs during the transition from VLDLs to LDLs.
- LDLs are cholesterol-rich particles, formed from IDLs by the removal of more triglyceride and apolipoprotein. Increased plasma LDL cholesterol, and hence plasma total cholesterol, is positively correlated with the incidence of ischaemic heart disease.

Table 12.4 **Properties of the five main classes of lipoproteins.**

Property	Chylomicrons	VLDL	IDL	LDL	HDL
Physical properties					
• Diameter (nm)	100–500	30–80	25–30	20–35	5–10
• Density (kg/L)	<0.95	<1.006	1.006–1.019	1.019–1.063	>1.063
• Electrophoresis	Stay at origin	Pre-β	β	β	α_1
Lipoprotein composition (approximate percentages)					
• Triglyceride	90	65	35	10	5
• Cholesterol	5	20	40	50	35
• Phospholipid	5	10	15	20	35
• Protein	1	5	10	20	25
Apolipoprotein composition*	C, B, E, (A)	C, B, E, (A)	B, (C, E, A)	B	A, C, E, (B)

*The main apolipoprotein components are listed in descending order of amount (trace components in parentheses).

- HDLs act as a means whereby cholesterol can be transported from peripheral cells to the liver, prior to excretion. Increased plasma HDL cholesterol is negatively correlated with the incidence of ischaemic heart disease, presumably explained by its role in transporting cholesterol from the periphery.
- A sixth type of lipoprotein particle, Lp(a), is synthesised in the liver and has approximately the same lipid composition as LDL (see further on). The physiological role of Lp(a) is not known, but its concentration is highly heritable. Plasma Lp(a) concentration is positively associated with the incidence of ischaemic heart disease, independently of other lipoprotein fractions. The effect may be due to competition between Lp(a) and plasminogen for endothelial cell receptors, thereby inhibiting thrombolysis.

The apolipoproteins

The protein components of the lipoproteins, the apolipoproteins, are a complex family of polypeptides that promote and control lipid transport through the circulation and lipid uptake into tissues. They are separable into four main groups (apoA, B, C and E), some of which may be subdivided, and apo(a).

- *ApoA* is synthesised in the liver and intestine. It is initially present in chylomicrons in lymph, but rapidly transfers to HDL.
- *ApoB* is present in plasma in two forms, $apoB_{100}$ and $apoB_{48}$. $ApoB_{100}$ is the protein component of LDL, and is also present in chylomicrons, VLDL and IDL. $ApoB_{48}$ (the N-terminal half of $apoB_{100}$) is only found in chylomicrons. $ApoB_{100}$ is recognised by specific receptors in peripheral tissues (see Chapter 12: LDL metabolism).
- *ApoC*. This family of three proteins (apoC-I, apoC-II and apoC-III) is synthesised in the liver and incorporated into HDL.
- *ApoE* is synthesised in the liver, incorporated into HDL and transferred in the circulation to chylomicrons and VLDL. There are three major isoforms (apoE2, apoE3 and apoE4) at a single genetic locus, giving rise to several genotypes (E3/3, E2/3, E2/4, etc.). ApoE is probably mainly involved in the hepatic uptake of chylomicron remnants and IDL; it binds to apoB receptors in the tissues.
- *Apo(a)* is present in equimolar amounts to $apoB_{100}$ in Lp(a). It has a high carbohydrate content and has a similar amino acid sequence to plasminogen. It varies in size due to a polymorphism causing variable numbers of repeats of part of its structure, resulting in a number of isoforms. There is an inverse correlation between the size of the isoform and the plasma Lp(a) concentration.

Enzymes involved in lipid transport

Four enzymes of relevance to clinical disorders are:

- *Lecithin cholesterol acyltransferase (LCAT)* transfers an acyl group (fatty acid residue) from lecithin to cholesterol, forming a cholesterol ester. In plasma, this reaction probably takes place exclusively on HDL, and may be stimulated by apoA-I.
- *Lipoprotein lipase* is attached to tissue capillary endothelium and splits triglycerides (present in chylomicrons and VLDLs) into glycerol and free fatty acids. Its activity increases after a meal, partly as a result of activation by apoC-II, which is present on the surface of triglyceride-bearing lipoproteins.
- *Hepatic lipase* has an action similar to that of lipoprotein lipase.
- *Mobilising lipase*, present in adipose tissue cells, controls the release of fatty acids from adipose tissue into plasma. It is activated by catecholamines, GH and glucocorticoids (e.g. cortisol), and inhibited by glucose and by insulin.

Metabolism of plasma lipoproteins

The above description of the lipoproteins and apolipoproteins is an oversimplification, and the following points should be emphasised:

- Plasma lipids and apolipoproteins exist in a dynamic state. There is interchange of lipids both between different lipoprotein particles and with tissues.
- There is considerable variation in the size and composition of individual lipoprotein particles within each lipoprotein class.

Chylomicron metabolism

Chylomicrons (Figure 12.2) are formed in the intestinal mucosa after a fat-containing meal, and reach the systemic circulation via the thoracic duct. They then transfer apoA to HDL and acquire apoC and apoE from HDL. The apoC-II activates lipoprotein lipase in

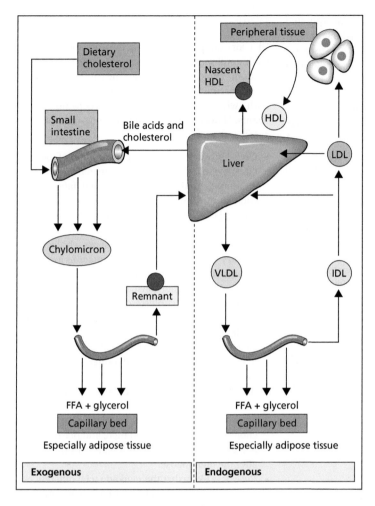

Figure 12.2 Endogenous and exogenous triglyceride metabolism (see text for details). FFA = free fatty acids.

the tissues, and triglycerides are progressively removed from the hydrophobic core of the chylomicrons. As the size of the particles decreases, the more hydrophilic surface components (apoC, unesterified cholesterol and phospholipid) transfer to HDL. The triglyceride-poor chylomicron remnants are taken up by the liver, where they are catabolised.

VLDL and IDL metabolism

Most VLDL is secreted into plasma by the hepatocytes ('endogenous' VLDL), but some originates from the intestinal mucosa ('exogenous' VLDL) (Figure 12.2). Hepatic VLDL synthesis is increased whenever there is increased hepatic triglyceride synthesis, for example when there is increased transport of fatty acids to the liver, or after a large carbohydrate-containing meal.

When first produced, VLDL consists mainly of triglycerides and some unesterified cholesterol, with apoB$_{100}$ and lesser amounts of apoE. ApoC-II is then acquired, mainly from HDL, and triglycerides are removed from the VLDL 'core' in a manner analogous to that for chylomicrons. The residual particles are known as 'VLDL remnants', or IDLs, which are either rapidly converted to LDL or removed from the circulation to the liver.

LDL metabolism

LDL probably all arises from VLDL metabolism in man. The LDL particles are rich in cholesterol esters, probably derived from HDL; apoB$_{100}$ is the only apolipoprotein. LDL is removed from the circulation by two processes; one regulated, the other unregulated.

- The *regulated mechanism* involves the binding of LDL to specific apoB$_{100}$ receptors present on the 'surface pits' of hepatocytes and other peripheral tissue cells. The entire LDL particle is incorporated into the cell by invagination of the cell membrane. Inside the cell, the particle fuses with lysosomes; apoB is then broken down and the cholesterol esters are hydrolysed, thereby making unesterified cholesterol available to the cell. The size of the intracellular cholesterol pool regulates:

- the rate of cholesterol synthesis in the cell, through the effect of cholesterol on HMG-CoA reductase;
- the number of LDL-apoB receptors on the cell surface.

The enzyme proprotein convertase subtilisin/kexin type 9 (PCSK9) plays a role in the metabolism of the LDL receptor. When the LDL receptor binds LDL and is internalised into the cell, if PCSK9 binds to the receptor the receptor is degraded and is not available for recycling to the cell surface to take up more LDL cholesterol from the circulation. Drugs that inhibit PCSK9 therefore increase the numbers of LDL receptors on the cell surface and lower cholesterol.

- The *unregulated mechanism* involves receptor-independent mechanisms of cholesterol uptake by cells; these are present particularly in macrophages. These mechanisms are brought into operation especially when plasma cholesterol is increased.

HDL metabolism

This heterogeneous group of particles is formed in the liver and intestinal mucosa. The HDL particles then undergo complex exchanges of lipid and protein with other plasma lipoproteins. However, the main point to note is that free cholesterol in tissues transfers to HDL in plasma. The cholesterol is then esterified by LCAT and transferred to LDL, which, in turn, is mainly taken up by the liver. Thus, HDL forms the principal route whereby cholesterol can return from peripheral tissues to the liver.

Investigation of plasma lipid abnormalities

Most laboratories measure plasma total cholesterol, HDL cholesterol and triglycerides. Further tests to characterise the lipoprotein abnormalities may be indicated in a few patients. The investigations are mainly of value in the investigation and assessment of cardiovascular risk.

Plasma total cholesterol

Diet, for example recent meals, does not affect plasma cholesterol much in the short term. This means that random cholesterol can be measured to assess cardiovascular risk. Plasma cholesterol is affected by both within-individual and between-individual factors. However, these tend to be long-term effects, as follows:

- *Diet:* The amount and the composition of dietary fat affect plasma cholesterol. In particular, fats containing mainly polyunsaturated fatty acids, such as those in fish and vegetable oils, tend to lower plasma cholesterol, whereas fats containing mainly saturated fatty acids, such as animal fat and butter, tend to raise plasma cholesterol. Dietary fibre may have a small effect in lowering plasma cholesterol. The consumption of 1–3 units of alcohol per day causes a significant rise in plasma HDL cholesterol. Dietary cholesterol intake has relatively little effect on plasma cholesterol.
- *Exercise:* Regular exercise tends to cause a rise in plasma HDL cholesterol and a small fall in plasma total cholesterol.
- *Age:* In developed countries, plasma cholesterol rises with age. This is probably related to diet.
- *Sex:* In pre-menopausal women, plasma total cholesterol is lower than in men, and plasma HDL cholesterol is higher. These differences disappear after the menopause.
- *Race:* It is likely that the marked racial differences, with particularly high plasma cholesterol in north Europeans, are mainly due to dietary and environmental factors rather than genetic differences.
- Numerous studies have shown that the incidence of ischaemic heart disease is directly correlated with plasma cholesterol, even within the 'reference range'. There is no clear cut-off between values for normal risk and increased risk, although risk rises particularly rapidly above about 6.5 mmol/L. Because of this association, it is inappropriate to employ reference ranges for plasma cholesterol concentration in the usual way, as these imply health without increased risk of disease. Instead, it seems more appropriate to define a desirable concentration (e.g. <5 mmol/L).

Plasma total cholesterol is a rather unsatisfactory measurement, because it represents the sum of the various ways in which cholesterol is transported in plasma. In fact, although raised plasma LDL cholesterol is associated with an increased risk of ischaemic heart disease, raised plasma HDL cholesterol is associated with a decreased risk of ischaemic heart disease and seems to have a protective effect.

Plasma triglycerides

Plasma triglycerides also show variations with age and sex, but more especially with diet. There is, in addition, considerable within-individual variation, which can make interpretation of a single result difficult.

Plasma LDL

Plasma LDL can be measured by ultracentrifugation, but this is not a practical technique for routine clinical laboratory use. The following equation can be used to calculate LDL cholesterol concentration if the measurements were made on a fasting sample:

LDL cholesterol = total cholesterol − HDL cholesterol
− triglyceride/2.2

where all measurements are in mmol/L. This is known as the Friedewald equation and assumes the absence of chylomicrons since the sample was taken in the fasting state, and therefore the total cholesterol is distributed between LDL, HDL and VLDL. The molar ratio of triglyceride to cholesterol in VDL is 2.2, as long as the triglyceride concentration is less than 4.5 mmol/L. The formula is therefore not valid if triglyceride is greater than 4.5 mmol/L, and has not been validated in patients on lipid-lowering drugs. However, it is convenient (and cheap).

LDL is predictive of cardiovascular risk, and strategies that reduce LDL provide cardiovascular benefit. Many guidelines for cardiovascular risk reduction recommend LDL levels as thresholds or targets for treatment.

LDL exists in a range of sizes and densities. There is evidence that the small dense subfractions of LDL are particularly atherogenic. There are no readily available routine laboratory methods for examining LDL subfractions, but a surrogate marker for the presence of these small dense LDL species is the combination of low or low-normal HDL and high or high-normal triglyceride. This pattern is sometimes referred to as an 'atherogenic lipid profile'. Measurement of apoB levels may provide similar information.

Plasma non-HDL cholesterol

The aim of lipid measurements is usually to enable an assessment of cardiovascular risk, and it would be useful to have a simpler approach to testing that avoids the need for fasting, that requires no assumptions about the lipoprotein species present in the sample, and which is valid whether the patient is taking lipid-lowering drugs or not. Non-HDL cholesterol is a candidate; this is simply the difference between total cholesterol and HDL cholesterol. It avoids the problems with the Friedewald equation and incorporates all the atherogenic lipoproteins, including LDL, IDL, VLDL, remnant particles and Lp(a). Its predictive value is at least as good in the non-fasting state as after an overnight fast. Triglyceride levels are increased in people who are obese or who have type 2 diabetes, and non-HDL cholesterol includes the contributions of these atherogenic triglyceride-containing lipoproteins. Many recent clinical trials have recognized the benefits of using non-HDL cholesterol rather than a calculated LDL. It is not yet in widespread routine clinical use, but its use is likely to increase in future.

Non-HDL is not suitable for pursuing a diagnosis of familial hypercholesterolaemia, or for LDL based cascade screening in relatives of an individual with familial hypercholesterolaemia.

Specimen collection

Blood specimens should ideally be collected after an overnight fast of 10–14 h, to reduce the variability in triglyceride concentration. This also ensures the absence of chylomicrons, meaning that the Friedewald equation for the calculation of LDL is valid. In fact there is evidence that the variability in triglyceride concentration is relatively minor and the effect on calculated LDL small. It is more convenient for patients to have blood taken on a random sample than after fasting, and the effect on prediction of cardiovascular disease is minimal. If triglyceride levels are raised on the non-fasting sample, then it would be appropriate to repeat the test on a fasting sample.

Results of plasma lipid and lipoprotein investigations can be misleading in specimens collected during or within a few weeks after a serious illness (e.g. an MI or a major operation). They often then show reduced plasma cholesterol and sometimes hypertriglyceridaemia. However, specimens collected within 24 h of an MI will still be representative of cholesterol levels before the infarction.

Routine investigations

One or more of the following investigations should be requested in patients suspected to be at increased risk of ischaemic heart disease or of a lipid disorder:

- *Plasma cholesterol.* This may be sufficient, if decisions about secondary prevention of cardiovascular disease are to be made.
- *Plasma HDL cholesterol,* if plasma cholesterol is raised or if additional risk factors are present. This can be used to calculate the cholesterol : HDL cholesterol ratio, which correlates well with cardiovascular risk and which is used in a number of methods developed to calculate overall cardiovascular risk in making decisions about primary prevention of cardiovascular risk. It is also needed for the diagnosis of hyper-α-lipoproteinaemia.
- *Plasma fasting triglycerides.* This is a weak independent risk factor for cardiovascular disease, a risk factor for acute pancreatitis if greater than 10 mmol/L, and is used in the calculation of LDL.

Specialised investigations

A number of specialised investigations, including ultracentrifugation, apolipoprotein and enzyme studies and molecular genetic studies, may occasionally be helpful.

The primary hyperlipoproteinaemias

The causes of hyperlipoproteinaemia (Table 12.5) are complex, and different disease mechanisms can give rise to similar lipid patterns. The approach adopted here is based on the observed lipid abnormalities.

Increased plasma lipid concentrations may be due to:

- genetic factors;
- environmental factors;
- a combination of the above;
- other diseases (secondary).

Primary hypercholesterolaemia

In about 95% of patients with primary hypercholesterolaemia, the abnormality is due to a combination of dietary factors and a number of yet to be identified genetic abnormalities in handling cholesterol.

In the minority of hypercholesterolaemic patients who have familial hypercholesterolaemia, there is usually a specific genetic defect in the production or nature of high-affinity tissue $apoB_{100}$ receptors. Occasionally the defect is in the structure of the $apoB_{100}$ itself, reducing recognition by the normal receptor. Heterozygotes have about 50% of normal receptor activity, and homozygotes have no receptor activity. Many heterozygotes have tendon xanthomas, and over 50% will have symptoms of coronary artery disease by the fourth or fifth decade. In homozygotes, heart disease often presents in the second decade. Plasma cholesterol is usually raised to 8–15 mmol/L in heterozygotes, and is even higher in homozygotes.

A rare mutation in the *PCSK9* gene can increase PCSK9 activity, reducing LDL receptor levels and causing an increase in LDL cholesterol. This causes a rare autosomal dominant form of familial hypercholesterolaemia.

Familial hypertriglyceridaemia

This group of conditions is associated with defects either in the production or in the catabolism of VLDL. Plasma triglycerides and VLDL are increased, plasma cholesterol is often also moderately increased, and plasma HDL is often reduced. Patients have an increased risk of ischaemic heart disease.

Table 12.5 **The primary hyperlipoproteinaemias (genetic classification).**

Hyperlipoproteinaemia	Concentrations in plasma		Lipoproteins mainly affected
	Cholesterol	Triglycerides (fasting)	
Familial hypercholesterolaemia	↑↑	N (or ↑)	LDL
Familial hypertriglyceridaemia	↑ or N	↑↑	VLDL (and chylomicrons)
Familial combined hyperlipidaemia	↑ or N	↑ or N	LDL and/or VLDL
Remnant hyperlipoproteinaemia	↑	↑	IDL and chylomicron remnants
Lipoprotein lipase deficiency (or apoC-II deficiency)	↑ or N	↑↑	Chylomicrons and VLDL

In some patients, there is chylomicronaemia in addition to increased plasma VLDL. This pattern may be brought on by alcohol excess, and is also seen in patients with diabetes. These patients may have eruptive xanthomas and attacks of acute pancreatitis.

Familial combined hyperlipidaemia

This disorder is difficult to classify, and the method of inheritance is unclear. Even in the same family, the gene does not always express itself in the same way, as there may be increased plasma LDL only, increased plasma VLDL only, or increases in both. The incidence of ischaemic heart disease is 3–4 times greater than in the general population.

 CASE 12.3

A 28-year-old man requested cholesterol testing because his father had died of an MI in his thirties, his paternal grandfather had developed angina in his early forties and died suddenly in his late forties, presumably of an infarction, and there was a further history of ischaemic heart disease at a young age in his more extended family. The GP noted that he had tendon xanthomas on his knuckles and on his Achilles tendons. He took plenty of exercise, followed a healthy diet and was not overweight, did not smoke and was normotensive.

Comment on the history and the following results:

Serum	Result	Reference ranges (adult male)
Cholesterol	10.6	mmol/L
Triglyceride	1.4	<1.7 mmol/L
HDL	1.9	0.9–1.4 mmol/L
Cholesterol : HDL	5.6	
LDL cholesterol	8.1	mmol/L

Comments: The family history and lipid results make familial hypercholesterolaemia the likely diagnosis here, and this is confirmed by the finding of tendon xanthomas. These are accumulations of cholesterol on the tendons, which are virtually pathognomonic of familial hypercholesterolaemia. The exercise he took probably accounted for the slightly high HDL. This, with his relatively young age, the fact he did not smoke and his normal blood pressure, would give him a relatively satisfactory calculated cardiovascular risk. However, these calculations do not apply in patients with familial hypercholesterolaemia, who are at a considerably higher than calculated risk. He merits treatment with lipid-lowering drugs.

Remnant hyperlipoproteinaemia

This is an uncommon disorder characterised clinically by cutaneous xanthomas and a high risk of premature ischaemic heart disease. In the plasma, there is an increase in cholesterol-rich but otherwise VLDL-like particles; these are probably IDLs (i.e. 'VLDL remnants'). Both plasma cholesterol and triglyceride concentrations are increased; plasma LDL is decreased.

This disorder is probably due to a combination of factors. There is abnormal conversion of VLDL to LDL. This is usually associated with the apoE2/2 genotype. As many as 1% of normal individuals have this genotype, but the incidence of remnant hyperlipoproteinaemia is only about 1 in 5000, so the genotype is insufficient in itself to cause remnant hyperlipoproteinaemia.

Remnant hyperlipoproteinaemia responds well to treatment with fibric acid derivatives (e.g. fenofibrate), so its recognition is important. Ultracentrifuge studies provide the definitive means of confirming the diagnosis.

Lipoprotein lipase deficiency

This is a rare autosomal recessive disorder causing hypertriglyceridaemia and chylomicronaemia. The incidence of ischaemic heart disease and acute pancreatitis is increased; eruptive xanthomas often occur. The primary defect is deficiency of either lipoprotein lipase or its activator, apoC-II.

Treatment involves restriction of normal dietary fat and replacement by means of triglycerides containing fatty acids of medium chain length (C8–C11); these are less prone to lead to chylomicron formation.

Other inherited defects

Hyper-α-lipoproteinaemia is an inherited abnormality that gives rise to increased plasma HDL and mildly increased plasma cholesterol. Patients have a *reduced* incidence of ischaemic heart disease. The only importance of hyper-α-lipoproteinaemia is that no treatment is required for the raised plasma cholesterol.

Raised Lp(a) is inherited and is a risk factor for ischaemic heart disease and thrombosis. None of the widely used lipid-lowering drugs, including statins, affect Lp(a) levels. Detection of a raised level can be used to justify the intensification of treatment of conventional risk factors.

Secondary hyperlipidaemia

Probably less than 20% of cases of hyperlipidaemia are secondary to other disease. Patterns of abnormality tend to vary, even within a single disease; plasma cholesterol or triglycerides, or both, may be affected.

- *Hypercholesterolaemia* is often a marked feature of hypothyroidism and of the nephrotic syndrome; in these two disorders, there is increased plasma LDL. The immunosuppressive drugs ciclosporin and tacrolimus, and the protease inhibitors used in the treatment of HIV infection, also cause hypercholesterolaemia. Coronary artery disease tends to develop in those patients with long-standing secondary hyperlipidaemia.
- *Lipoprotein X* is an abnormal discoid particle rich in phospholipid and unesterified cholesterol. It contains albumin within its core and apolipoprotein C on its surface, but unlike LDL contains no apolipoprotein B and is not removed by the LDL receptor. It is cleared by the reticuloendothelial system and the kidneys. Its precursor is bile lipoprotein, and in cholestasis this spills over into the plasma, binding to albumin to form lipoprotein X. Chronic cholestasis (for example due to primary biliary cirrhosis or cholestasis of pregnancy) thus causes the accumulation of lipoprotein X. This particle is probably not atherogenic.
- *Hypertriglyceridaemia* secondary to other disease is most commonly due to diabetes mellitus or to excessive alcohol intake, and is also a feature of HIV infection. It may occur in chronic renal disease and in patients on oestrogen therapy or retinoids. Protease inhibitors cause hypertriglyceridaemia as well as hypercholesterolaemia and this is superimposed on the dyslipdaemia seen in HIV infection.

The effects of alcohol on plasma lipids are complex. Regular drinking of small amounts increases plasma HDL without affecting other lipoprotein particles. Some heavy drinkers develop hypertriglyceridaemia due to increased plasma VLDL, possibly as a result of increased direction of fatty acid metabolism into triglyceride synthesis in the liver.

The hyperlipidaemia secondary to diabetes mellitus is also complex. Increased plasma VLDL is the usual finding, but often plasma LDL is also increased, whereas plasma HDL is reduced.

 CASE 12.4

A 33-year-old man was referred to the lipid clinic with a cholesterol of 10.2 mmol/L. He had a vague memory of having his cholesterol checked at a medical examination at work in his early twenties, and thought it had been normal at that time. He had been dieting for the last few months and had succeeded in losing ~3 kg, but his cholesterol had not changed. Over the preceding 2 years he had felt tired, and stressed by his work. His GP felt that he was depressed, and had been treating him with anti-depressants with little benefit. He had stopped playing football, and his muscles ached on exertion. He had put on 20 kg over this period.

Comment on the following results:

Serum	Result	Reference ranges (adult male)
Cholesterol	10.2	mmol/L
Triglyceride	1.1	<1.7 mmol/L
HDL	1.0	0.9–1.4 mmol/L
TSH	256	0.2–4.5 U/L
FT4	<6	9–21 pmol/L
CK	12 330	55–170 U/L
Na	129	135–145 mmol/L

Comments: He has an extremely high cholesterol that has not improved with diet; if his recollections were accurate, he had previously had a normal cholesterol. This raises the question of a secondary hypercholesterolaemia. He has certainly put on weight, which may increase lipids, but not usually to this extent. His symptoms of weight gain, tiredness and depression raised the possibility of hypothyroidism, and this was confirmed by his profoundly hypothyroid thyroid function tests. Hypothyroidism can also cause a myopathy, with aching muscles and very high CK, and a dilutional hyponatraemia. He thus had the full range of biochemical abnormalities that may be seen in hypothyroidism! Treatment with thyroxine resulted in a dramatic improvement in all his symptoms apart from the muscle aching, which still persisted 6 months later. Cholesterol came down to a satisfactory 4.6 mmol/L without the need for any lipid-lowering medication. CK and sodium returned to normal.

The primary hypolipoproteinaemias

Three rare familial diseases require brief mention. Their recognition has helped with the understanding of normal lipoprotein metabolism.

- *Tangier disease* is due to an increased rate of apoA-I catabolism. Only traces of HDL are detectable in plasma, and plasma LDL cholesterol is also reduced. Cholesterol esters accumulate in the lymphoreticular system, probably due to excessive phagocytosis of the abnormal chylomicrons and VLDL remnants that result from the apoA-I deficiency.
- *Abetalipoproteinaemia* is associated with a complete absence of apoB. The lipoproteins that normally contain apoB in significant amounts (i.e. chylomicrons, VLDL, IDL and LDL) are *absent* from plasma. Plasma cholesterol and triglycerides are very low.
- *Hypobetalipoproteinaemia* is due to decreased synthesis of apoB. Plasma VLDL and LDL, although reduced, are not absent.

Secondary hypolipidaemia

Greatly reduced plasma cholesterol concentration occurs whenever hepatic protein synthesis is depressed, as in protein-energy malnutrition (PEM; e.g. kwashiorkor in children), severe malabsorption or some forms of chronic liver disease.

Other biochemical cardiovascular risk factors or markers

Very high levels of homocysteine, up to 50-fold normal, are seen in homocystinuria, an inborn error of metabolism due to deficiency of the enzyme cystathionine β-synthase. Patients develop ocular, skeletal and vascular problems, with increased arterial and venous thrombotic events at an early age, and a markedly increased mortality. Lowering homocysteine in this group of patients has been demonstrated to lower the risk of cardiovascular disease.

Much lesser elevations in homocysteine levels are associated with an increased risk of cardiovascular disease, with patients in the upper quartile having twice the risk of patients in the lowest quartile, possibly through mechanisms involving endothelial damage and the promotion of thrombosis. However, the precise relationship remains unclear, and raised homocysteine may yet prove to be simply a marker of increased vascular risk rather than a causative risk factor. Homocysteine levels are strongly influenced both by genetic factors and by diet. Folic acid and vitamins B_6 and B_{12} are involved in the catabolic pathways of homocysteine; deficiencies of these vitamins can cause elevation of homocysteine levels and supplementation can cause its reduction. So far, controlled trials of the effect of supplementation of these vitamins on the development or recurrence of cardiovascular disease have had equivocal or negative results. Because of this the precise role of homocysteine measurement remains unclear. However, it may be measured in individuals with a personal or family history of cardiovascular disease in the absence of the conventional well-established risk factors such as hypercholesterolaemia or hypertension. Finding a high homocysteine under these circumstances provides a possible explanation, and can reinforce advice to ensure that the diet contains adequate amounts of folic acid and vitamins B_6 and B_{12}.

Patients with CRP, an inflammatory marker (see Chapter 16: C-reactive protein (CRP)) at the high end of the normal range (measured with a highly sensitive assay, hsCRP) have 1.5–4 times the cardiovascular risk of those with CRP at the low end of the normal range. Treatment of patients with statins results in a reduction of hsCRP. These observations have led to the investigation of hsCRP measurement for cardiovascular risk prediction or for guiding the intensity of lipid-modifying treatment. The available evidence has failed to establish a clinical role for hsCRP measurement.

Calculation of cardiovascular risk and its treatment by lipid lowering

It is possible to lower plasma LDL cholesterol by dietary and other lifestyle means, but the most effective therapy, usually leading to reductions of up to 30% or more, is with HMG-CoA reductase inhibitors ('statins'). It is this class of drug that has mainly been used in the clinical trials mentioned here.

It is conventional to consider cardiovascular risk reduction under the subdivisions of 'secondary prevention' (where the patient has established vascular disease, and the goal is to prevent recurrence), and 'primary prevention' (where the patient has no overt vascular disease, and the goal is to prevent its development). Multiple sets of guidelines have been published, differing to a greater or lesser extent in detail. These all essentially agree on the division into primary and secondary prevention, on the risk factors that should be treated, the concentration of primary prevention on those at greatest overall vascular risk, and the therapeutic options available. However, the precise thresholds and targets for treatment continue to evolve, and are partly influenced by economic issues. Guidelines continue to be produced as further clinical trials are published, and vary slightly in different countries. No specific guidelines are therefore referred to here, and readers should check their own national guidelines. In the UK this is likely to include guidelines produced by the National Institute for Health and Clinical Excellence (NICE).

In patients with previous MI or with angina, trial results are conclusive. Pre-existing vascular disease is the most potent risk factor for the development of further vascular disease, and the size of the population requiring treatment is relatively limited. Cholesterol reduction by about 25% reduces all-cause mortality by 30% and cardiac events by over 40%. Lifestyle interventions to discontinue smoking, adopt a healthy diet and take exercise are important, but should not delay lipid-lowering therapy. Guidelines suggest that virtually all patients with established vascular disease should be treated with lipid-lowering drugs, irrespective of baseline cholesterol levels. The goal is to achieve a cholesterol less than 4 mmol/L or an LDL cholesterol less than 2 mmol/L and if this is not achieved more potent statins or higher doses should be used.

In primary prevention, large-scale clinical trials have shown that cholesterol lowering (by an average 20%) in hyperlipidaemic men can reduce cardiovascular death and nonfatal MI by about 30%. The available evidence strongly supports the concept that those who will benefit most from treatment are those at greatest overall absolute risk. Someone with multiple modestly elevated risk factors may be at a greater risk than someone with a single markedly elevated risk factor. This means that there is a need for a means of calculating overall risk. The guidelines achieve this by the use of computer-based risk calculators or charts that stratify risk on the basis of sex, age, smoking, blood pressure and the cholesterol : HDL cholesterol ratio. An important caution is that these calculations do not apply to patients with inherited dyslipidaemias. Guidelines then specify the level of calculated risk that justifies treatment with cholesterol-lowering drugs. Guidelines disagree on whether there is a cholesterol target in primary prevention similar to that in secondary prevention, or whether the aim is simply to ensure that all eligible patients are treated.

 FURTHER READING

Thygesen, K., Alpert, J.S., Jaffe, S.A., Simoons, M.L., Chaitman, B.R. and White, H.D. (2012) Third Universal definition of myocardial infarction. *Circulation* **126**, 2020–35.

13

Liver disease

Learning objectives

To understand:

✔ the biochemical functions of the liver;

✔ the different reasons for jaundice and how the pattern of liver function tests can aid the differential diagnosis of liver disease;

✔ the more specialist biochemical tests that are available in the investigation of liver disease;

✔ that minor abnormalities in liver enzyme tests are common in relation to the problem of obesity.

Introduction

The liver plays a fundamental role in intermediary metabolism. It has a central position in carbohydrate and fat metabolism, storing glycogen at times of glucose repletion and converting excess carbohydrate to fat that it exports as VLDL (Chapter 12: Lipids). It is responsible for the synthesis of albumin and many other plasma proteins, as well as most of the coagulation factors. It synthesises bile acids, major constituents of bile, and is the key organ for detoxification, metabolism and inactivation of drugs and the metabolism and excretion of many endogenous compounds, including cholesterol, amino acids, steroid and other hormones. In this regard it also protects the body against potential carcinogens.

Liver disease is relatively common, and the measurements of serum levels of bilirubin, hepatic enzymes and albumin, as well as the prothrombin time (PT), provide simple tests to determine whether disease is present and give some guidance as to its nature.

This chapter outlines the principles governing the use and interpretation of the common liver function tests.

Structure of the liver

Only about 80% of the cells in the liver are hepatocytes (Figure 13.1); the remainder primarily consist of endothelial and stellate cells that line and support the hepatic sinusoids, alongside Kupffer cells, specialised macrophages that form part of the reticulo-endothelial system. The *functional unit* of each liver acinus consists of the portal tract, surrounded by radiating cords of hepatocytes. Blood enters the acinus via the portal tract and passes along the sinusoids towards the central vein. Hepatocytes in the periportal area receive relatively well-oxygenated blood, whereas the hepatocytes surrounding the central vein receive blood that has lost much of its oxygen and exchanged other substances with the cells of the periportal area. The cells surrounding the central vein are therefore the most susceptible to anoxia and injury by a wide range of toxic substances. Hepatocytes in the periportal area also have relatively high concentrations of the enzymes usually measured in blood for diagnostic purposes (e.g. ALP and the aminotransferases ALT and AST), while those surrounding the central vein are relatively deficient in

Clinical Biochemistry Lecture Notes, Tenth Edition. Peter Rae, Mike Crane and Rebecca Pattenden.
© 2018 John Wiley & Sons Ltd. Published 2018 by John Wiley & Sons Ltd.
Companion website: www.lecturenoteseries.com/clinicalbiochemistry

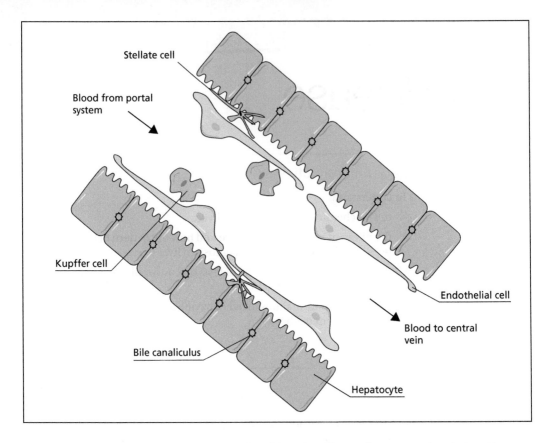

Figure 13.1 Ultrastructure of the liver. The hepatic sinusoid consists of layers of hepatocytes that sit alongside fenestrated endothelium. Kupffer cells and stellate cells have a role in phagocytosis of cellular debris and secreting supporting matrix, respectively. The bile canaliculus is formed by the plasma membrane of two hepatocytes. Blood flows from the portal system, allowing exchange with the hepatocytes, and out towards the central vein.

these enzymes. This may help to explain why some patients with centrilobular liver damage may have normal liver enzyme activities.

Liver function tests

Most laboratories perform a standard group of tests (Table 13.1), which do not assess genuine liver function but are useful for:

1   Detecting the presence of liver disease.
2   Placing the liver disease in the appropriate broad diagnostic category. This then allows the selection of further, more expensive and time-consuming investigations such as ultrasound, CT scanning, magnetic resonance spectroscopy, endoscopy and liver biopsy.
3   Following the progress of liver disease.

Table 13.1 Routine liver function tests (examples of widely performed groups of serum measurements).

Standard group of tests	Property being assessed
Serum albumin, PT	Protein synthesis
Serum bilirubin (total)	Hepatic anion transport
Serum enzyme activities:	
ALT, AST	Hepatocellular integrity
ALP, GGT	Presence of cholestasis

Hepatic anion transport: bilirubin

Measurement of bilirubin in blood and urine is usually used to assess hepatic anion transport, although other anions (such as bile salts) are also transported. Understanding the mechanisms by which bilirubin is formed and removed is essential for the diagnosis of patients with jaundice or liver disease given that abnormal levels of bilirubin in blood can occur in patients in whom there is no liver disease.

Bilirubin production and metabolism

The pathway of bilirubin production and excretion is shown in Figure 13.2.

Production

The body usually produces about 300 mg of bilirubin per day as a breakdown product of haem. About 80% arises from red cells, with the remainder coming from red cell precursors destroyed in the bone marrow ('ineffective erythropoiesis'), and from other haem proteins such as myoglobin and the cytochromes. Iron is removed from the haem molecule, and the porphyrin ring is opened to form bilirubin.

Transport in plasma and hepatic uptake

Bilirubin is insoluble in water and is carried in plasma bound to albumin, and is thus not filtered at the glomerulus unless there is glomerular proteinuria. On reaching the liver, the bilirubin is taken into the hepatocyte by a specific carrier mechanism.

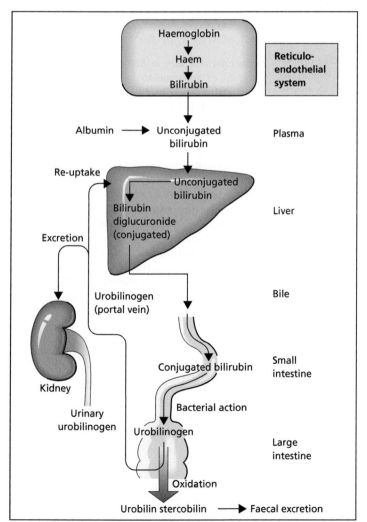

Figure 13.2 The formation and metabolism of bilirubin and its excretion into the intestine.

Conjugation of bilirubin and secretion into bile

In the endoplasmic reticulum of the hepatocyte, the enzyme *bilirubin UDP-glucuronyltransferase* conjugates bilirubin with glucuronic acid to produce bilirubin glucuronides which are water soluble and readily transported into bile. Secretion of bilirubin glucuronides into bile occurs against a high concentration gradient and is the rate-limiting step in removing bilirubin from the body. Secretion is a carrier-mediated, energy-dependent process.

Further metabolism of bilirubin in the gut

Bilirubin glucuronides cannot be reabsorbed from the gut and are degraded by bacterial action, mainly in the colon, to a mixture of colourless, water-soluble compounds collectively termed urobilinogen. These compounds oxidise to brown compounds known as urobilins and stercobilins and are excreted in the faeces. A small percentage of urobilinogen is absorbed and carried to the liver in the portal blood supply, that is, it undergoes an *enterohepatic circulation*. Most of this urobilinogen is cleared by the liver, but a proportion escapes clearance and is filtered at the kidney and appears in the urine, where it can be detected using point of care urine dipsticks.

Measurements of serum bilirubin

Normally, more than 95% of bilirubin in serum is unconjugated, but in liver disease the conjugated form may predominate. For most purposes, the measurement of serum total bilirubin (i.e. the sum of unconjugated and conjugated forms) is sufficient, particularly when results are interpreted in relation to the patient's history, findings on clinical examination and the results of urine urobilinogen and bilirubin measurements. Occasionally, it may be helpful to measure serum conjugated bilirubin and unconjugated bilirubin separately, especially in neonates (Chapter 22: Neonatal jaundice).

Hepatocellular damage: aminotransferase measurements

Soluble cytoplasmic enzymes and, to a lesser extent, mitochondrial enzymes are released into plasma in hepatocellular damage. The measurement of the activity of ALT or AST in serum provides a sensitive index of hepatocellular damage. Serum ALT measurements are more liver specific than those of AST. Cytoplasmic and mitochondrial isoenzymes of AST exist and, in chronic hepatocellular disease (e.g. cirrhosis), serum AST tends to be increased to a greater extent than ALT. The aminotransferases are mainly located in the periportal hepatocytes, and they do not give a reliable indication of centrilobular liver damage. As with all tests based on the release of enzymes from damaged tissue, there is a lag period of some 24 h from the initiation of tissue damage to the first appearance of increased enzyme levels in the plasma.

Cholestasis: alkaline phosphatase and γ-glutamyltransferase

Some enzymes, such as ALP and GGT, are normally attached, or 'anchored', to the biliary canalicular and sinusoidal membranes of the hepatocyte. For this reason, ALP and GGT tend to be released into plasma in only small amounts following hepatocellular damage. However, they are released in much greater amounts when there is cholestasis, since their synthesis is induced and they are rendered soluble – due, at least in part, to the presence of high hepatic concentrations of bile acids.

Changes in the activities of GGT and ALP often parallel each other in cholestatic liver disease. Serum GGT has the advantage of being more liver specific, as serum ALP may also be increased due to release from bone in bone disease. However, alcohol and many drugs such as anti-convulsants may induce the expression of GGT without causing cholestasis. An isolated increase in GGT should thus be interpreted with caution.

Hepatic protein synthesis

The measurement of certain plasma proteins provides an index of the liver's ability to synthesise protein.

Albumin

In chronic hepatocellular damage, there is impaired albumin synthesis with an accompanying fall in serum albumin. Albumin measurements provide a fairly good index of the progress of chronic liver disease. In acute liver disease, however, there may be little or no reduction in serum albumin, as the biological half-life is about 20 days and the fractional clearance rate is therefore low. Factors other than impaired hepatic synthesis may lead to a decreased serum albumin concentration. These include loss of albumin into the extravascular compartment, ascites, increased degradation, poor nutritional status and a fall as part of the acute-phase response.

Ascites

Increased portal venous pressure, a low plasma colloid oncotic pressure and Na⁺ retention due to secondary hyperaldosteronism combine to cause ascites in cirrhotic patients. This often develops when serum albumin falls below 30 g/L.

Coagulation factors

In liver disease, the synthesis of prothrombin and other clotting factors is diminished, leading to an increased *PT*. This may be one of the earliest abnormalities seen in patients with hepatocellular damage, because prothrombin has a short half-life (<6 h). The PT is often expressed as a ratio to a control value (the international normalised ratio, or INR).

Deficiency of *fat-soluble vitamin K*, due to failure of absorption of lipids, may also cause a prolonged PT. In vitamin K deficiency, the coagulation defect can often be corrected by parenteral administration of vitamin K, but this has no effect in patients with hepatocellular damage.

Immunoglobulins

Serum Ig measurements are of little value in liver disease because the changes are of low specificity. In most types of cirrhosis, serum IgA is often increased, while in primary biliary cirrhosis, serum IgM increases greatly. In chronic active hepatitis, serum IgG tends to be most increased.

Serological tests

Anti-mitochondrial antibodies (AMA) are present in over 95% of patients with primary biliary cirrhosis, and anti-smooth muscle and anti-nuclear antibodies are found in about 50% of patients with chronic active hepatitis. Viral antigens and antibody measurements are also important in detecting infective causes of liver disease.

Markers of fibrosis

A variety of markers have been described that may be of help in the assessment of hepatic fibrosis. Procollagen type III terminal peptide and hyaluronic acid (hyaluronan) are the most commonly used tests. These are discussed further in the section on NAFLD (Chapter 13: Nonalcoholic liver disease (NAFLD)).

Other liver function tests

A number of liver function tests have been described that give an indication of the functional liver mass. These tests are not often used but include the aminopyrine

---

 CASE 13.1

A 40-year-old housewife complained to her GP of generalised severe itching during the previous 9 months. She had no other symptoms, and she said that her alcohol consumption was small (2–3 U/week). On clinical examination, she was slightly jaundiced, and bilirubin was detected in the urine. The results of liver function tests were as follows:

Serum	Result	Reference range
Albumin	38	35–50 g/L
ALP activity	450	40–125 U/L
ALT activity	60	10–50 U/L

Serum	Result	Reference range
Bilirubin, total	60	3–21 μmol/L
GGT activity	150	10–55 U/L

Comments: This patient has cholestatic jaundice. Her pruritus is caused by the retention of bile salts. The presence of serum anti-mitochondrial antibodies in high titre indicated that the diagnosis was primary biliary cirrhosis, one of the causes of intrahepatic cholestasis. Retention of bile salts within the liver is liable to cause hepatocellular damage, which could account for the increased serum ALT activity in this patient.

breath tests, the galactose elimination test and the monoethylglycinexylidide (MEGX) test. The measurement of bile acids is primarily used for investigating hepatic dysfunction associated with pregnancy (Chapter 11: Obstetric cholestasis).

Disordered metabolism

Patients with severe liver disease may have:

1 significant *decreases in serum urea*, due to failure of the liver to convert amino acids and NH_3 to urea; these changes occur late in the disease. Note that there are other causes of a low serum urea (Table 4.2);

2 *increased plasma ammonia*, due to disruption of the urea cycle; this usually occurs late in disease;

3 *hypoglycaemia* due to impaired gluconeogenesis or glycogen breakdown, or both;

4 raised concentrations of all the *serum lipid fractions*, if cholestasis is present. An abnormal lipoprotein that contains high concentrations of phospholipid, *lipoprotein X*, is present in serum in nearly all the cases of cholestasis.

The place of biochemical tests in the diagnosis of liver disease

The jaundiced patient

Jaundice is due to hyperbilirubinaemia and becomes clinically apparent when the serum bilirubin exceeds about 50 μmol/L, although smaller degrees of hyperbilirubinaemia may be of diagnostic significance.

Measurements of serum bilirubin give a quantitative index of the severity of the jaundice; serum liver

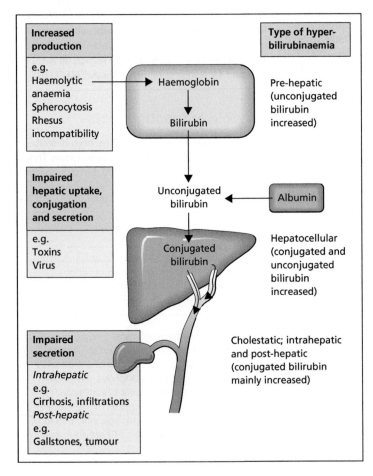

Figure 13.3 Types and causes of hyperbilirubinaemia.

Table 13.2 Bilirubin and urobilinogen measurements (examples of results in various conditions).

| Condition | Urine tests (point of care) | | Serum bilirubin | |
	Urobilinogen	Bilirubin	Total* (μmol/L)	Conjugated
Healthy individuals	Trace	Nil	2–21	About 5%
Gilbert's syndrome	Trace	Nil	<50	Below 5%
Haemolytic diseases	Increased	Nil	<60	Below 5%
Hepatitis:				
• Prodromal	Increased	Detectable	<35	Raised
• Icteric stage	Undetectable	Present	<250	Much raised
• Recovery stage	Detectable	Falling	Falling	Falling
Biliary obstruction	Undetectable	Present	<400	Much raised

*Values for serum total bilirubin are included so as to give indications of the order of severity of the hyperbilirubinaemia that may be observed in the various conditions listed.

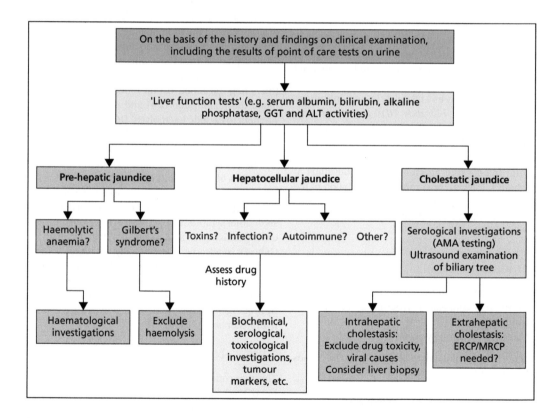

Figure 13.4 The investigation of jaundice. Dilated bile ducts in obstructive jaundice may be seen using ultrasonography. Further assessment is then possible using endoscopic retrograde cholangiopancreatography (ERCP) or magnetic resonance cholangiopancreatography (MRCP).

enzyme activity measurements and point of care tests on fresh urine specimens, for bilirubin and urobilinogen, usually allow the cause of jaundice to be defined as pre-hepatic, hepatocellular or cholestatic (Figure 13.3). Further appropriate tests can then be requested (Table 13.2).

Investigations of the jaundiced patient often use the strategy shown in Figure 13.4. Increased serum bilirubin can arise as a consequence of increased production, impaired metabolism or decreased biliary excretion.

Pre-hepatic hyperbilirubinaemia

This is due to overproduction of bilirubin causing an increase in serum unconjugated bilirubin. It occurs in

- haemolytic anaemia;
- haemolytic disease of the newborn, due to rhesus incompatibility;
- ineffective erythropoiesis (e.g. pernicious anaemia);
- gastrointestinal bleeding;
- extensive tissue bruising.

Hepatocellular hyperbilirubinaemia

This can arise from:

1   *hepatocellular damage* caused by infective agents, drugs/toxins, autoimmune and inherited disorders;
2   *cirrhosis* – usually as a relatively late complication;
3   *low activity of bilirubin UDP-glucuronyltransferase* in congenital deficiency (Gilbert's syndrome and Crigler–Najjar syndrome; see Chapter 13: The congenital hyperbilirubinaemias), premature infants (the enzyme normally develops at about full term), or competitive inhibition of the enzyme by drugs (e.g. due to novobiocin). This leads to increased serum unconjugated bilirubin only.

Cholestatic hyperbilirubinaemia

Cholestasis may be intrahepatic or extrahepatic. In both, there is conjugated hyperbilirubinaemia and bilirubinuria.
    Cholestasis commonly occurs in

- acute hepatocellular damage (e.g. due to infectious hepatitis);
- cirrhosis;
- intrahepatic carcinoma (most commonly secondary);
- primary biliary cirrhosis;
- drug toxicity (e.g. methyltestosterone, phenothiazines).

Extrahepatic cholestasis is most often due to

- gallstones;
- carcinoma of the head of the pancreas;
- carcinoma of the biliary tree;
- primary sclerosing cholangitis;
- bile duct compression from other causes.

The congenital hyperbilirubinaemias

These are all due to inherited defects in the mechanism of bilirubin transport and metabolism.

Gilbert's syndrome

This familial autosomal dominant trait is probably present in 5–10% of the population, with a relative preponderance in males. The unconjugated hyperbilirubinaemia that results is usually asymptomatic, and serum bilirubin fluctuates, with higher values tending to occur during intercurrent illness. Most patients have a serum bilirubin less than 50 μmol/L, but higher values are possible. Other commonly performed tests of 'liver function' are normal, and there is no bilirubinuria.

Gilbert's syndrome is caused by decreased expression of bilirubin UDP-glucuronyltransferase 1A1, due to a mutation in the promoter region of the gene. The syndrome can most easily be differentiated from the mild degree of hyperbilirubinaemia in haemolytic anaemia by analysis of red blood cell parameters (including full blood count, reticulocyte count and blood film), alongside LDH and haptoglobin measurement to exclude haemolysis. Determination of the proportion of conjugated bilirubin in serum is also useful in aiding the diagnosis; in Gilbert's syndrome, the proportion of conjugated bilirubin is usually below 30% of the total bilirubin.

In most cases, the finding of an isolated increase in unconjugated bilirubin, and the absence of haemolysis or other symptoms suggestive of hepatobiliary disease is sufficient to make a presumptive diagnosis of Gilbert's syndrome. Occasionally, in cases where unconjugated bilirubin is unusually high or when more than one cause of hyperbilirubinaemia is suspected, it may be necessary to confirm the diagnosis by sequencing of the promoter region of the glucuronyltransferase 1A1 gene.

Crigler–Najjar syndrome

This rare condition is due to a mutation in the bilirubin UDP-glucuronyltransferase gene *UGT1A1*, resulting in low enzyme activity. Individuals demonstrate severe unconjugated hyperbilirubinaemia in the neonatal period, leading to kernicterus and often to early death.

Dubin–Johnson syndrome and Rotor syndrome

These rare disorders are characterised by a benign conjugated hyperbilirubinaemia, accompanied by bilirubinuria. In both, there is a defect in the transfer of conjugated bilirubin into the biliary canaliculus. Urinary coproporphyrins are normal in patients with Dubin–Johnson syndrome, but increased in Rotor syndrome.

Acute hepatitis

This is usually caused by viruses (hepatitis A, B, C, D and E, cytomegalovirus or Epstein–Barr). Toxins such as ethanol and paracetamol can also damage the liver. There is often a pre-icteric phase when increases in ALT and AST activities and in urobilinogen in urine occur. By the time clinical jaundice appears, serum ALT and AST activities are usually more than six times, and occasionally more than 100 times, the upper reference value. The stools may be very pale, due to impaired biliary excretion of bilirubin, and urobilinogen then disappears more or less completely from the urine. ALP activity is usually only slightly increased, up to about twice the upper reference value, but it may be considerably raised in cases (relatively uncommon) in which there is a marked cholestatic element, as occurs in acute alcoholic hepatitis.

 CASE 13.2

A 13-year-old boy was taken by his mother to see the GP because he had been feeling hot for the previous 2 days and had been complaining that his muscles ached. He had eaten little for the previous 2 days. On examination, the doctor found that the boy was pyrexial (38.4 °C) and appeared jaundiced.

There was no abdominal pain or tenderness, lymphadenopathy or enlargement of the spleen or liver. Urobilinogen was within normal limits in urine, and there was no detectable bilirubin in the specimen. The doctor requested liver function tests, which were as follows:

Serum	Result	Reference range
Albumin	45	35–50 g/L
ALP activity	180	40–125 U/L
ALT activity	30	10–50 U/L
Bilirubin, total	60	3–21 μmol/L
GGT activity	35	10–55 U/L

Five days later, the boy had recovered. He had no fever and his jaundice had gone, but serum bilirubin was still elevated at 30 μmol/L, as was the ALP activity at 175 U/L. The reticulocyte count and other

haematological investigations had all been normal on both occasions. What is the most likely diagnosis, and how would you explain the abnormal results among the liver function tests?

Comments: This patient has Gilbert's syndrome. This was revealed when he developed a flu-like illness and went off his food. Caloric restriction in these patients can be used as a test to unmask the latent mild hyperbilirubinaemia. The absence of bilirubin in the urine showed that the hyperbilirubinaemia was due to increased plasma unconjugated bilirubin, and the normal reticulocyte count excluded haemolytic anaemia as the cause.

The raised ALP activity was of bone origin, expected in a child of this age entering puberty when there is rapid bone turnover. The serum GGT activity was normal, which helped to confirm this explanation.

Acute viral hepatitis due to hepatitis A virus usually resolves quickly, and biochemical indices of abnormality revert to normal within a few weeks. A chronic carrier state after hepatitis A infection is not described. The virus is spread through the faecal–oral route. In contrast, hepatitis B and C are transmitted through blood products or other infected body fluids. Hepatitis B can give rise to an acute hepatitis, but this is less common with hepatitis C. However, between 50 and

 CASE 13.3

A GP was called to see a 21-year-old female student who had been complaining of a flu-like illness for 2 days. The illness had become worse, with symptoms of fever, vomiting and abdominal tenderness in the right upper quadrant. On examining the patient, the doctor found that she was pyrexial and jaundiced. The liver was enlarged and tender. On questioning her, the doctor found that she had recently returned from a long holiday in Asia.

A sample of urine appeared dark, and bilirubin was present and urobilinogen was increased. A blood sample was taken for liver function tests, the results of which were as follows:

Serum	Result	Reference range
Albumin	40	35–50 g/L
ALP activity	190	40–125 U/L
ALT activity	560	10–50 U/L
Bilirubin, total	110	3–21 μmol/L
GGT activity	60	5–35 U/L

> **What is the most likely diagnosis?**
>
> **Comments:** The results and presenting features are characteristic of hepatitis caused by an infective agent. The presence of bilirubin in the urine showed that there was a conjugated hyperbilirubinaemia, and the markedly elevated serum ALT activity and increased urinary urobilinogen indicated that the jaundice was hepatocellular in origin.
>
> Both serum ALP activity and GGT were slightly elevated, indicating that there was some degree of intrahepatic cholestasis.
>
> Possible causes could include hepatitis A, B, C, Epstein–Barr virus, etc. In this case, the serum contained a high titre of antibodies to hepatitis A.

80% of individuals infected with hepatitis C become chronically infected and develop chronic liver disease. In the case of hepatitis B, less than 5% of infected individuals typically go on to develop a chronic infection.

Poisoning and drugs

Many drugs are capable of inducing acute hepatitis similar to that seen in viral hepatitis. In its severest form, the hepatitis can lead to acute hepatic failure; in the UK and USA up to 50% of cases of acute hepatic failure are caused by drug-induced liver injury.

The most commonly implicated agents in liver dysfunction include paracetamol (see Chapter 21: Specific drugs and poisons), nonsteroidal anti-inflammatory agents (NSAIDs), statins and antimicrobials, and the mechanisms involved are diverse. Some agents primarily exert an acute hepatitis (e.g. paracetamol, NSAIDs), whereas others may predominantly cause cholestasis (e.g. chlorpromazine and tricyclic antidepressants). The chronic use of some agents may cause chronic hepatitis (e.g. methyldopa, diclofenac) or long-term risk of fibrosis and cirrhosis (e.g. methotrexate). The toxicity demonstrated will depend on both the individual patient and the dose and duration of therapy. Importantly, some agents (e.g. phenytoin, ethanol) can induce GGT synthesis without necessarily causing liver damage.

Acute liver failure

This condition is usually caused by paracetamol poisoning or viral infection causing severe hepatitis. It is accompanied by major metabolic disturbances including hyperammonaemia, hyponatraemia, hypocalcae-mia, hypoglycaemia and a lactic acidosis often masked by respiratory alkalosis. The levels of the aminotransferases do not correlate well with the severity of the disease. In severe cases, the prognosis is poor unless treated by transplantation. Survival rates of 60% at 1 year following transplantation for acute liver failure are reported.

Chronic hepatitis

Hepatic inflammation that persists for more than 6 months is regarded as 'chronic hepatitis'. It may be due to chronic infection with hepatitis virus, alcohol abuse or be autoimmune in origin. Often such patients have an isolated elevation in serum aminotransferase or GGT, unless the disease has progressed to cirrhosis. Autoimmune hepatitis is frequently treated with azathioprine. The therapeutic action of azathioprine depends on the production of active metabolites. Toxicity can occur in patients who have low activities of the enzyme thiopurine methyl transferase (TPMT). There is a genetic polymorphism in the *TPMT* gene, and genotyping or phenotyping for *TPMT* is advisable before initiating therapy with azathioprine (Chapter 21: Pharmacogenomics).

Cholestatic liver disease

Both extrahepatic (e.g. gallstones) and intrahepatic (e.g. tumours, certain drugs) causes of obstruction cause cholestasis. The distinction between the two is often clinically important from the point of view of further investigation and treatment, but it can rarely be made by biochemical testing.

Serum bilirubin is often greatly increased, and there is marked bilirubinuria; urobilinogen often becomes undetectable in urine. Serum ALP and GGT activities are considerably increased, often to more than three times the upper reference values, but serum ALT and AST activities are usually only moderately raised. In long-standing cholestatic jaundice, hepatic protein synthesis may be impaired and serum ALP activity may start to fall as a result, and even return to normal; this emphasises the importance of performing a baseline set of investigations as early as possible in patients with liver disease.

Serum ALP and GGT activities may be markedly increased in patients with partial biliary obstruction, due to local obstruction in one of the smaller biliary ducts, such as often occurs in both primary and secondary carcinoma of the liver. Partial biliary obstruction may have little or no effect on the capacity of the liver to excrete bilirubin, so there may be no evidence

Table 13.3 Abnormalities in liver function tests that may help to differentiate cause.

| Investigation | Hepatocellular damage | | Cholestasis | Cirrhosis | Tumours |
	Acute	Chronic			
Albumin	N or ↓	N to ↓↓	N or ↓	N or ↓	N or ↓
Bilirubin (total)	N to ↑↑	N or ↑	N to ↑↑	N or ↑	N
Aminotransferases	↑↑ or ↑↑↑	N or ↑	N or ↑	N or ↑	N or ↑
ALP	N or ↑	N or ↑	↑↑	N to ↑↑	↑
GGT	N or ↑	N or ↑	↑↑	N or ↑	↑
Igs	N or ↑	↑‡	↑†	N or ↑*	N
PT	N or ↑	N or ↑	N or ↑	N or ↑	N
Effect of parenteral vitamin K on PT	None	May correct	May correct	None	

N = normal; ↑ = increased; ↑↑ = much increased; ↑↑↑ = very much increased; ↓ = decreased; ↓↓ = much decreased. N indicates that serum bilirubin is often normal when cholestasis is localised, as it often is with secondary deposits in the liver.
*Serum IgA is particularly increased in cirrhosis.
†Serum IgM is increased in primary biliary cirrhosis.
‡Serum IgG is increased in chronic active hepatitis.

of jaundice in these patients, at least initially; bilirubin excretion in the other parts of the liver may be capable of fully compensating for the sector affected by the local biliary obstruction.

Biochemical features that may help to distinguish cholestasis from hepatocellular damage are summarised in Table 13.3. These are 'typical' findings, and many cases do not follow these patterns exactly. The distinction between intrahepatic and extrahepatic cholestasis is usually made by radiological investigations, for example ultrasound for initial assessment of dilated bile ducts followed by endoscopic retrograde cholangiopancreatography (ERCP) or magnetic resonance cholangiopancreatography (MRCP). Liver biopsy may be required.

Infiltrations of the liver

The liver parenchyma may be progressively disorganised and destroyed in patients with primary or secondary carcinoma, lymphoma, amyloidosis, reticuloses, tuberculosis, sarcoidosis and abscesses. These diseases often lead to partial biliary obstruction, with the associated biochemical changes described above. Serum α-foetoprotein (AFP) is often greatly increased in hepatocellular carcinoma (Chapter 17: Tumour markers commonly used in clinical practice) but it can also be moderately increased in chronic hepatitis and cirrhosis. Regular monitoring of serum AFP is also useful for monitoring patients who are at increased risk of developing hepatocellular carcinoma (e.g. those with

 CASE 13.4

A 68-year-old retired labourer presented complaining of loss of weight, tiredness and loss of appetite. He had lost 19 kg during the previous 3 months, but had been eating normally up until 3 weeks previously. He had experienced no pain, but on questioning admitted to drinking moderately for most of his life. He also stated that he had been passing dark urine for some time and that his stools were quite pale.

The examination showed a tired, thin man with jaundice. There was a palpable mass in the right upper quadrant of the abdomen, with no tenderness. The results of the liver function tests were

Serum	Result	Reference range
Albumin	32	35–50 g/L
ALP activity	632	40–125 U/L
ALT activity	55	10–50 U/L
Bilirubin, total	90	3–21 μmol/L
GGT activity	200	10–55 U/L

Urine analysis showed the presence of bilirubin, and urobilinogen was undetectable. AFP in plasma was not increased.

What is the most likely diagnosis?

Comments: The pale stools, presence of bilirubin and lack of urobilinogen in the urine, accompanied by high serum activities of ALP and GGT, suggest that the patient has cholestatic jaundice. The abdominal mass suggested that a tumour of the biliary tract or the pancreas may be responsible. Hepatocellular carcinoma was unlikely, as AFP was negative.

Ultrasound showed a large abdominal mass and dilated intrahepatic and extrahepatic bile ducts. A CT scan suggested that there was a tumour at the head of the pancreas that was obstructing the common bile duct.

chronic hepatitis C infection). Patients with liver tumours often have elevated ALP and GGT as the only abnormality due to localised obstruction.

Cirrhosis of the liver

Alcoholism, viral hepatitis, autoimmune disease and prolonged cholestasis are the most frequent known causes of cirrhosis in the UK, although in half the cases no obvious cause is found. There is increasing concern that the obesity epidemic associated with NAFLD in industrialised nations (see Chapter 13: Nonalcoholic liver disease (NAFLD) etc.) may lead to increasing cases of cirrhosis in the small proportion of NAFLD patients who progress to cirrhosis via the development of non-alcoholic steatohepatitis (NASH). Less often, cirrhosis is associated with metabolic disorders such as Wilson's disease (see Chapter 13: Copper in liver disease), cystic fibrosis (Chapter 22: Cystic fibrosis), α_1-antitrypsin deficiency (Chapter 16: α_1-Antitrypsin (AAT) (α_1-anti-protease)), or haemochromatosis (Chapter 18: Iron overload).

Mild cirrhosis In these cases, no clinical abnormalities may be apparent, due to the reserve functional capacity of the liver. Serum GGT measurements provide a sensitive means of detecting mild cirrhosis, but most heavy drinkers (many of whom do *not* have cirrhosis of the liver) have raised serum GGT activity; this usually declines within 2 months of stopping drinking. Marked abnormalities in liver function tests are rarely present.

Severe cirrhosis The following clinical features may occur, either alone or in combination: haematemesis, ascites and acute hepatic decompensation, often fatal. Jaundice may develop, serum albumin falls and the PT becomes abnormal. Clinical deterioration accompanied by prolonged PT, a generalised aminoaciduria, increased plasma ammonia and reduced serum urea may herald the development of acute hepatic failure.

A number of biochemical markers have been proposed, either alone or in combination, to provide a noninvasive estimate of hepatic cirrhosis. Examples include AST : ALT ratio, N-terminal peptides of procollagen type III (PIIINP), and hyaluronic acid amongst others, although as yet none can surpass histological assessment. The use of fibrosis testing panels such as the European liver fibrosis panel (ELF; consisting of hyaluronic acid, PIIINP and tissue inhibitor of matrix metalloproteinase 1) can further increase diagnostic accuracy.

Amongst the more useful of the biochemical markers is hyaluronic acid, a glycosaminoglycan synthesised by hepatic stellate cells and degraded by sinusoidal endothelial cells by a specific receptor-mediated process. Elevated hyaluronic acid is associated with the sinusoidal capillarisation that is seen in cirrhosis, and values are significantly higher in patients with liver cirrhosis compared with hepatic fibrosis, chronic hepatitis and fatty liver. Measurement of fasting serum hyaluronic acid can reliably differentiate cirrhotic from noncirrhotic liver disease and can be regarded as a useful test in the diagnosis of liver cirrhosis, particularly when a liver biopsy is contraindicated.

The AST:ALT ratio has long been established as a marker of hepatic fibrosis; in cirrhotic patients, the concentration of AST predominates such that an AST : ALT ratio >1 is predictive of cirrhosis. False positives are, however, known to occur in patients with alcoholic hepatitis.

Copper in liver disease

The liver is the principal organ involved in copper metabolism. The amount it contains is maintained at normal levels by excretion of copper in bile and by incorporation into caeruloplasmin (see Table 16.1). The liver's copper content is increased in Wilson's disease, primary biliary cirrhosis, prolonged extrahepatic cholestasis and intrahepatic bile duct atresia in the neonate.

Wilson's disease (hepatolenticular degeneration) is a rare, hereditary, autosomal recessive disorder with a prevalence of about 1 in 30 000, although this is probably an underestimate. The defective gene codes for a Cu^{2+} transporter protein called ATP7B (ATPase, Cu^{2+} transporting, β-polypeptide), present predominantly in the liver but also kidney and brain. In the liver it transports Cu^{2+} in the Golgi apparatus, allowing it to be incorporated into caeruloplasmin. At times of Cu^{2+} excess, the Cu^{2+} is moved into vesicles in the Golgi that are then extruded from the liver cell into the bile, allowing Cu^{2+} excretion from the body to take place. In Wilson's disease, copper is deposited in many tissues, including the liver, brain, eyes and kidney.

Symptoms are primarily due to liver disease and to degenerative changes in the basal ganglia. Serum caeruloplasmin is nearly always low.

The diagnosis may be suspected from the family history or on clinical grounds, such as liver disease in patients less than 20 years old, or based on characteristic neurological disease. Kayser–Fleischer rings, due to the deposition of copper in the cornea, can be detected in most, but not all patients. The following biochemical tests are usually useful:

- *Serum caeruloplasmin:* This is usually less than 0.16 g/L (reference range 0.16–0.47 g/L).
- *Serum copper:* This is usually less than 10 μmol/L (reference range 10–22 μmol/L).
- *Urinary copper output:* This is always more than 1.0 μmol/24 h (normally <0.6 μmol/24 h).
- *Liver copper* is always greater than 250 μg/g dry weight (reference range 50–250 μg/g dry weight). This is the most sensitive test, but it involves liver biopsy.

These tests are not 100% specific for Wilson's disease. For example, serum caeruloplasmin may occasionally be low in severe cirrhosis, and urinary copper output and liver copper may be raised in biliary cirrhosis. However, urinary copper output is valuable for case-finding among relatives, because a normal result virtually excludes Wilson's disease. Full DNA sequencing of the gene is possible in the context of family screening and assessment (more than 500 mutations in the gene have been reported so there is no single locus that can be used for diagnostic testing). Scoring systems that combine clinical findings with laboratory findings can be used to improve diagnostic accuracy.

Abnormalities of other biochemical tests are often present in Wilson's disease. There is usually evidence of renal tubular damage, with a generalised (overflow) aminoaciduria, glycosuria and phosphaturia and, in advanced cases, renal tubular acidosis.

 CASE 13.5

A 23-year-old man was admitted to hospital with fulminant hepatorenal failure. He was jaundiced, with marked abnormalities in his liver function tests. There was also clear evidence of intravascular haemolysis. He had been experiencing vague abdominal discomfort over the past 3 years and, over this time, his liver function tests had been normal with the exception of ALT, which was found to be consistently elevated at 80 U/L (reference range 10–50 U/L).

Abdominal ultrasound showed a picture consistent with cirrhosis, with no evidence of biliary obstruction. Blood cultures, anti-mitochondrial and anti-nuclear antibodies were negative, as were tests for hepatitis virology. There was no history of drug abuse, and paracetamol was not detected in the serum.

A liver biopsy revealed inflammatory and fatty changes, and stained heavily for copper. Serum caeruloplasmin was low at 0.11 g/L (reference range 0.16–0.47 g/L).

What is the likely diagnosis? How would you confirm this?

Comments: The man has Wilson's disease (Chapter 13: Copper in liver disease). The diagnosis was confirmed by finding a decreased serum caeruloplasmin of 0.11 g/L (reference range 0.16–0.47 g/L). The usual clinical manifestations of the disease are caused by excessive copper deposition, particularly in the liver and brain. The biochemical defect is present at birth, but symptoms typically appear in older children, adolescents and young adults. Most patients present with hepatic or neurological dysfunction. The haemolysis is thought to be due to the sudden release of copper from the liver, which damages the erythrocytes. About 30% of patients present with features of chronic hepatitis. Most, but not all, patients have Kayser–Fleischer rings. About 15% of patients with active hepatic involvement have normal serum caeruloplasmin concentrations; this is thought to be due to hepatic inflammation, which leads to an increase in caeruloplasmin production as part of the acute-phase response that may be sufficient to bring values into the reference range.

Patients presenting with fulminant hepatic failure usually die unless a liver transplant can be performed. In other patients, treatment with a low copper diet and penicillamine to chelate and increase urinary copper excretion usually leads to a good prognosis.

Alcoholic liver disease

Chronic over-indulgence in ethanol is a common cause of liver disease including fatty liver, cirrhosis and alcoholic hepatitis.

The diagnosis of alcohol abuse can be difficult, with accurate patient history and physical examination of central importance. The following tests may help provide objective evidence of excess alcohol consumption:

1 *GGT and mean cell volume (MCV) of erythrocytes:* Alcohol induces the synthesis of GGT by the liver, but as a single test for the recognition of chronic alcohol abuse serum GGT lacks sensitivity. The

diagnostic value of serum GGT measurements can be increased by measuring the MCV of erythrocytes as well, and the finding of both a slight macrocytosis and an increased serum GGT activity provides probably the best routinely available combination of measurements for detecting alcohol abuse.

2 *Carbohydrate-deficient transferrin (CDT):* In patients with alcohol-induced liver disease, transferrin in serum has a reduced carbohydrate (sialic acid) content. Serum CDT is increased in about 90% of patients who drink more than 60 g of alcohol per day.

3 *Blood ethanol.*

Nonalcoholic fatty liver disease (NAFLD) and nonalcoholic steatohepatitis (NASH)

The increasing worldwide problem of obesity (see Chapter 15: Obesity) has led to an increase in the problem of fatty injury to the liver, a condition termed nonalcoholic fatty liver disase (NAFLD). The condition is estimated to affect 20–30% of the adult population in developed countries. NAFLD covers a spectrum of pathology from simple fatty change or steatosis through to nonalcoholic steatohepatitis (NASH) and on to more severe fibrosis and cirrhosis. Most individuals with NAFLD have steatosis but a small percentage will have NASH or more serious problems; up to 20% of patients with NASH go on to develop cirrhosis.

Steatosis is characterised by fatty change in the hepatocytes, without significant inflammation or fibrosis. Diagnosis is typically made on the basis of mild elevations in serum ALT and GGT, the former typically less than three times the upper reference range, in the presence of other evidence of insulin resistance (raised or high normal fasting glucose; obesity with central adiposity; typical lipoprotein changes of insulin resistance (Chapter 12: Secondary hyperlipidaemia)). The diagnosis is assisted by imaging studies such as upper abdominal ultrasound scanning which confirms fatty change to the liver. A diagnosis of NAFLD depends upon careful history and examination to exclude alcoholic liver disease and liver disease due to medication, infective and metabolic causes, etc.

Biopsy is the only proven method for accurate diagnosis and to allow simple steatosis to be clearly differentiated from NASH or more severe liver disease. Biopsy is not without risk and careful clinical judgement is needed to consider which individuals this should be reserved for. Older individuals (>45 years) with type 2 diabetes, severe obesity or where the AST : ALT ratio is >1 or there is uncertainty about the underlying liver disease might, for example, fall into the biopsy group. Although individuals with NAFLD may not be strictly diabetic, the condition is associated with future increased risk of diabetes and is likely to be a marker for cardiovascular disease. Accordingly, therapies to reduce the problem, including lifestyle issues such as weight loss and raising exercise levels, should be stressed. The place of drug treatment, as distinct from managing cardiovascular risk, diabetes itself or drugs for weight management (e.g. orlistat), is not entirely clear.

The precise reason why a small percentage of patients with steatosis progress to NASH or more serious liver disease is unclear. A favoured hypothesis at present is the so-called two-hit model, whereby the first hit is the insult of fatty change, principally as a result of insulin resistance and the metabolic derangements that follow. A second hit or insult is then hypothesised to promote inflammation and oxidant damage. It seems that steatosis itself can provoke chronic inflammation, probably by increased NF-κB (nuclear factor-κB) transcription factor activation with release of inflammatory cytokines such as tumour necrosis factor-α. Identifying individuals with NASH requires liver biopsy, and attempts have been made to identify the higher risk patient with fatty change who may have progressed to NASH and where biopsy may be indicated.

Other causes of liver disease

These include haemochromatosis (Chapter 18: Iron overload), paracetamol poisoning (Chapter 21: Specific drugs and poisons) and pregnancy (Chapter 11: Preeclampsia and Obstetric cholestasis).

Ascites

Liver disease is the most common cause of ascites. If a diagnostic paracentesis is performed, the appearance of the fluid (blood-stained, bile-stained, milky, etc.) should be noted, and fluid total protein and albumin should be determined. Results should also be interpreted alongside findings obtained from cell count and white cell differential to help establish the cause.

Transudates and exudates

Ascites with a fluid protein less than 30 g/L is called a *transudate*. It is usually associated with noninfective causes such as uncomplicated cirrhosis, in which there is a combination of back-pressure effects and low serum albumin. However, the fluid protein concentration may be greater in some of these patients, and 30 g/L is not a reliable diagnostic cut-off point.

Ascites with a fluid protein concentration much in excess of 30 g/L is called an *exudate*. It usually indicates the presence of infective conditions such as tuberculous peritonitis, malignant disease or pancreatic disease. If pancreatic disease is thought to be the cause, fluid amylase activity should be measured; a serosanguinous fluid with a high amylase activity will help to confirm the diagnosis.

Measurement of the serum-ascites albumin gradient (SAAG) is useful in the diagnosis of portal hypertension, which often occurs in patients with cirrhosis. SAAG is calculated by subtracting the ascitic fluid albumin concentration from the serum albumin concentration; a gradient >11 g/L is highly suggestive of portal hypertension.

Other biochemical tests that are useful in determining the cause of ascites include:

- *Glucose:* Ascitic fluid glucose concentration usually matches plasma glucose concentration; disproportionately low ascitic fluid glucose suggests consumption by white blood cells, bacteria or malignant cells
- *LDH:* Lactate dehydrogenase is usually disproportionately low in ascitic fluid compared to serum in patients with uncomplicated ascites. However, LDH increases where there is an infective or malignant process, such that the ratio of ascitic fluid LDH : serum LDH approaches 1.0 or greater.

14

Gastrointestinal tract disease

Learning objectives

To understand:

✔ laboratory assessment of gastric and pancreatic disorders;

✔ tests of intestinal function;

✔ the investigation of malabsorption and diarrhoea.

Introduction

This chapter discusses the principles and limitations of laboratory tests that are currently available for the investigation of GI tract disease. These tests complement the use of radiological, endoscopic and biopsy procedures which are now in widespread use and may often provide the primary diagnosis. The laboratory tests that have proved most valuable are given in Table 14.1.

Stomach

Peptic ulcer

Most disorders of gastric function are best assessed initially using radiological investigations and endoscopy. Most peptic ulcers are associated with *Helicobacter pylori* infection which weakens the protective mucous coating of the stomach and duodenum. The organism is present in the mucosa and is protected from stomach acidity by the creation of a more neutral microenvironment through the secretion of large amounts of urease and the subsequent conversion of urea to ammonia

and carbon dioxide. This reaction forms the basis of the urea breath test to detect *H. pylori* infection. In the few patients who present with atypical or recurrent peptic ulceration that is resistant to treatment with H_2 antagonists, proton pump inhibitors and antibiotics to eradicate *H. pylori*, biochemical tests to quantify plasma gastrin may be of value.

Tests for *H. pylori* infection

Urea breath test

This noninvasive test relies on the urease activity of *H. pylori* to detect active infection. The patient ingests either ^{13}C- or ^{14}C-labelled urea, and urease, if present, hydrolyses urea into ammonia and isotopically labelled carbon dioxide. Carbon dioxide is absorbed from the gut and subsequently expired in the breath where it can be trapped and quantified. This breath test is used both for the identification of patients with active infection and for establishing the effectiveness of treatment.

Serological tests

Patients infected with *H. pylori* develop antibodies to the organism that can be detected by serological testing. Although serological tests are used to identify patients who have been infected with the organism, they are

---

Clinical Biochemistry Lecture Notes, Tenth Edition. Peter Rae, Mike Crane and Rebecca Pattenden.
© 2018 John Wiley & Sons Ltd. Published 2018 by John Wiley & Sons Ltd.
Companion website: www.lecturenoteseries.com/clinicalbiochemistry

Table 14.1 **Biochemical tests described in this chapter for the investigation of GI tract disease.**

Condition to be investigated	Biochemical investigations
Peptic ulcer	
• *Helicobacter pylori*	^{13}C urea breath test
	Antibodies to *H. pylori*
Zollinger–Ellison syndrome	Plasma gastrin
Acute pancreatitis	Serum amylase activity
Chronic pancreatic insufficiency	Faecal elastase
Intestinal malabsorption	
• Coeliac disease	Anti-tissue transglutaminase IgA
• Bacterial colonisation	Glucose hydrogen breath test
• Bile acid malabsorption	Serum 7α-OH-cholestenone
Inflammation (any cause)	Faecal calprotectin
Verner–Morrison syndrome	Plasma vasoactive intestinal peptide (VIP)
Carcinoid syndrome	Urinary 5-hydroxyindoleacetic acid
Laxative abuse	Urine laxative screen

less helpful in confirming its eradication because of the slow reduction in antibody titres.

Faecal antigen testing

Enzyme immunoassays can be used to detect the presence of *H. pylori* in stool specimens.

Gastrin

Gastrin is a polypeptide released by the G cells in the gastric antrum and duodenum and is a potent stimulator of gastric acid production. Its release is normally inhibited if the gastric pH is low, but circulating levels are increased in patients with chronic hypochlorhydria. Thus, plasma gastrin may be elevated as a physiological response to achlorhydria or hypochlorhydria due to gastritis, treatment with H_2 antagonists, proton pump inhibitors, pernicious anaemia or previous vagotomy. Increased plasma gastrin may also be found in patients with hypercalcaemia or following gastric surgery, as a result of which the antral mucosa may have become isolated from gastric contents. The most important clinical application for the measurement of gastrin is in the investigation of patients with gastric acid hypersecretion thought to be caused by a gastrinoma (Zollinger–Ellison syndrome).

Zollinger–Ellison syndrome

This syndrome is caused by a gastrinoma, that is, neoplasia of gastrin-producing cells either in the pancreas or the stomach, the former being the more common site. Approximately 60% of gastrinomas are malignant and 30% occur as part of the MEN syndrome (type I). Increased gastrin production leads to chronic hypersecretion of gastric acid, which in turn causes peptic ulceration and sometimes diarrhoea and fat malabsorption leading to steatorrhoea. The steatorrhoea is thought to be due to high H^+ in the intestinal lumen; this inhibits the action of pancreatic lipase. In some patients, an isolated simple duodenal ulcer or diarrhoea may be the presenting feature.

The diagnosis of gastrinoma is based on the detection of an unequivocally elevated fasting plasma gastrin in the presence of gastric acid hypersecretion. Patients should not be receiving proton pump inhibitors or H_2 receptor blockers at the time of measurement. Provocative testing may be necessary in about 15% of patients where the basal plasma gastrin concentration is normal or only slightly increased and gastrinoma is suspected. The preferred test involves the IV injection of secretin which usually produces a 2-fold increase in plasma gastrin in patients with gastrinoma, while no change occurs in patients with G-cell hyperplasia.

The pancreas

The pancreas is a complex gland with important endocrine and exocrine functions. Its principal endocrine role relates to the regulation of glucose metabolism through the secretion of insulin and glucagon from the islets of Langerhans, and is discussed elsewhere in this volume (Chapter 6). Pancreatic juice is produced by the exocrine tissue and released into the duodenum where it is mixed with partially digested food. It is an alkaline fluid that contains a mixture of enzymes essential for protein, carbohydrate and lipid digestion. Secretion is induced in response to nervous stimuli, but mainly by the hormones secretin and cholecysto-kinin-pancreozymin (CCK-PZ). These are secreted by the small intestine in response to the entry of food.

Acute pancreatitis

Acute pancreatitis is commonly associated with gallstones or alcoholism; vascular and infective causes have also been recognised. Confirmation of the clinical diagnosis mainly depends on serum amylase activity measurements. Serum lipase is also a highly sensitive and specific diagnostic marker for acute pancreatitis, with some studies suggesting it is superior to serum amylase for this purpose. Serum calcium may fall considerably in severe cases of acute pancreatitis, but sometimes not for a few days; it probably falls as a result of the formation of insoluble calcium salts of fatty acids in areas of fat necrosis.

Serum amylase

Amylase in serum arises mainly from the pancreas (P-isoamylase) and the salivary glands (S-isoamylase). Serum P-isoamylase activity is a more sensitive and more specific test than total amylase for the detection of acute pancreatitis, but total serum amylase activity is most often measured and is usually, but not always, greatly increased in acute pancreatitis.

Serum amylase activities greater than 10 times the normal value are virtually diagnostic of acute pancreatitis. Maximum values of more than five times the upper reference limit are found in about 50% of cases, but are not pathognomonic of acute pancreatitis, because similarly high values sometimes occur in the afferent loop syndrome, mesenteric infarction and acute biliary tract disease, as well as in acute parotitis.

Smaller and more transient increases may occur in almost any acute abdominal condition (e.g. perforated peptic ulcer, ruptured ectopic pregnancy), or after injection of morphine and other drugs that cause spasm of the sphincter of Oddi. Moderate increases have also been reported in patients with DKA. In patients with acute pancreatitis, serum amylase activity usually returns to normal within 3–5 days.

Macro-amylasaemia

In this rare disorder, part of the serum amylase activity circulates as a high molecular weight form which, unlike normal amylase, is not cleared by the kidney.

The diagnosis may be made when the increased serum amylase activity is found to be persistent and, in the absence of renal impairment, accompanied by a normal urinary amylase activity.

Chronic pancreatitis

Impaired secretion of pancreatic enzymes may not be evident until the disease is advanced, but may then give rise to malabsorption, especially steatorrhoea. Tests involving the analysis of bicarbonate and enzyme activity in duodenal aspirate were previously regarded as the gold standard for assessing exocrine pancreatic function. However, they require a high degree of technical expertise and are time consuming, expensive and uncomfortable for the patient, and have now been replaced by pancreatic imaging techniques. The direct measurement of pancreatic elastase in faeces is now regarded as the most useful biochemical test of exocrine pancreatic secretion.

Faecal elastase

Elastase is a pancreas-specific enzyme that is not degraded during intestinal transport. Concentrations in faeces are 5–6 times higher than those of duodenal fluid, and low levels are associated with pancreatic insufficiency. Although patients with modest degrees of pancreatic insufficiency cannot be reliably identified, its diagnostic sensitivity in patients with severe disease is high. False-positive results may be observed in some patients with watery diarrhoea.

Faecal elastase is not affected by pancreatic enzyme replacement therapy and is a convenient test to perform

---

 CASE 14.1

A 25-year-old woman in the first trimester of pregnancy presented with acute abdominal pain. Initial biochemistry results revealed a serum amylase result of 2500 U/L (reference range <100 U/L).

What is the differential diagnosis?

Comments: With an amylase result elevated to this degree, the most likely diagnosis is acute pancreatitis. However, other possible differential diagnoses include ruptured ectopic pregnancy and obstruction.

An obstetric referral ruled out ruptured ectopic pregnancy as the cause and further investigations revealed the presence of gallstones. The diagnosis was confirmed as acute pancreatitis secondary to cholelithiasis.

CASE 14.2

A 49-year-old man presented with a history of weight loss and chronic abdominal pain which was sometimes exacerbated by eating. He had experienced episodes of diarrhoea and had been passing greasy foul-smelling stools, which were difficult to flush. He consumed up to a bottle of whisky per day. Biochemical testing showed that U&Es were within reference limits. Other results were as follows:

Serum	Result	Reference range
Calcium	1.83	2.20–2.60 mmol/L
Albumin	29	36–47 g/L
ALP	183	40–125 U/L
ALT	36	0–50 U/L
Bilirubin	16	3–21 µmol/L
GGT	269	10–55 U/L
Amylase	251	<100 U/L
Random glucose	16	<11.1 mmol/L

Comment on these results. What is the most likely diagnosis?

Comments: When a patient presents with chronic abdominal pain associated with steatorrhoea but without a previous history of acute pancreatitis, the usual diagnostic problem is to distinguish between chronic pancreatitis and carcinoma of the pancreas. The modestly raised serum amylase is not diagnostic of pancreatic disease because similar levels may be found in other abdominal disorders such as perforated peptic ulcer or cholecystitis.

An ultrasound examination and CT scan revealed dilation and calcification of the main pancreatic duct and was consistent with the diagnosis of chronic pancreatitis. The subsequent demonstration of a low level of faecal elastase (76 µg/g faeces; reference range >200 µg/g faeces) confirmed that the exocrine pancreatic secretory function was inadequate. It is likely that the cause of this patient's disease was long-term alcohol abuse and that this was responsible for the elevation of serum GGT through hepatic enzyme induction. The elevation of ALP was found to be due to the bone isoenzyme, suggesting that fat malabsorption had led to vitamin D deficiency, osteomalacia and low serum calcium. The elevated random plasma glucose is consistent with clinical diabetes that tends to occur relatively late in the course of chronic pancreatitis.

because only a single stool sample is required. It is recommended as the test of first choice in the investigation of patients presenting with diarrhoea thought to be of pancreatic origin.

Small intestine and colon

Tests of absorptive function

Carbohydrate absorption

With the widespread availability of small bowel histology, previously established noninvasive tests for investigating the absorptive capacity for carbohydrates have been discontinued in many centres. For example, the xylose absorption test, which was used to investigate the ability of the intestine to absorb monosaccharides, is now available only in a minority of laboratories. Similarly, the measurement of intestinal permeability by quantifying the absorption and urinary excretion of an oral mixture of disaccharide (lactulose) and monosaccharide (rhamnose) is now rarely performed in routine clinical practice. Other than demonstrating that an abnormality may exist, these tests are nonspecific and nondiagnostic and will not be considered further.

Disaccharidase deficiency

Disaccharidase deficiency may be exhibited as intolerance to one or more of the disaccharides – lactose, maltose or fructose. The defect may be congenital or acquired. The most reliable way of specifically diagnosing disaccharidase deficiency is to measure enzyme activity in small intestinal biopsy specimens. Many gastroenterologists advocate monitoring the symptomatic response to a low dairy diet as the most reliable test for lactase deficiency, which is the most common of the disaccharidase deficiencies.

Amino acid absorption

Certain specific disorders of amino acid transport affect both intestinal and renal epithelial transport. In Hartnup disease, there is impaired transport of neutral amino acids, and deficiency of some essential amino acids (especially tryptophan) may occur. In cystinuria (Chapter 4: Tests of tubular function/The aminoacidurias), the dibasic amino acids (cystine, ornithine, arginine and lysine) are affected; however, there is no associated nutritional defect, despite the fact that lysine is an essential amino acid. These disorders are investigated by examining the pattern of amino acids excreted in the urine by chromatography.

Fat absorption

The faecal fat test, which involves 3- or 5-day collections of stools for the measurement of unabsorbed fat, has traditionally been used to assess fat absorption. However, due to difficulties relating to the inherently unpleasant nature of the test, inadequate sample collection, lack of analytical quality control and standardisation, and the limited diagnostic information provided by a positive result, many laboratories have abandoned the use of this test and it can no longer be recommended.

Triglyceride (triolein) breath test

This test avoids the difficulties and unpleasantness of collecting faeces over several days. Following digestion and absorption of an oral dose of ^{14}C-triolein (the marker is in the fatty acid component), part of the fatty acid is metabolised to $^{14}CO_2$, which is then excreted in expired air. A high $^{14}CO_2$ excretion is associated with normal fat absorption, whereas $^{14}CO_2$ excretion is low in patients with fat malabsorption. Despite the simplicity of this test, it is rarely requested and is not widely available. Breath tests have a low sensitivity for mild or moderate malabsorption.

Bile acid absorption

Bile acids are essential for the absorption of dietary fats. The primary bile acids are formed in the liver, conjugated with glycine and taurine, and then excreted in bile. Together with phospholipids, bile salts form micelles, which render dietary fats soluble; bile salts also promote the action of pancreatic lipase and co-lipase, and solubilise the products of lipolysis and allow them to be absorbed. Insufficiency of bile acids may give rise to malabsorption of fat (Table 14.2).

Bile salts are mostly reabsorbed in the terminal ileum through an active process and then transported back to the liver where they are re-excreted in bile, completing the enterohepatic circulation. Disease or resection of the terminal ileum results in a reduction of absorptive capacity and a loss of bile acids into the colon where they may inhibit sodium reabsorption and cause water secretion and diarrhoea.

Evidence of bile acid malabsorption can be obtained by the measurement of the serum metabolite 7α-OH-cholestenone, an intermediate in the bile acid biosynthetic pathway (Figure 14.1), which is increased in the presence of increased bile acid turnover. This test is not widely available; an alternative is the ^{75}Se homotaurocholate (75Se-HCAT) test in which the percentage retention of an oral dose of this synthetic γ-emitting bile salt is estimated by whole body scanning, 7 days after its administration.

Bacterial colonisation of the small intestine

The small intestine is usually sterile. However, when there is stasis (e.g. blind loop, stricture) or a colonic fistula or, occasionally, when immune mechanisms are impaired, anaerobic bacteria colonise the intestine. This often causes fat malabsorption, due at least partly to excessive deconjugation of bile acid conjugates by the bacteria and the premature passive reabsorption of the resulting unconjugated bile acids. This leads to a relative deficiency of bile salts in the intestinal lumen and decreased micelle

Table 14.2 Malabsorption due to insufficient bile salts.

Reason for bile salt insufficiency	Examples of causes of the insufficiency
Impaired synthesis of bile acids	Cirrhosis of the liver
Impaired delivery of bile acids to the intestine (due to obstruction to the outflow of bile)	Gallstones, carcinoma of the head of the pancreas
Impaired delivery of bile acids to the enterohepatic circulation	
Impaired absorption of bile acid conjugates from the terminal ileum	Ileal disease (e.g. Crohn's disease), resection of the terminal ileum
Impaired ability of the liver to clear bile acid conjugates from the portal blood and to secrete them again into the bile	Cholestasis associated with hepatic cirrhosis
Deconjugation of bile acid conjugates in the upper small intestine (reducing their effective concentration at the site of fat absorption)	Bacterial colonisation of the upper small intestine (the 'stagnant gut syndrome')

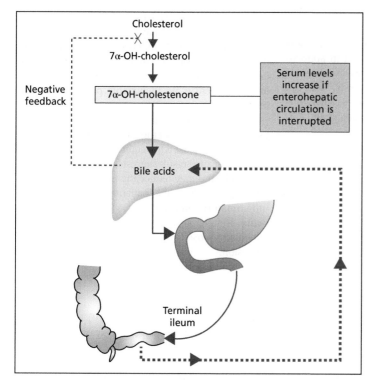

Figure 14.1 Bile acid biosynthesis increases if its enterohepatic circulation is interrupted, leading to an increase in the serum concentration of the biosynthetic intermediate 7α-OH-cholestenone.

formation. Vitamin B_{12} deficiency may also develop due to its consumption by the bacteria.

Investigations

- *Culture of small bowel aspirate:* The definitive diagnosis of bacterial colonisation of the small intestine requires intubation for the collection of specimens, on which microbiological procedures are then performed.
- *Glucose hydrogen breath test:* This is based on the ability of some bacteria to ferment carbohydrates with an end-product of hydrogen, which is not produced by mammalian cells. The hydrogen produced in the gut by bacterial action following an oral glucose load is absorbed from the intestine and transported to the lungs where it is excreted in expired air and can be measured. While the sensitivity of the test is poor compared with the culture of a small bowel aspirate, it is of value if a positive result is obtained.

Serological tests for coeliac disease

Coeliac disease is an autoimmune disorder triggered by a sensitivity to gliadin and is the most common small bowel enteropathy in the Western world. Screening studies indicate that the overall prevalence in European populations is approximately 1% although many cases may remain undiagnosed because of the diversity of symptoms associated with the disease. First-degree relatives of an affected patient have an increased risk of the disease and there is also an association with other autoimmune disorders such as type 1 diabetes and autoimmune thyroiditis.

Serological testing for coeliac disease is now the most frequently requested laboratory investigation in patients with GI disturbances. It is also included in practice guidelines for the investigation of iron deficiency anaemia and in some clinical protocols for monitoring patients with other autoimmune disorders.

Circulating antibodies to tissue transglutaminase (tTG) are found in patients with coeliac disease and testing for anti-tTG IgA is the first-line investigation of choice. The assay is readily automated and has superseded the more technically demanding test for anti-endomysium IgA which is also present. Anti-tTG IgA has a high sensitivity and specificity for coeliac disease and is useful both in screening and in monitoring the response to treatment. A small intestinal biopsy remains the gold standard in making the final diagnosis.

IgA deficiency

It should be noted that selective IgA deficiency occurs in 1:500 of the general population and in approximately 2–3% of patients with coeliac disease. To avoid false-negative serum IgA antibody tests, total IgA levels should be measured in all patients undergoing initial screening. In IgA-deficient patients, anti-tTG IgG should be measured.

 CASE 14.3

A 12-year-old boy who had been diagnosed with type 1 diabetes 6 years earlier was generally unwell and now complained of intermittent episodes of diarrhoea. Initial biochemical investigations did not reveal any electrolyte disturbances or abnormalities of liver function, and haematological parameters were within reference limits. Coeliac serology results were as follows:

Serum	Result	Reference range
Anti-tTG IgA	<0.07	0.1–5.0 AU
Total IgA	<0.1	0.8–4.5 g/L
Anti-tTG IgG	>100	0.1–10.0 U/mL

Comments: This case illustrates the importance of checking total IgA levels when anti-tTG IgA is requested. Here the anti-tTG IgA result was unreliable because the patient was IgA deficient and it was essential that anti-tTG IgG antibodies were measured. The elevated anti-tTG IgG result suggested a diagnosis of coeliac disease which was confirmed by duodenal biopsy showing severe flattening of the villi and extensive loss of the brush border. The co-existence of coeliac disease and type 1 diabetes in this patient is consistent with the recognised increase in the prevalence of coeliac disease in patients with other autoimmune disorders.

Gastrointestinal inflammation

Calprotectin

Calprotectin is a calcium-binding protein derived from activated neutrophils as a result of inflammation and is released into the faeces when pathology resulting in an inflammatory process occurs in the intestine. It is resistant to degradation in the gut and its measurement in faeces has a high sensitivity and specificity for organic disease. Highest levels are found in inflammatory bowel disease (e.g. Crohn's disease and ulcerative colitis) and bacterial infection, but faecal calprotectin may also be increased in cancer of the colon and stomach, colonic polyps and diverticular disease. In contrast, faecal calprotectin is normal in patients with irritable bowel syndrome in which there is no identifiable pathology in the intestine.

The measurement of faecal calprotectin provides a useful noninvasive method of identifying patients with organic disease who require further GI investigations. A negative result suggests that organic disease is unlikely and may reduce the need for endoscopic investigations in some patients. In patients with inflammatory bowel disease faecal calprotectin concentrations correlate with disease activity and may also be used to predict relapse in patients in remission.

Faecal occult blood

Testing for faecal occult blood (FOB) is now firmly established as a tool for screening asymptomatic populations for bowel cancer, and it results in a 16% reduction in the relative risk of colorectal cancer mortality. The success of screening programmes depends on the standardisation of specimen collection and the optimisation of laboratory analysis, which is performed in specialist screening centres only. It is now recommended that for bowel cancer screening a faecal immunochemical test (FIT) for human blood should replace the widely used guaiac FOB test. FIT has fewer false positives and is more acceptable to patients. There is also a growing body of evidence suggesting that quantitative FITs for haemoglobin have a role in the referral pathway and investigation of symptomatic patients presenting to primary care. In contrast, FOB testing using guaiac testing methods is regarded as too insensitive for use in the investigation of patients with iron deficiency anaemia or with symptoms of bowel cancer.

The investigation of malabsorption and diarrhoea

Efficient digestion and absorption require the stomach, pancreas, hepatobiliary system and small intestine all to be functioning normally. Severe defects in the function of any one of these organs may cause intestinal malabsorptive disease; the patient may complain

Table 14.3 Examples of the ways in which GI diseases cause malabsorption.

Dietary constituent	Disease of the GI tract	Why malabsorption may occur
Generalised malabsorption	Coeliac disease	Villous atrophy
Polysaccharides	Chronic pancreatitis	Amylase deficiency
Disaccharides	Intestinal mucosal defect	Disaccharidase deficiency
Proteins	Chronic pancreatitis	Pancreatic peptidase deficiency
Amino acids	Intestinal mucosal defect	Specific amino acid transport abnormalities
Lipids	Chronic pancreatitis	Lipase and/or co-lipase deficiency
	Insufficient bile salts	Micelle formation impaired
	Gastrinoma	High intestinal H^+ inhibits pancreatic lipase
	A β-lipoproteinaemia	Transfer of lipids to plasma impaired

In addition to the above, any generalised intestinal disease is liable to cause malabsorption of all dietary constituents.

of diarrhoea or weight loss. The causes of carbohydrate, protein and amino acid, and lipid malabsorption are summarised in Table 14.3. Most of these have been referred to in this chapter, but a few are considered elsewhere in this volume.

Clinical diagnosis

First, it is important to consider the history of the patient's illness and the findings on physical examination, and to formulate a provisional diagnosis and list the differential diagnoses.

- *Pancreatic disease* may cause malabsorption of protein, fat or carbohydrate, due to deficiency of digestive enzymes.
- *Biliary disease* may cause malabsorption of fat and fat-soluble vitamins, due to lack of bile acids.
- *Intestinal mucosal disease* may affect digestion or transport, or both, of many dietary constituents, and reabsorption of bile acids. The effects may be general, or relatively specific.
- *Bacterial colonisation of the small intestine* may cause a functional deficiency of bile acids, and so interfere with absorption of fats. It may also interfere with the digestion of protein or absorption of amino acids, and decrease the availability of water-soluble vitamins.

Initial investigations

- *Microbiological examination*, including stool microscopy and culture, should always be performed before biochemical tests are requested whenever an infectious cause of a GI disorder needs to be excluded.

- *A faecal specimen* should be inspected; this may suggest that the patient has steatorrhoea.
- *Preliminary biochemical investigations on blood specimens* should include urea and electrolytes, albumin and other 'liver function tests', calcium and CRP. Preliminary haematological investigations (Hb, full blood count, vitamin B_{12}, folate and ferritin) should also be performed.

Further investigations

- *Radiology* (e.g. barium meal, barium enema), *endoscopy* (e.g. gastroscopy, duodenoscopy, ERCP, colonoscopy) and *mucosal biopsy* (e.g. duodenal biopsy) may be indicated.
- *Coeliac serology:* Anti-tTG IgA.
- *Tests of pancreatic function*, for example faecal elastase.

Several other biochemical abnormalities may occur in association with intestinal malabsorption, and require appropriate investigation and treatment. These include:

- *Vitamin deficiency:* Fat-soluble vitamins (A, D, E and K) share absorptive mechanisms with other dietary lipids. Malabsorption of fat-soluble vitamins, which is most commonly manifest as vitamin D deficiency (Chapter 5: Hypocalcaemia/Vitamin D deficiency), occurs in conditions causing fat malabsorption.
- *Defects in calcium absorption* that may cause rickets or osteomalacia.
- *Malabsorption of iron:* This may cause iron deficiency anaemia. Mixed deficiencies of vitamin B_{12}, folate and iron may also occur.
- *Malabsorption of protein:* Reduction in serum albumin most often results, but hypogammaglobulinaemia may be marked.

Factitious diarrhoea

Factitious diarrhoea is becoming increasingly common in tertiary referral centres, and a high index of clinical suspicion may be necessary to prevent extensive needless investigation. Possible laxative abuse should be investigated in a specialist laboratory by screening a random urine sample for over-the-counter laxatives including the colonic stimulants bisacodyl and senna. If possible, the urine sample should be collected at a time when the patient is known to have diarrhoea. It should be remembered that patients may use laxatives intermittently and that a single negative result does not exclude this diagnosis.

Osmotic laxatives such as magnesium sulphate also may cause diarrhoea when used inappropriately, and an elevated faecal osmotic gap may provide a clue to their use. The faecal osmotic gap is calculated by measuring the sodium and potassium concentrations in faecal water and then doubling their sum to account for anions. This figure is then subtracted from an assumed osmolality of 290 mosm/kg, which has been shown to give a close approximation to intracolonic osmolality.

CASE 14.4

A 26-year-old woman was referred to the GI clinic with a 3-month history of abdominal discomfort and intermittent watery diarrhoea. Initial blood tests, including U&Es, liver function tests and CRP, did not show any significant abnormality although it was noted that the serum potassium was at the lower limit of the reference range. Haematological indices were normal. A screen for coeliac disease involving the measurement of anti-tTG IgA was also negative, as was a stool culture.

Measurement of electrolytes in the faecal water and calculation of the faecal osmotic gap (290 − 2 × (faecal sodium + faecal potassium)) yielded the following results:

Faecal	Result
Sodium	17 mmol/L
Potassium	12 mmol/L
Osmotic gap	232 mmol/kg

What conclusions may be drawn from these results?

Comments: A faecal sodium concentration of <60 mmol/L and a faecal osmotic gap >100 mmol/kg suggests that the diarrhoea was due to the presence of an osmotically active substance. Further investigation

demonstrated that the concentration of magnesium in the faecal water was 63 mmol/L (reference cut-off 45 mmol/L), indicating that the diarrhoea was likely to be factious in origin and due to the ingestion of a magnesium-containing laxative.

In secretory diarrhoea associated with colonic stimulants or hormonal causes (e.g. a VIP-producing tumour), the osmotic gap is low (<50 mmol/kg) and the faecal sodium is generally >90 mmol/L.

Carcinoid tumours and the carcinoid syndrome

Carcinoid tumours arise in the gut or in tissues derived from the embryological foregut (e.g. thyroid, bronchus). The most common sites are the terminal ileum and the ileocaecal region. The tumours produce vasoactive amines which, because of the venous drainage of the tumours, are usually carried directly to the liver and there inactivated. Symptoms are only likely to occur either when the tumour has metastasised to the liver, or when the tumour drains into the systemic circulation (e.g. bronchial adenoma of the carcinoid type).

Most carcinoid tumours secrete excessive amounts of 5-hydroxytryptamine (5-HT; serotonin), which is metabolised and excreted in urine as 5-hydroxyindoleacetic acid (5-HIAA). Atypical carcinoid tumours secrete excessive amounts of 5-hydroxytryptophan (5-HTP) and relatively little 5-HT; they may also secrete histamine. Whereas only about 1% of dietary tryptophan is normally metabolised to 5-HTP, 5-HT and 5-HIAA, in the carcinoid syndrome as much as 60% of dietary tryptophan is metabolised along this hydroxyindole pathway.

The *carcinoid syndrome* is usually associated with tumours of the terminal ileum and extensive secondary deposits in the liver. The main presenting features include flushing attacks, abdominal colic and diarrhoea, and dyspnoea, sometimes associated with asthmatic attacks. Valvular disease of the heart is often present. Carcinoid tumours can give rise to severe hypoproteinaemia and oedema, even in the absence of cardiac complications. There may also be signs of niacin deficiency, due to major diversion of tryptophan metabolism away from the pathway leading to niacin production (Chapter 15: Principal dietary constituents/Vitamins/Niacin). Some carcinoid tumours produce ACTH or ACTH-like peptides, and may cause Cushing's syndrome (Chapter 9: Investigation of suspected adrenocortical hyperfunction/

Table 14.4 **Examples of GI peptides.**

Peptide and GI location	Probable functions
Gastric antrum and duodenum	
• Gastrin (in cells called the G cells)	Stimulates gastric H^+ production. Also trophic to gastric mucosa
Duodenum and jejunum	
• Secretin	Stimulates water and HCO_3^- secretion from the pancreas
• CCK*	Stimulates secretion of enzymes by the pancreas, and contraction of the gallbladder
• Glucose-dependent insulinotrophic peptide (GIP)[†]	Stimulates post-prandial release of insulin, inhibits gastric acid secretion
• Motilin	Stimulates intestinal motor activity
Pancreas	
• Pancreatic polypeptide	Inhibits enzyme release from the pancreas, and relaxes the gallbladder
Ileum and colon	
• Enteroglucagon	Increases small intestinal mucosal growth and slows the rate of intestinal transit
All areas of the GI tract	
• VIP*	Secretomotor actions, also vasodilatation, and relaxation of intestinal smooth muscle

*CCK and VIP are examples of peptides found both in the GI tract and in the CNS.
[†]GIP is also known as gastric inhibitory polypeptide.

Cushing's syndrome) in the absence of the symptoms commonly associated with the carcinoid syndrome.

Biochemical investigation of 5-HT metabolism

Measurement of 5-HIAA excretion in a 24-h urine specimen is the most widely performed investigation; the output is usually greatly increased. Bananas and tomatoes contain large amounts of 5-HT; they should not be eaten the day before or during the urine collection.

Timing of urine collection If attacks are frequent, the time of starting the collection is unimportant. If attacks are less often than daily, the patient should be instructed to wait and begin the collection when the next attack occurs.

GI hormones and Verner–Morrison syndrome

A number of GI hormones with various hormonal and local effects have been identified (Table 14.4). Excess amounts of these GI peptides are secreted by rare tumours. These tumours can often be identified by finding raised levels of the corresponding peptide in plasma. For example, in the Verner-Morrison syndrome, hypersecretion of vasoactive intestinal peptide (VIP) causes severe watery diarrhoea and hypokalaemia.

 FURTHER READING

NICE (2013) DG11 Faecal calprotectin diagnostic tests for inflammatory diseases of the bowel. NICE, London.

15

Nutrition

Learning objectives

To understand:

✔ the nutritional requirements that comprise a healthy, balanced diet;

✔ the concepts of malnutrition, undernutrition and obesity and how these arise;

✔ the macronutrient and micronutrient components of nutrition and the effects of micronutrient deficiencies;

✔ the principles of nutritional support and the distinction between enteral and parenteral nutrition.

Introduction

In worldwide terms, nutritional problems are responsible for much morbidity and mortality. *Malnutrition* is a generic term for a diet that is unbalanced and that can lead to illness. Although it is often equated with undernutrition and starvation it also encompasses over-nutrition and obesity at the other end of the spectrum. Individuals may also become malnourished through lacking one or more micronutrients in the diet although this problem often accompanies undernutrition. *Obesity* is an excess of body fat arising from an excess of calorie intake over expenditure. The term *nutritional disorder* is often used more specifically to describe eating disorders such as anorexia nervosa, bulimia nervosa or binge eating (Table 15.1).

Nutritional issues, directly or indirectly, impinge upon many of the tests undertaken in clinical biochemistry. Many analytes are altered by nutritional status. For example, diet exerts important short-term effects on blood triglyceride and glucose levels, and longer-term effects on cholesterol levels. Certain inborn errors of metabolism may demand special diets, which are monitored biochemically (e.g. phenylalanine in PKU). Less obviously, diagnostic tests may only be valid if certain nutritional requirements are met. For example, measurement of 5-HIAA requires exclusion of rich sources of serotonin from the diet (Chapter 14: Carcinoid tumours and the carcinoid syndrome), screening for hypercalciuria requires an adequate calcium intake, etc. Laboratory measurements are also necessary in the management of patients receiving nutritional support, especially total parenteral nutrition (TPN), and in the assessment of malabsorption (e.g. faecal elastase). Suspected nutritional deficiencies, ranging from possible iron deficiency to vitamin or trace metal deficiencies, also require specialist laboratory tests.

Principal dietary constituents

The nutrients in food can be subdivided into the following categories:

- energy (in the form of carbohydrate and fat);
- protein (as a source of nitrogen and essential amino acids);
- major minerals (notably potassium, sodium, magnesium, calcium);

Clinical Biochemistry Lecture Notes, Tenth Edition. Peter Rae, Mike Crane and Rebecca Pattenden.
© 2018 John Wiley & Sons Ltd. Published 2018 by John Wiley & Sons Ltd.
Companion website: www.lecturenoteseries.com/clinicalbiochemistry

Table 15.1 Causes of nutritional problems.

Causes of undernutrition	
Sociopolitical	Poverty, lack of access to food, disease, conflict, lack of safe drinking water, social isolation, alcohol or drug dependency
Physical	Physical disability (difficult to shop or cook), teeth in poor condition
Medical	Condition causing lack of appetite – cancer, liver disease, persistent pain, nausea
	Mental health problems affecting self-care – depression, schizophrenia
	Inability to digest and absorb nutrients – Crohn's disease, ulcerative colitis
	Dementia – unable to communicate needs
	Dysphagia
	Eating disorders – anorexia nervosa

Causes of obesity	
• Poor diet	Processed or fast food high in fat and sugar, larger portions than required, sugar-containing drinks, alcohol, comfort eating
• Lack of physical activity	Sedentary job, lack of regular exercise, inactive lifestyle
• Genetics (rare)	Prader–Willi syndrome
• Medical	Hypothyroidism, Cushing's syndrome
• Drugs	Corticosteroids, some anti-convulsants, anti-depressants and anti-psychotics

- micronutrients (essential vitamins and trace elements).

Food also contains non-nutrients. These include, for example:

- fibre;
- non-nutritive naturally occurring substances which may add flavour, smell, colour, etc. to food.
- substances present as additives or arising from food production (e.g. preservatives, colouring, fungicides used to preserve fruit, growth hormones used in animal husbandry).

Carbohydrates

The major source of dietary energy is normally provided by carbohydrate, in the form of free sugars (e.g. sucrose, lactose) or digestible polysaccharides; the major food polysaccharide is starch, found in cereals, root vegetables and legumes. Nondigestible polysaccharides contribute to dietary fibre. The energy content of carbohydrate amounts to 4 kcal/g. The current WHO recommendation is that free sugar intake should contribute no more than 10%, and ideally less than 5%, of total energy intake. Carbohydrates are not essential nutrients, but insufficient carbohydrate intake leads to ketosis.

Stored carbohydrate is limited to muscle and liver glycogen, with the latter's store depleted 18–24 h after starvation. Dietary carbohydrate that exceeds the body's energy requirements and storage capacity can be converted by the liver to fat.

Fats

Dietary fat consists largely of triglycerides, with small amounts of other constituents (e.g. cholesterol). Triglycerides contain saturated or unsaturated fatty acids, or both. Saturated fats are typically animal in origin, and unsaturated fats are principally of plant or fish origin. In terms of daily intake, the current recommendation in the UK is that energy intake from fat should ideally be no more than 30% of total calorie intake with no more than a third provided as saturated fat. The energy density of fat is greater than that of carbohydrate at about 9 kcal/g. In Britain, on average, 35% of total energy is taken as fat and 48% as carbohydrate, so the weight of fat eaten is substantially less than that of carbohydrate on this diet.

Linoleic and linolenic acids comprise the 'essential' free fatty acids required for membrane synthesis and serving as precursors for prostanoid biosynthesis. Arachidonic acid is also essential but can be made *in vivo* from linoleic acid.

Table 15.2 Trace elements essential to the human body.

Essential trace element	Approximate total adult body content	Daily oral intake (recommended for adults)*	Serum
Chromium	<6mg	0.1mg	<40nmol/L
Cobalt	1mg	As vitamin B_{12}	<50nmol/L
Copper	100mg	1.2mg	10–22µmol/L
Iodine	10–20mg	0.15mg	<5nmol/L[†]
Iron	4–5g	Males: 10mg	14–32µmol/L
		Females: 10–50mg[‡]	10–28µmol/L
Manganese	10–20mg	3mg	70–280nmol/L
Molybdenum	10mg	0.2mg	<15nmol/L
Selenium	15mg	0.1mg	0.75–1.50µmol/L
Zinc	1–2g	7–10mg	10–18µmol/L

*Much smaller amounts of inorganic trace elements are required if these are being provided as part of TPN.
[†] The total concentration in iodine-containing compounds in serum, mainly contained in the thyroid hormones, is 250–600nmol/L; only 5nmol/L is present as inorganic iodide.
[‡] 10–20mg/day in the reproductive period; 20–50mg/day during pregnancy.

Proteins

Dietary protein from both animal and plant sources is required as a source of nitrogen and the essential amino acids (8 of the 20 amino acids used in protein synthesis are essential). The carbon skeleton of the amino acids can also be a source of energy, and protein normally provides about 11–14% of total calories on a 70–100g protein diet; the minimum requirement is 40g of protein of good biological value. Vegetable protein may be deficient in one or more of the eight essential amino acids, but this deficiency can be overcome by complementation, whereby a combination of cereals and legumes together provides protein of good biological value. As with carbohydrate, the energy supplied is 4kcal/g.

Trace elements

More than 20 elements are known to be essential in animal nutrition. Of these, seven are 'bulk' elements (Na, K, Ca, Mg, Cl, S and P) and the rest are referred to as trace elements, present in tissues at less than 100ppm. Table 15.2 lists some data about those that are known as essential trace elements.

The clinical importance of iron (e.g. in haem), iodine (in thyroid hormones) and cobalt (in cobal-

amin) is well established. Clinical syndromes associated with deficiency of copper, selenium, zinc, chromium, manganese and molybdenum have all been described. The effects of iodine and iron deficiency are described elsewhere (Chapter 8: Thyroid hormone synthesis, action and metabolism and Chapter 18: Iron deficiency). Deficiency of inorganic cobalt has not been reported in man.

Deficiencies of essential trace elements usually arise in association with inadequate intake in malnutrition, or with other abnormal nutritional states (e.g. total parenteral nutrition, neonatal feeds, synthetic diets). Excessive losses, especially due to severe and chronic GI diseases, may also cause deficiency. Specific inherited disorders in trace element handling are rare.

Methods of assessing essential trace element deficiency are not straightforward and depend upon specialised techniques available in a limited number of laboratories. Moreover, plasma concentrations may not necessarily reflect actual nutritional status for a particular trace element, where intracellular levels may be more relevant. Changes in concentration may also reflect changes in concentration of plasma proteins that bind these elements. Despite these limitations, plasma values are often taken to indicate a specific deficiency.

Table 15.3 **Known functions of zinc, copper and selenium, and causes and consequences of deficiency.**

Micronutrient	Function	Reason for deficiency	Clinical consequences (where known)
Zinc	Structural/co-factor role for several enzymes (e.g. alkaline phosphatase, carbonic anhydrase, enzymes of nucleic acid synthesis)	Dietary deficiency uncommon but observed with poor intake, malabsorption. Acrodermatitis enteropathica is a rare inherited deficiency of a membrane Zn-transport protein (*SLC39A4* gene). Levels may fall as part of acute phase response (Zn partly albumin-bound; increased incorporation into metallothionein)	Dermatitis, immune deficiency, poor wound healing
Copper	Required for the action of several enzymes: superoxide dismutase (anti-oxidant); tyrosinase (melanin synthesis); dopamine hydroxylase (synthesis of noradrenaline); cytochrome *c* oxidase (energy generation); lysyl oxidase (cross-linking collagen). Circulates on caeruloplasmin which can increase as part of the acute phase response (see also Wilson's disease – Chapter 13: Copper in liver disease)	Rare but in association with long-term artificial feeding and malnutrition in infants fed exclusively cow's milk. High Zn intake can precipitate Cu deficiency (via metallothionein synthesis, which chelates Cu)	Microcytic anaemia, neutropenia. Osteoporosis
Selenium	Structural component of several enzymes where it is incorporated into protein as selenocysteine. Includes anti-oxidant enzymes such as glutathione peroxidase and thioredoxine reductase, and other enzymes such as type I iodothyronine 5-deiodinase. Se deficiency is often assessed by measurement of glutathione peroxidase activity of red cells	Rare but found in association with low Se content in soil, possibly artificial nutrition	Cardiac and skeletal myopathy. Possible increased risk of atheroma and some cancers

Diagnosis may only be made retrospectively on the basis of a clinical condition likely to have given rise to deficiency that can be attributed to the lack of trace elements, and which responds to treatment with the appropriate supplementation.

Zinc, copper and selenium

These micronutrients are more commonly monitored than other trace elements in the assessment of nutritional status, largely because of established deficiency syndromes associated with them.

Table 15.3 summarises some of the known functions of these micronutrients and the causes and consequences of deficiency.

Other trace elements

Chromium may be involved in glucose homeostasis. A chromium complex present in brewer's yeast ('glucose tolerance factor') may improve glucose tolerance in some subjects with diabetes. Malnourished infants may develop glucose intolerance that improves with chromium supplementation. In adults, a syndrome presenting with weight loss, peripheral neuropathy and marked insulin-insensitive glucose intolerance has been described that improves with chromium supplementation.

Manganese is a co-factor for many enzymes, for example those involved in the synthesis of glycosaminoglycans, cholesterol and prothrombin. Despite this, true deficiency of manganese in humans appears to be very rare.

CASE 15.1

A 3-month-old baby boy developed a red rash around his mouth, on the scrotum and on the elbows and knees. His parents reported him to be very irritable and to have developed diarrhoea. Hair loss was also reported. The GP noted that the problem coincided with weaning onto cow's milk. Examination of the child confirmed a sharply demarcated, red, scaly rash and also a red tongue with several mouth ulcers. The child himself appeared well nourished. Laboratory investigations carried out on the child included a plasma zinc level of 3 μmol/L (age-related reference range 10.0–18.0 μmol/L). What is the diagnosis and treatment?

Comments: The child's nutritional status appeared to be satisfactory, both in terms of dietary history and anthropometric measurements. Despite this, the low plasma zinc suggested a specific deficiency of this trace element. It was also noted that the problem coincided with the introduction of cow's milk.

The child has an inherited condition called acrodermatitis enteropathica in which there is a mutation in a gene called *SLC39A4* that codes for a zinc transporter protein called ZIP4. Zinc is more readily assimilated from human milk and the problem can often manifest itself on introducing cow's milk. The condition is recessively inherited and was formerly serious and potentially fatal until the nature of the defect in zinc absorption was discovered. It responds readily to zinc supplementation.

Table 15.4 The vitamins.

Vitamin	Outline of the principal functions	Recommended daily intake	Some effects of deficiency
Fat-soluble vitamins			
• Vitamin A (retinol)	Vision, epithelial cell function	0.7 mg (males) 0.6 mg (females)	Night blindness, keratomalacia
• Vitamin D (cholecalciferol)	Intestinal absorption of calcium, bone formation	8.5–10 μg for children 10 μg for adults	Rickets and osteomalacia
• Vitamin E (tocopherols)	Anti-oxidant, membrane stability	4 mg (male) 3 mg (female)	Haemolytic anaemia
• Vitamin K (phytomenadione)	Hepatic synthesis of prothrombin	1 μg per kg body weight	Coagulation defects
Water-soluble vitamins			
• Thiamin (vitamin B_1)	All the vitamins that comprise the group of B vitamins act as co-enzymes or prosthetic groups for various enzymes that are important in intermediary metabolism	1.0 mg (males) 0.8 mg (females)	Beri-beri, cardiac myopathy
• Riboflavin (vitamin B_2)	See above	1.3 mg (males) 1.1 mg (females)	Cheilosis, stomatitis (as for vitamin B_1)
• Niacin	See above	17 mg (males) 13 mg (females)	Pellagra
• Pyridoxine (vitamin B_6)	See above	1.4 mg (males) 1.2 mg (females)	Dermatitis, stomatitis, CNS symptoms
• Biotin	See above	<0.9 mg	Anorexia, dermatitis
• Folic acid	See above	200 μg (400 μg in pregnancy)	Megaloblastic anaemia
• Cyanocobalamin (vitamin B_{12})	See above	1.5 μg	Megaloblastic anaemia
• Vitamin C (ascorbic acid)	Collagen formation	40 mg	Scurvy, anaemia

Molybdenum is a component of xanthine oxidase and some other metallo-enzymes. Its deficiency has been reported to cause xanthinuria, with low serum urate and low urinary uric acid output.

Cobalt is necessary for vitamin B_{12} metabolism.

Vitamins

Vitamins are all organic compounds that, as originally defined, cannot be synthesised in the human body and must be provided in the diet. They are essential for the normal processes of metabolism, including growth and maintenance of health. It is now known that the body is able to produce part or even all of its requirements for some of the vitamins, for example vitamin D from cholesterol and niacin from tryptophan. Table 15.4 summarises some data concerning both water-soluble and fat-soluble vitamins.

Deficiency may arise from inadequate diet, impaired absorption, insufficient utilisation, increased requirement or increased rate of excretion. Toxicity due to excess vitamin intake of A and D has also been described. Vitamin deficiency develops in stages:

1 *Subclinical deficiency*, in which there is depletion of body stores. These are normally relatively large in the case of fat-soluble vitamins (e.g. A and D) and vitamin B_{12}, but small in the case of other water-soluble vitamins.
2 *Overt deficiency*, which is usually accompanied by other evidence of malnutrition (e.g. protein-energy malnutrition).

Biochemical investigations help to confirm the diagnosis of some overt vitamin deficiency diseases, and may allow the diagnosis to be made at an earlier stage. Several types of biochemical tests are available, of which only some will be applicable to the investigation of suspected deficiency of a particular vitamin. The vitamin may be directly measured in whole blood, plasma or serum, erythrocytes, leucocytes or tissue biopsy specimens. Alternatively, direct measurement of the vitamin or one of its major metabolites in urine is possible. In general, plasma concentrations of vitamins do not necessarily reflect the vitamin status of the body. Measurements of vitamins in cells generally give a much better indication of the body's vitamin status. Plasma levels usually fall before cellular and tissue levels fall, but low or undetectable plasma levels can occur in the absence of deficiency. Conversely, recent dietary intake can cause the plasma concentrations of vitamins to fluctuate markedly, even in severe deficiency. However, a sustained high plasma vitamin usually excludes a deficiency state.

Clinical suspicion of a vitamin deficiency can also be corroborated by observing a response to the relevant vitamin supplementation; however, in the absence of measurements, the level of certainty is lower.

Deficiency of fat-soluble vitamins

Vitamin A

This vitamin is present in the diet as retinol. It can also be derived from dietary β-carotene, some of which is hydrolysed in the intestine to form retinol. A rich source is liver, although leafy vegetables and some fruits also provide the vitamin in large amounts. After absorption, followed by esterification in the mucosal cells, the ester is transported in the blood bound to retinol-binding protein (RBP) and pre-albumin. Specific binding proteins on cell membranes are involved in the uptake of vitamin A ester from plasma into the tissues. The vitamin is stored in the liver, mainly as its ester.

The active form of vitamin A, 11-*cis*-retinal, is necessary for rod vision, and its deficiency can cause night blindness. Another form, retinoic acid, induces differentiation of epithelial cells. Vitamin A deficiency predisposes to GI and respiratory tract infections and leads to night blindness and, if severe, to keratinisation of the cornea, corneal ulceration and, ultimately, blindness. In developing countries, those at risk include premature infants, infants and young children and pregnant and lactating women.

Laboratory measurement is carried out by assessment of plasma retinol concentration. Low RBP levels are found during a systemic inflammatory response. This can cause up to a 50% reduction in measured retinol concentration, even in the absence of any nutritional deficiency. Similarly RBP synthesis is decreased in liver disease and in malnutrition. Plasma vitamin A levels do not start to fall until hepatic stores are significantly depleted, so normal plasma levels do not necessarily reflect adequate body stores, but reduced stores are reflected in low plasma levels.

Vitamin D

The formation and metabolism of vitamin D are described in Chapter 5: Control of calcium metabolism. Rickets in infancy and childhood, and osteomalacia in adults are the main forms of vitamin D deficiency (Chapter 5: Vitamin D deficiency).

Vitamin E

Eight related tocopherols and tocotrienols possess vitamin E activity; they have anti-oxidant properties, and protect against oxidant (free radical) damage to polyunsaturated fatty acids in cell membranes. The active form in humans is alpha-tocopherol. The vitamin is found in oils, nuts, seeds and leafy green vegetables.

Vitamin E deficiency is a rare complication of prolonged and severe steatorrhoea, and of prolonged parenteral nutrition. Altered red cell membrane stability can lead to haemolytic anaemia in children, while skeletal muscle breakdown may be responsible for the raised serum CK activity observed in both adults and children. Neurological consequences have also been described.

The main circulating form of vitamin E is α-tocopherol, which is bound to lipoproteins and therefore influenced by the cholesterol concentration. Measurement is best expressed as a ratio of α-tocopherol to cholesterol. Both α-tocopherol and cholesterol fall in the inflammatory response, and the ratio is unaffected.

Vitamin K

Vitamin K is not only found in liver and leafy vegetables (as K_1 or phylloquinone) but is also synthesised by colonic bacteria (as K_2 or menaquinone). It is necessary for the post-translational modification in proteins of glutamate side chains by γ-carboxylation. The presence of a second carboxyl group on the glutamate side chain confers phospholipid-binding properties on the modified protein in the presence of Ca^{2+}. Proteins containing γ-carboxyglutamate include certain clotting factors (II, VII, IX and X) and the bone matrix protein, osteocalcin. Oral anti-coagulants such as warfarin act by antagonising the metabolism of vitamin K.

Vitamin K deficiency is most often caused by long-term treatment with broad-spectrum antibiotics, long-term artificial feeding, chronic liver disease and fat malabsorption. Levels may be low in the newborn (leading to haemorrhagic disease of the newborn).

Phylloquinone status can be assessed by functional assays such as the prothrombin time (PT) – an important test in the investigation and management of jaundiced patients (Chapter 13: Coagulation factors) and of those on anti-coagulant treatment. It can also be directly measured in plasma. Most of the circulating phylloquinone is bound to VLDL, so the result is best expressed as a plasma phylloquinone : triglyceride ratio. Plasma phylloquinone falls in the inflammatory response but the phylloquinine : triglyceride ratio is unchanged so remains a reliable indicator of vitamin K status.

Deficiency of water-soluble vitamins

Ascorbic acid (vitamin C)

Vitamin C deficiency leads to scurvy, characterised by perifollicular haemorrhages, swollen gums with loosened teeth, bruising, spontaneous haemorrhages and anaemia. Frank scurvy rarely occurs nowadays, but its subclinical form is not uncommon, especially among elderly people living alone. Ascorbic acid is a water-soluble anti-oxidant which maintains iron in the reduced (ferrous) form and which is essential to the activity of lysine and prolyl oxidase which cross-link collagen. Rich sources include citrus fruits, blackcurrants and potatoes.

Vitamin C status is assessed by its measurement in plasma. This may not provide a good index of tissue stores; it is affected by recent dietary intake and by the systemic inflammatory response. It is therefore useful to check simultaneously for an inflammatory response by measuring CRP. In clinical practice, suspicion of vitamin C deficiency may prompt a trial of vitamin C supplementation without formal measurement of vitamin C status.

Thiamin (vitamin B_1)

Rich sources of dietary thiamin include wheat germ, yeast, legumes, nuts and some meats. It is readily absorbed, and the main circulating form is thiamin diphosphate (TDP), found almost entirely within the red blood cells. It is phosphorylated to its active form, thiamin pyrophosphate (TPP), in the liver. It is important as a co-enzyme in carbohydrate metabolism, being necessary for oxidative decarboxylation reactions (e.g. conversion of pyruvate to acetyl-CoA) and transketolation reactions. Deficiency is associated with generalised malnutrition and is also found in chronic alcoholism; it can lead to mood changes (depression, irritability), defective memory, peripheral neuropathy and, in more extreme cases, to beri-beri with cardiac failure. Severe and acute deficiency leads to Wernicke's encephalopathy, with memory loss and nystagmus; it is essential to supply adequate amounts of thiamin during re-feeding when requirements are increased.

Red blood cell TDP concentration is a good indicator of tissue thiamin stores. Assessment of status is by measurement of TDP in either whole blood or packed red cells.

Riboflavin (vitamin B_2)

Dietary sources of vitamin B_2 include liver, kidney and milk products. Vitamin B_2 circulates as riboflavin, flavin mononucleotide (FMN) and flavin adenine dinucleotide (FAD), both in the plasma and the red blood cells. The predominant form is red cell FAD. The nucleotides of riboflavin are the prosthetic groups of many enzymes involved in electron transport, and riboflavin is essential for normal oxidative metabolism (e.g. as a co-factor for cytochrome c reductase and succinyl-CoA dehydrogenase).

Deficiency occurs typically in association with other nutrient deficiencies, due to poor diet, alcoholism or malabsorption. The findings include angular stomatitis,

CASE 15.2

A 56-year-old female with chronic alcoholism is admitted for observation after sustaining a head injury in a fall. She is confused, and examination reveals peripheral oedema and tachycardia. Sensation is markedly reduced in all limbs distally in a glove and stocking distribution and the patient is ataxic, with a slight horizontal nystagmus.

What type of nutritional deficiency might account for the findings in this woman and how might you confirm your suspicions?

Comments: This woman displays the clinical features of thiamin deficiency. This is a recognised complication in a proportion of alcoholics and reflects low thiamin intake, impaired absorption and possibly accelerated destruction of thiamin diphosphate. The principal manifestations of thiamin deficiency affect the cardiovascular and nervous systems. Patients may develop peripheral vasodilatation, retention of water and sodium, and a biventricular heart failure. The tachycardia and peripheral oedema are expected findings in relation to the cardiovascular problems of thiamin deficiency. In the nervous system, a peripheral neuropathy may be found and is shown in this patient in the reduced sensation. The CNS may also be involved, and the clinical features of ataxia and nystagmus support CNS involvement. Confirmation of the diagnosis is best made by measuring whole blood or packed red cell TDP concentration.

cheilosis and skin and eye lesions. Deficiency usually occurs as part of a mixed state involving several vitamins of the B complex, often including thiamin.

Vitamin B_2 status is best assessed by measurement of red cell FAD concentration. This is unaffected by the systemic inflammatory response.

Niacin (vitamin B_3)

This term includes nicotinic acid and its amide (collectively referred to as niacin). Nicotinamide is a component of nicotinamide–adenine dinucleotide (NAD) and its phosphate (NADP); these are co-enzymes for many dehydrogenases. The body's requirements for nicotinamide are met partly by dietary niacin, but a substantial part normally comes from metabolism of tryptophan.

Deficiency can be caused by an inadequate dietary intake. It may also be caused by conditions in which large amounts of tryptophan are metabolised along abnormal pathways (e.g. carcinoid syndrome, Chapter 14: Carcinoid tumours and the carcinoid syndrome), and an acute deficiency can be precipitated

by isoniazid treatment. Severe deficiency leads to pellagra, characterised by dermatitis (typically exposed skin parts), diarrhoea and mental changes, including dementia in chronic deficiency.

Although it is possible to assess niacin status by measuring urinary metabolites or plasma tryptophan, these lack sensitivity and specificity for niacin deficiency. Niacin status is usually assessed by the clinical response to a therapeutic trial of niacin administration.

Folic acid and vitamin B_{12}

Folate is often considered alongside vitamin B_{12} or the cyanocobalamins (there are a number of dietary forms) because both are required as co-enzymes in nucleic acid biosynthesis. The body stores of these vitamins are very different, with folate stores being sufficient to last up to about 4 months, while vitamin B_{12} stores can last for 2–4 years.

The active form of folate is tetrahydrofolic acid, which functions as a co-enzyme in the transport of one-carbon units from one compound to another and is essential for nucleic acid synthesis. Good sources are liver, kidney and fresh vegetables. Deficiency leads to impaired cell division, especially manifest as pancytopenia, with defective red cell maturation (megaloblastic anaemia); folate deficiency is one of the common vitamin deficiency states in humans arising from malabsorption, increased requirement (e.g. pregnancy) or excessive losses (e.g. dialysis) or a combination. Folic acid supplementation reduces the occurrence (or recurrence) of foetal neural tube defects (spina bifida, anencephaly and encephalocoele) by about 70%; the vitamin should be started by the mother before conception. Folate status is assessed by measurement of serum or red cell folate concentration.

Vitamin B_{12} serves as a co-factor for the enzymes methionine synthase and L-methylmalonyl CoA mutase. Methionine synthase converts homocysteine to methionine such that homocysteine levels increase and methionine levels fall in B_{12} deficiency. High homocysteine in plasma is associated with increased cardiovascular risk and the low methionine levels can lead to a deficiency of the methyl donor S-adenosyl-methionine required for nucleic acid synthesis. The mutase enzyme converts methylmalonyl CoA to succinyl CoA which is necessary for haemoglobin synthesis.

Dietary deficiency of cyanocobalamins is rare but is found in vegans (the vitamin is largely obtained from animal sources). The usual cause is pernicious anaemia, in which autoimmune disease causes loss of intrinsic factor that is required for absorption of the vitamin in the terminal ileum. Deficiency leads to megaloblastic anaemia and pancytopenia. Additionally, B_{12} deficiency may lead to demyelination, particularly of the spinal cord, with neurological defects. High folate levels in the presence of vitamin B_{12} deficiency may correct the megaloblastic anaemia but fail to correct the neurological problems. Indeed, in combined folate and B_{12} deficiency, replacement of folate without B_{12} can precipitate subacute combined degeneration of the spinal cord. Deficiency of B_{12} is usually diagnosed by serum levels of B_{12} and haematological examination of blood and bone marrow specimens; it is confirmed by measuring anti-intrinsic factor antibodies (parietal cell antibodies are often present but are less specific). Where B_{12} deficiency appears to be present but there are no anti-intrinsic factor antibodies, vitamin B_{12} absorption can be assessed before and after the administration of intrinsic factor (the Schilling test). This can demonstrate impaired intestinal absorption due, for example, to coeliac disease. It is now only very rarely performed.

Other water-soluble vitamins

The term vitamin B_6 includes pyridoxine, pyridoxal, pyridoxamine and their 5-phosphate derivatives. Good sources are liver and cereals (whole grain). The active form of the vitamin, pyridoxal 5′-phosphate (PLP), is the prosthetic group of more than 100 enzymes largely involved in protein and amino acid metabolism. These enzymes include the aminotransferases – ALT and AST – and amino acid decarboxylases. Deficiency of vitamin B_6 is rare and nearly always occurs as part of a mixed deficiency of the B vitamins. Isoniazid, used in the treatment of tuberculosis, is reported to lead to deficiency possibly by metabolic competition. Body stores are low, so deficiency can develop relatively rapidly.

Plasma PLP is mainly bound to albumin and is therefore reduced by a systemic inflammatory response. Red cell PLP concentration is not affected so is a better means of assessing vitamin B_6 status.

Biotin serves as a co-enzyme for carboxylase reactions, including those catalysed by pyruvate carboxylase and acetyl-CoA carboxylase. Deficiency in man has been reported during TPN, and very rarely in association with excessive consumption of raw egg white, which contains the biotin-binding protein, avidin. Deficiency symptoms include dermatitis, alopecia, mental depression, nausea and vomiting.

Assessment of nutritional status

Malnutrition is an independent risk factor for patient morbidity and mortality, and is associated with increased healthcare costs, so the nutritional status of all patients should be assessed. All hospital inpatients should be screened using the Malnutrition Universal Screening Tool ('MUST'), which takes into account the patient's BMI, any unplanned weight loss, and the presence of acute illness (Table 15.5). High-risk patients are identified by their MUST score and can be more comprehensively assessed, usually by a dietitian. This assessment depends upon a combination of history, clinical examination and biochemical results. The history and clinical examination alone, without biochemical measurements, are often sufficient. A good dietary history, which may require detailed recording of food and drink intake over a 7-day period, is very valuable and may identify generalised malabsorption or a specific nutritional problem.

Physical examination can reveal signs of malnutrition (e.g. bleeding gums in scurvy; dermatitis in niacin deficiency). Nutritional measures include body weight and height (for determination of BMI). Less frequently, skin-fold thickness as a measure of subcutaneous fat, and mid-arm muscle area (derived from mid-arm muscle circumference and triceps skin-fold thickness) as a measure of skeletal muscle mass can be measured, but these are subject to error and do not respond rapidly to changes in nutritional status. Bioelectrical impedance can be measured to determine total body water content, fat and fat-free mass, and is quick, easy and relatively cheap, but subject to errors. Estimates of muscle mass can be made from 24-h urinary creatinine or 3-methylhistidine excretion and of nitrogen losses by measurement of 24-h urinary urea excretion. These are prone to a variety of errors and are essentially obsolete.

Biochemical tests to assess overall nutritional status are of very limited value. Serum albumin concentration is sometimes used but is a poor measure of nutritional state as it is affected by renal and liver disease as well as nutrition. Moreover, levels can fall rapidly as part of the acute-phase response, while malnourished patients may display acceptable albumin levels for weeks (because reduced formation is accompanied by reduced catabolism). Other 'nutritional' proteins such as retinol-binding protein or transferrin offer little advantage over albumin.

In contrast, specific biochemical measurements of vitamins or trace elements may be helpful in nutritional assessment and confirm an underlying deficiency suspected on clinical grounds.

Nutritional support

A spectrum of problems require nutritional support, ranging from specific nutritional support (e.g. avoiding phenylalanine in phenylketonuria (Chapter 22: Phenylketonuria)) to more global nutritional support.

Table 15.5 **Malnutrition Universal Screening Tool (MUST).**		Score
Step 1 BMI score		
• BMI (kg/m²)*	>20	0
	18.5–20	1
	<18.5	2
Step 2 Weight loss score		
• Unplanned weight loss in past 3–6 months	<5%	0
	5–10%	1
	>10%	2
Step 3 Acute disease effect score		
• Acutely ill, no nutritional intake >5 d		2
Step 4 Overall risk of malnutrition		
• Add scores from above steps	**Low risk** – Routine clinical care	0
	Repeat as required	
	Medium risk – Observe	1
	If improved or adequate intake, no clinical concern; if no improvement, clinical concern	
	High risk – Treat	2 or more
	Refer to dietitian or nutrition support team, improve overall nutritional intake, monitor and review	

*Body mass index (BMI) is the weight (kg) divided by the height (m) squared.

The aim of nutritional support in the latter group is to prevent the complications of undernutrition. In hospital patients these will include an impaired immune response, impaired thermoregulation, muscle wasting (contributing to falls and respiratory infection), inactivity (contributing to venous thromboembolism and pressure sores) and impaired wound healing.

Patients who would benefit from nutritional support include those who may be undernourished or may not be able to feed normally for a more extended period of time; those who are severely ill with sepsis, multiple trauma or extensive burns, who may develop a marked negative nitrogen balance. Other indications include unconsciousness, clinical cachexia, radiotherapy or chemotherapy, major resection for malignancy, renal failure, postoperative management of major surgery and complications of surgery, or any circumstances in which the GI tract is not available or is unable to support nutrition (e.g. severe inflammatory bowel disease, gut resection, fistula).

As long as the GI tract is functioning, the preferred route for nutrition is the enteral one. For some patients this may be as basic as attention to an adequate, balanced oral diet, possibly with the addition of dietary supplements. Although oral feeding is the most desirable (and safest) route it may not be possible in the presence of oral pathology, with swallowing difficulties (most commonly as a consequence of a stroke), or in the anorexic or unconscious patient. In this situation, tube feeding provides a good alternative – it is cheaper and safer than parenteral nutrition, while allowing delivery of all nutritional requirements. It is also physiological, in the sense that nutrients are absorbed into the portal circulation. It also helps maintain the integrity of the gut. In the short term a nasogastric or nasojejunal tube can be used, but possible problems include discomfort, aspiration, incorrect placement and dislodgement. For longer-term enteral feeding a percutaneous endoscopic gastrostomy (PEG) tube should be considered. When enteral feeding is not possible – for example, if the GI tract is not functioning – then it may be necessary to provide nutrition parenterally (see Chapter 15: Parenteral nutrition).

Energy requirements vary depending upon build, level of activity and, in sick patients, on whether they are pyrexial or catabolic (e.g. after trauma or major surgery). Basal energy requirements can be calculated on the basis of sex, weight, height and age, and adjusted for activity, hypercatabolism, etc. Energy is provided by a mixture of carbohydrate and fat. The calorific value of carbohydrate of 4 kcal/g contrasts with the 9 kcal/g of fat, so inclusion of fat means that a smaller volume can be used

Nitrogen is provided by protein and/or amino acids in the diet, and a balanced feed should provide the essential amino acids required for health. Protein also has a calorific value similar to that of carbohydrate. In general, protein intake should normally provide 10–15% of the energy requirements. Utilisation of amino acids also depends upon the overall adequate provision of calories to meet energy requirements.

Micronutrients will also be needed and are provided on the basis of the recommended dietary allowance (RDA), either as a balanced diet or as actual constituents of defined feeds.

Water requirements must also be met, taking into account insensible losses plus the minimal volume to allow adequate renal excretion. In general, around 2 L will be required, but the actual figure will vary depending on other potential fluid losses, the presence of pyrexia, renal function, etc. Similarly, basic electrolyte requirements will vary depending upon actual daily losses, renal function, baseline deficiencies, etc.

Parenteral nutrition

Some of the indications for parenteral (intravenous) nutrition are listed in Table 15.6. It is particularly indicated in the short bowel syndrome or in the presence of fistula formation involving the GI tract. Short bowel syndrome is a malabsorption disorder caused by a lack of functional small intestine, usually due to Crohn's disease in adults and to necrotising enterocolitis in children. It causes diarrhoea, malnutrition and weight loss. In general, there is not much to be gained in using parenteral nutrition if this is considered to be likely for less than a week because of the balance between benefits and potential complications.

Most parenteral feeding is complete, providing all essential nutrients exogenously, and it is then known as total parenteral nutrition (TPN). Nutrients are delivered (typically via a central vein) at a pre-defined rate using an appropriate pump and delivery set, usually from a large bag containing all the prescribed ingredients and over a 24-h (or near 24-h) period. Administration of parenteral nutrition via a peripheral vein is possible for short periods, but unusual. The hyperosmolar glucose and amino acid solutions used are irritants and can lead to thrombophlebitis, limiting the energy that can be delivered by the peripheral route. For this reason administration via a central vein is usually chosen. TPN is also used in the home in some patients who require constant ongoing support through this route (e.g. short bowel syndrome) and may then be delivered during the overnight period.

Composition of the complete intravenous feed

Table 15.7 lists the typical composition of an adult feed over a 24-h period. More accurate assessment of energy requirements depends upon estimated expenditure, which relates to height, weight and age, as well as factors such as pyrexia, mobility and whether or not the patient is hypercatabolic. The electrolyte requirements illustrated are typical and can be adjusted according to individual need. They may, for example, be increased in the presence of excessive electrolyte losses (e.g. diarrhoea) or reduced with renal disease, cardiac failure or advanced liver disease. Micronutrient requirements would vary less on an individual basis but could be adjusted to meet specific deficiencies.

Table 15.6 **Principal indications for total parenteral nutrition.**

- Short bowel syndrome
- Radiation enteritis
- Acute pancreatitis
- Prolonged ileus
- Severe inflammatory bowel disease (especially fistula formation)
- Hypermetabolic states (e.g. severe burns, sepsis)

Table 15.7 **Total parenteral nutrition: typical composition of a standard feed.**

Nitrogen	12–14 g (as amino acids)
Fat	900 kcal (as 500 mL of 20% fat emulsion)
Glucose	1000 kcal (as 1.25 L of 20% dextrose)
Sodium	70–100 mmol
Potassium	60–100 mmol
Calcium	5–10 mmol
Magnesium	5–10 mmol
Phosphate	30 mmol
Trace elements	Present
Vitamins	Present (water soluble and fat soluble)
Volume	2.5–3 L

1 *Energy content:* The complete IV feed must provide adequate calories, typically 1800–2000 kcal/24 h. More may be required in some circumstances (e.g. after severe burns). Calories are normally provided as a mixture of carbohydrate (glucose) and fat. In order to provide 1000 kcal as glucose, it is necessary to use hypertonic solutions, because about 5 L of 5% dextrose would be needed in order to provide 1000 kcal, whereas the same amount of energy could be provided with 1.25 L of 20% dextrose. Fat, administered as an emulsion, has a higher energy content than glucose, such that 500 mL of a 20% fat emulsion provides about 900 kcal. The fat emulsion should also provide essential fatty acids.

2 *Nitrogen content:* The usual adult nitrogen requirement is 9 g per day. Commercially available solutions contain all the essential amino acids (arginine, histidine, leucine and isoleucine, lysine, methionine, phenylalanine, tryptophan, valine) with a prescription normally in the range 12–14 g nitrogen/24 h. Some patients require less nitrogen (e.g. small, elderly patients), while others require more (e.g. hypercatabolic patients with severe burns, multiple trauma).

3 *Electrolyte content:* Typically, the Na^+ requirement will be 70–100 mmol/24 h, but more will be needed in the event of excessive losses of Na (e.g. severe diarrhoea, fistula), and less where there is Na^+ retention (e.g. renal disease, congestive cardiac failure). Potassium requirements are more variable. Intracellular repletion, or the administration of glucose and insulin, may increase demands for K^+, whereas requirements will be very small in renal failure or where there is extensive tissue breakdown. A stable patient probably requires 60–100 mmol K^+/24 h.

4 *Vitamins and minerals:* The requirements for calcium and phosphate depend on individual needs of patients, but average requirements are about 5–10 mmol/24 h for calcium and 30 mmol/24 h for phosphate. The magnesium requirement is normally about 5–10 mmol/24 h. Trace metals and both water-soluble and fat-soluble vitamins are also added to the feed.

5 *Fluid volume:* This is dictated by clinical circumstances, but 2.5–3 L/24 h meets the requirements for most patients (less in the elderly). Depending upon the particular energy prescription, a certain minimum volume will be required to deliver the prescribed number of calories.

It is emphasised that the above description represents a suitable standard regime only. Individual patients may have requirements that differ considerably from those listed above.

Biochemical monitoring of patients on total parenteral nutrition

The proper monitoring of patients on TPN starts with attention to routine observations such as temperature, heart rate, blood pressure, fluid balance and regular weighing (where feasible). It is important to regularly inspect the site of insertion of the intravenous line. Regular biochemical and haematological measurements (the latter include full blood count and clotting measurements) are required. Biochemical measurements that should be made are as follows:

- Serum urea, creatinine, Na^+, K^+ and total CO_2 concentrations daily until the patient is stable, with accurate records of fluid balance, because large volumes are administered. Where there are potentially large electrolyte losses (e.g. via a fistula after surgery on the GI tract, the diuretic phase of acute renal failure), knowledge of the fluid Na^+ and K^+ concentrations and the volume of the fluid lost can assist in the interpretation of abnormal serum electrolyte values, and help decide on the amounts of Na^+, K^+ and water to be administered.
- Capillary glucose should be measured 6-hourly until stable and then at least daily, with laboratory glucose measurement as required.
- CRP measurement twice weekly can be useful on account of the infection risks associated with the feeding line.
- Serum calcium (and albumin, to assist interpretation of the calcium; Chapter 13: Albumin), phosphate and magnesium should be measured about 2 or 3 times weekly until stable and in the absence of severe derangements of these analytes.
- Mild derangements in 'liver function tests' are sometimes observed during TPN, and these tests (Chapter 13: Liver function tests) should also be carried out twice weekly.
- Trace element monitoring (principally copper, zinc and selenium) requires baseline measurement and every 2–3 weeks initially. Iron, ferritin, vitamins B_{12} and folate are also measured at about the same frequency as the trace elements. Individuals on longer-term nutrition – including home TPN – also have assessment of the status of vitamins and other trace elements such as manganese.
- Regular measurement of other proteins (i.e. in addition to albumin) can be used to assess nutritional status but is of limited value.

Complications of total parenteral nutrition

Complications of TPN include hunger and gut atrophy (because no nutrition is being received by the stomach and the GI tract), and problems related to the TPN delivery system itself (sepsis, including infection at the catheter insertion site, phlebitis and thrombosis). Blood and other cultures may be required. Catheter care and the stipulation that, except in extreme emergencies, the catheter must be used exclusively for the administration of the feed are important concepts in feeding patients by the parenteral route. Cholecystitis, fatty liver and liver failure are also possible complications.

The principal biochemical complications are:

- Electrolyte disturbances. These are the same as those arising in any patient receiving intravenous fluids and electrolytes (see Chapter 2: Disturbances of water, sodium and potassium balance).
- Glucose intolerance is a relatively common problem, especially in the older individual, and often reflects the high glucose content of feeds and an imbalance arising from a lack of insulin exacerbated by an increase in stress hormones causing insulin resistance (e.g. associated with sepsis and the catabolic state), which favours hyperglycaemia. Insulin infusion is often necessary. Conversely, sudden cessation of the high-glucose feed can lead to a rebound hypoglycaemia.
- Liver function test abnormalities are also described. Fatty liver disease and steatohepatitis are recognised with associated liver function test abnormalities and may reflect increased fat production within the liver from carbohydrate. A cholestatic picture is also possible, especially in the absence of any enteral feeding. In general, the liver function test and liver changes appear to be reversible, although children are more susceptible to longer-term problems, as are adults on longer-term TPN.
- Hypocalcaemia and hypomagnesaemia can reflect inadequate intake; magnesium, in particular, can be lost with sodium and potassium if fluid losses are excessive. Low phosphate frequently reflects the increased phosphate requirements associated with tissue growth and repair (see the next paragraph).

The re-feeding syndrome

This is a potentially serious condition that especially arises when a more severely malnourished patient is re-fed too quickly. It is not restricted to parenteral nutrition. In a malnourished individual there is an adaptation to poor carbohydrate supply that includes increased ketone body formation and utilisation, low insulin and low basal metabolic rate (BMR). The sudden availability of plentiful glucose will stimulate insulin and a switch to glucose utilisation, with increased requirements for phosphate, potassium and magnesium that move into the cell under the influence of insulin. Thiamin requirements are also raised (e.g. for pyruvate dehydrogenase activity on the glucose oxidation pathway). The consequences can be life-threatening, with hypokalaemia, hypophosphataemia and hypomagnesaemia, and neurological and cardiovascular problems associated with thiamin deficiency.

Patients at risk include those with:

- low BMI ($<16 \, kg/m^2$);
- chronic malnutrition (including kwashiorkor and marasmus);
- anorexia nervosa;
- undernutrition with pre-existing hypomagnesaemia, hypokalaemia (e.g. severe, chronic alcoholism).

To prevent re-feeding syndrome attention should be paid to fluid resuscitation, electrolyte replacement, and micronutrients before starting nutritional support. In particular thiamin replacement should commence prior to feeds, to prevent Wernicke's encephalopathy and other complications of thiamin deficiency. Calories should be introduced gradually, with careful monitoring of fluid balance and biochemistry.

The nutrition team

It cannot be emphasised too strongly that nutritional support is a multidisciplinary affair. Clinical biochemistry has a crucial role to play in advising on the selection of tests, recording the results and advising on the metabolic complications that might arise. Ideally, a nutrition team includes representatives from clinical biochemistry, microbiology, pharmacy, dietetics and nursing, in addition to one or more clinicians (often general surgeons), all of whom should have a special interest in nutrition. As well as advising on policy in this costly area, such a team should be able to offer expert advice and be competent to audit nutritional care.

Major nutritional problems

This section will consider two contrasting nutritional problems that, on a worldwide scale, are both common and important. These are undernutrition and obesity.

Undernutrition

Undernutrition remains a serious problem on a global scale. A group comprising UNICEF, the WHO and the World Bank estimated that in 2015 156 million children under 5 were affected by undernutrition, although the rates are steadily falling. Nearly half of all deaths in children under 5 are attributable to undernutrition, amounting to 3 million deaths per year. In Africa 32% of children under 5 are stunted and in Asia 24%. Stunted is defined as being short for age, due to the failure to grow because of chronic or recurrent malnutrition; this can have devastating lifelong consequences.

The BMI or body mass index is defined as weight/height^2 (expressed in kilograms and metres, respectively), and is a simple and widely used method of estimating body fat mass. The acceptable range of BMI in adults is 18.5–24.9 (Table 15.8). In children the classification depends on sex- and age-specific centiles. Undernourished individuals suffer from a broad range of problems that include failure of growth, lack of resistance to infection, and impact on learning and physical activity. In turn, these problems in adults can limit the actions needed to overcome the problems of inadequate food supply.

Table 15.8 WHO Classification of body mass index (BMI).

BMI (kg/m²)	Classification
<18.5	Underweight
18.5–24.9	Healthy weight
25.0–29.9	Overweight
30.0–34.9	Class I obesity
35.0–39.9	Class II obesity
>39.9	Class III obesity

 CASE 15.3

A 53-year-old female with a BMI of 21 undergoes small bowel resection for a volvulus after an acute surgical admission and subsequently requires parenteral nutrition to meet her nutritional needs. A feed is prescribed which takes into account her calorie and nitrogen requirements, and provides suitable daily amounts of electrolytes and water as well as micronutrients. Despite this, biochemical monitoring of serum reveals a phosphate of 0.3 mmol/L, a magnesium of 0.4 mmol/L and a potassium of 3.0 mmol/L. The sodium is 132 mmol/L with a creatinine of 38 µmol/L. Plasma glucose is 8.2 mmol/L.

Can you explain these findings? What changes would you make to her feed, if any? Are there any other biochemical measurements which might be helpful at this stage, bearing in mind that she has short bowel syndrome and is likely to require home parenteral nutrition?

Comments: The patient already has a low BMI prior to her surgery. Her reduced muscle bulk is reflected in the low serum creatinine of 38 µmol/L. The introduction of nutrients by means of parenteral nutrition will stimulate the laying down of new cellular material which requires electrolytes such as phosphate, magnesium and potassium to be incorporated into the new cell structure. This anabolic utilisation of these electrolytes is stimulated by the simultaneous infusion of glucose and the insulin response elicited. The low serum levels of these electrolytes almost certainly reflect their incorporation into cellular material and indicate that the parenteral feed should be adjusted to provide more of these electrolytes. Mild hyponatraemia is quite a common finding in patients undergoing parenteral nutrition and is not, in itself, an indication to increase the sodium content of the feed. Assessment of the urine sodium excretion in a 24-h urine collection can establish whether or not sodium administration is adequate. Similarly, a raised plasma glucose is also not an uncommon finding in the face of the high glucose load administered as a component of the parenteral feed. Levels would need to be monitored, although a value of 8.2 mmol/L would not necessarily be an indication for insulin administration on the basis of a single, isolated reading. Baseline micronutrient assessment should also be considered.

In general terms, the problem of undernutrition can arise from insufficient food, anorexia, persistent vomiting or regurgitation, or malabsorption. It may also be seen where the basal metabolic rate is increased (severe infections, thyrotoxicosis), in cancer cachexia and other illnesses. The severity of undernutrition is assessed by clinical and dietary history, supplemented by appropriate anthropometric measurements and biochemical tests (see section on Nutritional assessment).

A range of biochemical abnormalities may be found. Blood glucose may be low, with a corresponding increase in plasma free fatty acids and ketone bodies (with associated mild metabolic acidosis). Plasma glucagon and cortisol levels increase, increasing insulin resistance, while insulin secretion is reduced, impairing glucose tolerance. Reverse T3 increases at the expense of normal T3. Creatinine excretion diminishes, reflecting a reduced muscle mass.

Protein-energy malnutrition (PEM) in children leads to a spectrum of diseases. Nutritional marasmus is the childhood version of severe starvation, and is typically found in cases where the child is weaned early onto dilute cow's milk formula. Weight is less than 60% of the standard weight, and there is often evidence of vitamin and other nutrient deficiencies, with associated chronic infections. In kwashiorkor, the diet is low in protein but may be relatively satisfactory in carbohydrate intake (e.g. a child weaned onto diets such as yam, cassava or diluted cereal). The insulin levels may be less affected (because carbohydrate is present), with diversion of amino acids from the viscera to muscles, leading to impaired albumin synthesis by a fatty liver (with reduced lipoprotein export). The low albumin leads to the characteristic hypoalbuminaemic oedema found in this condition.

Obesity

The most common nutritional disorder in affluent societies is defined as an excess of body fat. In 2015 42 million children were overweight, an increase of around 15 million over the previous 15 years. Adults with a BMI over 25 are considered overweight and over 30 are considered obese (Table 15.8). Different thresholds apply in South Asia and China, because the harmful consequences of obesity in these ethnic groups occur at lower thresholds. In the UK, about 25% of adults are clinically obese, with over 60% of adults being either overweight or obese. The prevalence of obesity is similar in men and women, but men are more likely to be overweight. Worldwide, obesity is replacing malnutrition and infectious diseases as the most significant health problem. In general, it arises from an excess of calorie intake over expenditure. The problem may be multifactorial, with socioeconomic factors, age, sex and heredity all contributing. Susceptibility to obesity may have a polymorphic genetic component accounting for 25–70% weight variation. It may arise in conjunction with disorders such as hypothyroidism or Cushing's syndrome, for example, and may be a consequence of drug treatment (e.g. steroids, sulphonylurea drugs). There are also some rare genetic forms of obesity that arise from single gene disorders that affect neurohumoral control of appetite and weight. Nevertheless, the great majority of obesity reflects lifestyle patterns of excess calorie intake and reduced physical activity. The lack of education on nutritional matters has also been highlighted.

Biochemical measurements may all be normal, but simple obesity shows an association with type 2 diabetes (Chapter 6: Diabetes mellitus), hyperlipidaemia (typically a mixed hyperlipidaemia), hyperuricaemia and fat deposition in the liver (NAFLD), sometimes with mild derangements in liver function tests.

The metabolic and other problems associated with obesity have led to the concept of a condition termed the metabolic syndrome that carries increased risk of cardiovascular disease. There are various definitions of this condition that differ in detail but are broadly similar. For example, the International Diabetes Federation defines the condition on the basis of central adiposity plus any two of four factors (fasting triglyceride ≥1.7 mmol/L; HDL-cholesterol <1.03 in males or <1.29 in females; a blood pressure of ≥130/85; a fasting glucose of ≥5.6 mmol/L). Central adiposity is determined by the waist circumference (generally >90 cm in men and >80 cm in women). The precise aetiology of the metabolic syndrome is unknown, but central adiposity and insulin resistance are certainly key factors. The clinical utility and pathogenesis of the condition have been questioned and its recognition may offer no benefit over and above established means of cardiovascular risk estimation and it may simply reflect the metabolic derangements on the pathway to type 2 diabetes.

 CASE 15.4

A 42-year-old male visits his GP with a history strongly suggestive of angina on exertion. The GP records a weight of 125 kg and a height of 1.6 m. Waist circumference is 120 cm. His blood pressure is elevated at 175/105. A blood sample is sent to the laboratory and shows a fasting glucose of 6.8 mmol/L, cholesterol of 7.2 mmol/L, triglycerides of 6.2 mmol/L and HDL of 0.6 mmol/L.

What is the likely condition in this man which underlies his ischaemic heart disease? What are the criteria used to diagnose this particular condition?

Comments: This patient has the features of the metabolic syndrome (see Chapter 15: Obesity). Although the fasting glucose does not reach a level diagnostic for diabetes mellitus, a glucose tolerance test would be recommended. His problem of angina and probable ischaemic heart disease is likely to progress unless attention is paid to correcting these problems, by a combination of lifestyle or drug-related means. In this type of patient, a lifestyle approach that concentrates on weight loss and nutrition can have a major impact on successfully managing his ischaemic heart disease.

In recent years, there has been increasing research in the area of obesity and appetite control, and this has revealed some very rare monogenic forms of obesity. Severe early-onset obesity can be due to mutations in genes of the leptin/melanocortin axis involved in regulation of food intake. Leptin is a 16-kDa hormone that is secreted by adipose tissue, and may act as a sensor of peripheral nutrient stores and have a role in appetite control. Early theories that this may have a more general role in obesity have not been borne out. Other rare causes of monogenic obesity include mutations in the melanocortin-4 receptor (MC4R). This is the receptor for α-melanocyte–stimulating hormone whose action on the hypothalamus is to reduce appetite and increase energy expenditure. Obesity may also be associated with a number of other genetic syndromes which are additionally characterized by mental retardation, dysmorphic features and organ-specific developmental abnormalities. Prader–Willi syndrome is probably the best known of these but there are many others, all individually rare.

The treatment of obesity, in the absence of rare genetic causes or when secondary to other illnesses or drugs, is directed at individual lifestyle issues of food intake and activity levels, and the social and cultural determinants of these. Targeted use of anti-obesity drugs (such as the pancreatic lipase inhibitor, orlistat) or bariatric surgery (such as gastric-banding) has a place in some individuals but cannot be the answer at a population level. Population-based strategies that promote healthy eating and encourage exercise through education are undoubtedly increasingly important along with political influence on the food industry and agriculture.

 FURTHER READING

Ayling, R. and Marshall, W. (2007) *Nutrition and Laboratory Medicine*. ACB Venture Publications, London.

British Heart Foundation Statistics website: http://www.bhf.org.uk/research/heart-statistics

Levels and Trends in Child Malnutrition UNICEF/WHO/World Bank Group Joint Child Malnutrition Estimates. Key Findings of the 2016 Edition. http://www.who.int/nutrition/publications/jointchildmalnutrition_2016_estimates/en/

Office of Dietary Supplements, NIH (USA) website: http://ods.od.nih.gov

16

Inflammation, immunity and paraproteinaemia

Learning objectives

To understand:

✔ that failure to express functional plasma proteins may manifest itself as specific clinical conditions;

✔ that plasma protein concentrations are modified by trauma, inflammation and sepsis (the acute-phase response) without any clinical sequelae;

✔ which functional plasma proteins are measured for diagnostic purposes;

✔ the causes of hypoalbuminaemia;

✔ the clinical conditions that are associated with aberrant expression of immunoglobulins;

✔ the investigations performed in patients with suspected paraproteinaemias.

Introduction

Plasma contains over 300 proteins. Many of these have a specific biochemical role, and organic disease may result when their concentration in plasma is reduced. Conversely, disease processes such as trauma, infection and inflammation may themselves lead to changes in the concentration of a wide range of plasma proteins but without any clinical sequelae. Many plasma proteins, including most enzymes and tumour markers, have no known function in blood, and arise as a result of cell death, tissue damage or over-expression by malignant cells. The measurement of some specific proteins, however, may have a valuable clinical role in monitoring progression of a disease or response to therapy. Table 16.1 lists

examples of commonly measured plasma proteins that can be crudely assessed by protein staining following separation using electrophoresis (EPH). Electrophoresis separates these proteins into the broad groups of α1, α2, β1 β2 and γ globulins, together with an albumin band (Figure 16.1, centre lane). Currently, most of the proteins listed in Table 16.1 are quantified using immunoassay rather than EPH. EPH is now used mainly to detect over-expression of monoclonal paraproteins that may not be accurately quantified by the antibodies used in immunoassay (see Chapter 16: Myeloma, lymphoid malignancies and paraproteinaemia; and Figure 16.1, right lane).

Total protein in serum is often measured, although a fall in the concentration of one protein may be masked by a coincident or compensatory increase in

---

Clinical Biochemistry Lecture Notes, Tenth Edition. Peter Rae, Mike Crane and Rebecca Pattenden.
© 2018 John Wiley & Sons Ltd. Published 2018 by John Wiley & Sons Ltd.
Companion website: www.lecturenoteseries.com/clinicalbiochemistry

Table 16.1 Examples of plasma proteins commonly measured for the diagnosis and monitoring of specific diseases.

Proteins and their electrophoretic mobility	Principal function(s)	Used in the detection or investigations of disease
Albumin	Colloid oncotic pressure, transport functions	Malnutrition, malignancy, liver, kidney and GI disease
α_1-Globulins		
• α_1-Foetoprotein	Foetal form of albumin	Neural tube defects, tumour marker, antenatal screening
• α_1-antitrypsin	Anti-protease	α_1-antitrypsin deficiency
• Prothrombin	Blood clotting	Coagulation screen; liver function test
α_2-Globulins		
• Caeruloplasmin (Chapter 13)	Copper transport	Wilson's disease
• Haptoglobin	Haemoglobin binding	Haemolytic disorders
• α_2-Macroglobulin	Anti-protease, transport	Proteinuria (e.g. selectivity investigations)
β-Globulins		
• C-reactive protein	Activates complement system	Infection, inflammation, cardiovascular risk
• β_2-Microglobulin	Regulates immune response	Monitoring myeloma, renal failure
• Transferrin (Chapter 18)	Iron transport	Iron deficiency/excess
γ-Globulins		
• Igs (IgG, IgA, IgM, etc.)	Immune response	Liver disease, infections, autoimmune disease, paraproteinaemias, etc.

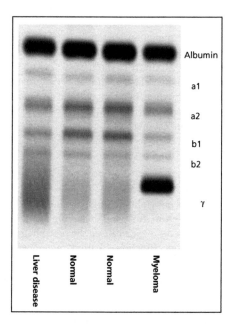

Figure 16.1 Separation of serum proteins by electrophoresis. The pattern in a normal serum sample (centre lanes). The discrete band of a paraprotein found typically in the γ globulin region in patients with myeloma (right lane) and diffuse increase in γ-globulin as can be seen in infection or liver disease (left lane).

another. Elevated total protein can be a useful early clue in the diagnosis of myeloma (see Chapter 16: Investigation of suspected myeloma).

Changes in plasma proteins in trauma, infection and inflammation – 'the acute-phase response'

Following trauma, infection, inflammation, burns, etc., the body responds by initiating a series of mechanisms that lead to:

- acute haemodynamic changes;
- a rapid fall in the concentration of some plasma proteins (e.g. albumin, transferrin);
- an increase in the concentration of several specific proteins some hours after the injury. These proteins are the acute-phase proteins, and are listed in Table 16.2.

The cytokines and a host of vasoactive substances are important mediators of the acute-phase response.

Table 16.2 **Examples of plasma proteins that change during the acute-phase response.**

Increase	Decrease
C-reactive protein	Albumin
α_1-Antitrypsin	Transferrin
Caeruloplasmin	Pre-albumin
α_1-Acid glycoprotein	
Fibrinogen	
Ferritin	
Haptoglobin	

Table 16.3 **Causes of hypoalbuminaemia.**

Artefact
- Dilution of sample (e.g. taken from arm during intravenous infusion)

Physiological
- Pregnancy (haemodilution)
- Recumbency
- Genetic (analbuminaemia)

Pathological
- Impaired synthesis – chronic liver disease, malnutrition, malabsorption, inflammation
- Increased metabolism – injury, surgery, sepsis, malignancy
- Increased loss – hypoxia, sepsis, skin lesions, burns, protein-losing enteropathy, nephrotic syndrome
- Increased volume of distribution – overhydration, cardiac failure, acites

The rapid decrease in concentration of certain proteins appears to result from loss of plasma protein into the extravascular space, due to increased vascular permeability caused by cytokines, prostaglandins and histamine. The increase in the acute-phase plasma proteins results from increased synthesis and release, which appears to be mediated mainly by interleukin-6.

Albumin

Albumin is quantitatively the most important contributor towards maintaining the colloid oncotic pressure of plasma, and hypoalbuminaemia may lead to the development of oedema. Albumin also accounts for more than 50% of the total plasma protein concentration. Albumin variants occur in the healthy population, and heterozygotes for some variant albumins may express two gene products, which appear as two bands on electrophoresis. This is known as *bisalbuminaemia*, and has no pathological significance.

Increased albumin concentration is found in dehydration and if excessive venous stasis is applied during venepuncture.

Hypoalbuminaemia

Low albumin may arise as a consequence of a number of conditions, including cirrhosis, nephrotic syndrome, heart failure and malnutrition, although inflammation leading to the acute-phase response is the most common cause (Table 16.3). Hypoalbuminaemia is an important prognostic indicator of poor outcome in hospitalised patients.

Investigation into the cause of low serum albumin should be guided by clinical suspicion of the underlying disease process. Tests performed may include liver function tests, serum creatinine, electrolytes and C-reactive protein (or erythrocyte sedimentation rate; ESR), alongside consideration of nutritional status. Measurement of urinary protein or albumin concentration is important to exclude a renal cause of protein loss.

Very rarely hypoalbuminaemia is caused by a genetic mutation in the albumin gene, termed analbuminaemia. Albumin is often very low in such patients (usually <1 g/L) and they are usually asymptomatic, often being diagnosed in later life with features of mild oedema, hypotension and hypercholesterolaemia.

C-reactive protein (CRP)

This protein is a β-globulin, originally named after a property of serum that had been obtained from acutely ill patients, which caused the precipitation of a polysaccharide (fraction C) from pneumococcal extracts. CRP binds strongly to phosphocholine on dying cells and appears to activate the complement system.

CRP can markedly increase in infection and inflammatory disease processes. CRP appears to provide a sensitive but nonspecific test for organic illness and is widely measured as an alternative or adjunct to the less sensitive ESR. CRP measurements using a sensitive assay have been advocated as a marker for coronary risk but have not been widely adopted for this purpose.

Erythrocyte sedimentation rate (ESR)

This common inexpensive haematology test provides a nonspecific test for inflammation. The ESR is the measure of the rate at which erythrocytes sediment in anti-coagulated blood. ESR essentially is an indirect measure of the acute-phase proteins (mainly fibrinogen). The high fibrinogen levels that occur in inflammation cause red cells to aggregate and form stacks called 'rouleaux', which settle faster than dispersed red cells. ESR may also be increased in patients who have high concentrations of immunoglobulins but no inflammation (e.g. in the paraproteinaemias) and also in patients who have anaemia or renal failure.

CRP vs ESR measurements

CRP concentrations change more quickly and to a greater extent than ESR. Thus CRP may be more useful as an early marker of acute disease and in monitoring response to therapy in acute illness. CRP is also useful for differentiating acute infection from inflammation in patients with autoimmune conditions such as lupus.

Conversely, changes in ESR occur more slowly than those in CRP. ESR is most often used to investigate patients with unexplained symptoms when chronic inflammation or neoplasia is suspected. ESR is also useful for monitoring chronic inflammatory states including rheumatoid arthritis, polymyalgia rheumatica and temporal arteritis.

α_1-Antitrypsin (AAT) (α_1-anti-protease)

Proteases such as trypsin, chymotrypsin, elastase and thrombin are continually being released into the blood in small amounts from a number of sources, including the pancreas, leucocytes and intestinal bacteria. AAT is one of several plasma proteins that inhibit the activity of these proteases, particularly neutrophil elastase, and may function to limit proteolytic activity at sites of inflammation. Interest in AAT principally relates to the association between certain diseases of the lung and liver and AAT deficiency due to genetic polymorphisms. Genetic alterations in the protein prevent its release from hepatocytes where it is synthesised. As a result unopposed protease action in alveoli may lead to damage and emphysema, while accumulation of AAT in heptocytes may cause liver disease by inducing apoptosis. AAT deficiency affects around 1:3000–1:5000 of the population, putting it in the top three of the lethal genetic diseases (cystic fibrosis and Down's syndrome being the other two). Not all patients with AAT deficiency develop significant clinical problems.

Clinical consequences of the genetic polymorphism of AAT

AAT production is controlled by the *SERPINA1* gene (previously known as PI; protease inhibitor) on chromosome 14, and more than 150 genetic variants have been described. The most common allele has been named M, with the usual homozygote being PI^{MM} (the MM type). The two most common mutations that give rise to AAT deficiency are the PI^Z and PI^S alleles; more rarely is deficiency associated with a null allele. Individuals that are homozygous or compound heterozygous for the PI^Z or PI^S alleles are prone to both pulmonary and hepatic disease.

Pulmonary emphysema

About 1% of patients with emphysema have AAT deficiency PI^{SZ} or PI^{ZZ}, but the percentage is much higher in young patients. When associated with AAT deficiency, emphysema tends to manifest itself in the 20–40 year age group. Smoking appears to be a strong predisposing factor for the development of the disease in these patients, possibly because particles in smoke stimulate phagocytic activity, with the local release of proteases.

Hepatic disorders

Most children with the Z phenotype demonstrate abnormal liver function tests during the first year of life. Neonatal jaundice, usually presenting as a predominantly cholestatic picture, occurs in approximately 10% of PI^{ZZ} individuals. Although the jaundice may resolve, subsequent progression to hepatic cirrhosis can occur. Approximately 20% of childhood cases of cirrhosis can probably be attributed to AAT deficiency; individuals with the Pi^{ZZ} phenotype continue to carry an increased risk of cirrhosis and hepatocellular carcinoma into adulthood.

Investigation

Phenotyping of AAT is desirable in all patients in whom plasma AAT concentrations are low or borderline, so that appropriate genetic counselling can be given to affected individuals or their family members. Genotyping can also be used to investigate relatives of patients with AAT deficiency and for antenatal screening purposes.

CASE 16.1

A 73-year-old retired male civil servant with a 12-month history of increasing shortness of breath and recurrent lung infections presented to his GP complaining of recent onset of lower back pain. He had also developed a wheeze. He had been a lifelong nonsmoker.

His electrolytes, albumin immunoglobulins, full blood count and PSA were normal.

A serum electrophoresis was also requested to exclude myeloma. This showed no evidence of a paraprotein (Chapter 16: Myeloma, lymphoid malignancies and paraproteinaemia) but from the serum EPH the laboratory noted a marked decrease in the α1-globulin band prompting quantification of serum α$_1$-antitrypsin; this was found to be low at 0.4 g/L (reference range 1.1–2.1 g/L) with a Pi^{ZZ} phenotype. Chest X-ray showed evidence of basal bullous emphysema.

Comment: The patient had developed emphysema caused by α$_1$-antitrypsin deficiency of the Pi^{ZZ} phenotype. In smokers, emphysema due to α$_1$-antitrypsin deficiency usually presents in younger patients, but the condition may manifest itself in the elderly who have been lifelong nonsmokers. Subsequent investigations of his liver function suggested no significant liver problems. PSA and serum EPH had been requested to exclude prostatic malignancy or myeloma as a cause of the lower back pain. The back pain later resolved and no further investigations were required.

The immunoglobulins and disease

The immunoglobulins (Igs) are synthesised by the plasma cells of the lymphoreticular system.

The basic Ig molecule consists of a pair of identical heavy chains (M_r 50–75 kDa each) and a pair of identical light chains (M_r 22 kDa each) linked by disuphide bridges. There are five principal types of heavy chain (γ, α, μ, δ and ε) and two types of light chain (κ and λ); thus every Ig can be assigned a formula that indicates its composition (e.g. $\gamma_2\kappa_2$). The antigen-combining sites sit between the adjacent light and heavy chains (Figure 16.2).

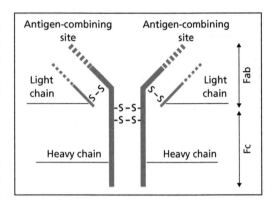

Figure 16.2 The Ig protein consists of two identical pairs of heavy and light chains, held together by disulphide bonds (shown as –S–S). The molecules can be split by papain into three components: two antigen-binding fragments (Fab), each of which has one binding site, and the crystallisable fragment (Fc). The variable regions of the Ig molecule are shown as interrupted lines. The heavy chains are one of five types (γ, α, μ, δ or ε), and the light chains are one of two types (κ or λ).

The immunoglobulin classes

Three major classes of Ig (IgG, IgA and IgM) and two minor ones (IgD and IgE) have been recognised; the type of heavy chain determines the class. Table 16.4 lists several features of the major classes.

- *IgG immunoglobulins* are the major antibody of the secondary immune response and are formed particularly in response to soluble antigens such as toxins and the products of bacterial lysis. They are widely distributed in the ECF, and cross the foetoplacental barrier.
- *IgM immunoglobulins* are pentamers of the basic Ig structure linked around a J chain polypeptide. They tend to be formed especially in response to particulate antigens, such as those on the surface of bacteria. In the presence of complement, IgMs are very effective in producing lysis of these cells. IgM formation usually precedes IgG formation, and IgMs are thus thought to provide an early defence.
- *IgA immunoglobulins* in plasma exist in monomeric form. However, more than 50% of IgA synthesis occurs in lymphoreticular cells under the mucosa of the respiratory and alimentary tracts. Here, dimeric 'secretory IgA' is synthesised and secreted into the alimentary or respiratory tract, giving defence against local infections.
- *IgD immunoglobulins* are present in minute amounts in plasma with monomer IgM, on the surface of B lymphocytes. They are probably

Table 16.4 **Some features of the major classes of the Igs.**

Feature	IgG	IgA	IgM
Average molecular mass	146 kDa	160 kDa	875 kDa
Plasma concentration	5.0–13.0 g/L	0.5–4.0 g/L	0.3–2.5 g/L
Light chain type	κ or λ	κ or λ	κ or λ
Heavy chain type	γ	α	μ
Structure of protein	$\gamma_2\kappa_2$ or $\gamma_2\lambda_2$	$\alpha_2\kappa_2$ or $\alpha_2\lambda_2$	$(\mu_2\kappa_2)_5$ or $(\mu_2\lambda_2)_5$
Plasma half-life	21 days	6 days	5 days
Immune response	Secondary	Local, secretory	Primary
Present in secretions	Trace	Yes	Trace
Transplacental passage	Yes	No	No

concerned with antigen recognition and with the development of tolerance.

- *IgE immunoglobulins* bind to cells such as the mast cells of the nasopharynx. In the presence of antigen (allergen), an antigen–antibody reaction leads to the release of histamine and other amines and polypeptides from the mast cell, giving rise to a local hypersensitivity reaction.

Immunoglobulin deficiencies

Physiological causes

The concentration of IgM and IgA in serum is low at birth and gradually rises until adult levels are achieved at approximately 1 year and 10 years, respectively. In contrast, IgG is high at birth due to transplacental passage of maternal IgG. After birth, IgG falls due to loss of maternal IgG but gradually rises again until adult values are found after 1 year.

Inherited deficiencies of immunoglobulin synthesis

Hypogammaglobulinaemia and the more rare *agammaglobulinaemia* are conditions in which there is defective production of IgG, IgA and IgM. Children develop severe, recurrent bacterial infections when over the age of 1. The most common is IgA deficiency, which has an incidence of approximately 1:400.

Acquired deficiencies of immunoglobulin synthesis

Secondary hypogammaglobulinaemia is much more common than the inherited deficiencies. It may occur in lymphoid neoplasia (e.g. chronic lymphatic leukaemia, Hodgkin disease, multiple myelomatosis),

following immunosuppressant therapy (e.g. glucocorticoids, sulfasalazine), and secondary to protein-losing syndromes (e.g. nephrotic syndrome).

Polyclonal hypergammaglobulinaemia

Liver disease, infection and autoimmune disease give rise to stimulation of B lymphocytes and an increased production of γ-globulin, which on serum protein EPH is revealed as a broad (diffuse) band (Figure 16.1, left lane). The increase may affect all the Ig classes, or it may affect predominantly one class. Quantitation of the separate Ig classes is only occasionally helpful in diagnosis because in most cases the cause of the hypergammaglobulinaemia is apparent. The measurement of antibodies to specific antigens is of value (e.g. hepatitis surface antigens). Multiple discrete bands (oligoclonal bands) or, rarely, a single discrete band may occur in the λ-globulin region in response to an antigenic stimulus and need to be distinguished from paraproteinaemia.

Monoclonal hypergammaglobulinaemia (paraproteinaemia)

Paraproteins are monoclonal Ig or light chains produced by a clonal population of B cells. They are often identified as a discrete Ig band on electrophoresis of serum (Figure 16.1, right lane). Plasma cell disorders are often associated with multiple myeloma and malignant lymphoid tumours, but benign causes are also described. The detection of a paraprotein in blood or urine requires further investigation to determine whether the paraproteinaemia is malignant or benign (see next paragraph).

Myeloma, lymphoid malignancies and paraproteinaemia

Malignant paraproteinaemias are found in multiple myeloma, plasmacytoma, malignant lymphoid tumours and heavy chain disease. The prevalence of paraproteinaemia rises with age, and is about 3% in the geriatric population.

Multiple myeloma is the most common disorder associated with a paraprotein (M- protein) and is due to malignant proliferation of plasma cells which leads to bone destruction, impaired immune function, hyperviscosity and renal impairment. The presenting features are listed in Table 16.5.

Most myelomas produce complete Ig molecules, usually IgG, and the amount produced is often proportional to the tumour mass. Excessive amounts of light chains or parts of heavy chains are also produced in about 85% of cases. Dimers of light chains (M_r 44 kDa) are usually found in urine, and are called 'Bence Jones' protein. In about 10–20% of cases of myeloma (usually the less differentiated – termed 'light-chain disease' or 'Bence Jones myeloma'), excess light chains may be the only abnormality in serum.

Waldenström macroglobulinaemia usually follows a more prolonged course than multiple myeloma. There is proliferation of cells that resemble lymphocytes rather than plasma cells. They produce complete IgM molecules and often an excess of light chains. Increased plasma IgM causes increased plasma viscosity, which tends to make the circulation sluggish, and thromboses are common.

Heavy-chain disease (Franklin disease) comprises a group of rare conditions in which heavy-chain fragments corresponding to the Fc portion of the Igs are synthesised and excreted in urine. Abnormal production of α and γ heavy chains is the most common derangement.

Amyloidosis is a heterogeneous group of clinical conditions characterised by systemic deposition of protein fibrils. Amyloid fibrils may occur as a secondary complication of plasma cell malignancies (see Chapter 16: Amyloidosis).

Investigation of suspected myeloma

The tests used to diagnose and monitor patients with myeloma are shown in Tables 16.6 and 16.7. Patients in whom a paraproteinaemia has been identified should be referred for specialist review.

Serum protein electrophoresis shows a single or multiple discrete band(s), usually in the γ-globulin region but occasionally in the β-globulin or α_2-globulin region. In patients in whom there is over-production of monoclonal Ig, the concentration of the other Igs may be reduced (immune paresis). Occasionally, a band due to the presence of light chains may be observed. Serum rather than plasma must be used, because the fibrinogen band present in plasma may obscure or mimic paraproteins. Quantification of serum free light chain concentration and the κ:λ ratio may also be helpful.

Urine protein electrophoresis on a fresh early morning urine sample is needed to detect Bence Jones protein; its small size (M_r 44 kDa) means that it is cleared

---

Table 16.5 Clinical presentation in myeloma.

- Bone pain (with lytic areas on X-ray)
- Impaired renal function
- Anaemia
- Hypercalcaemia
- Recurrent infection
- Hyperviscosity

Table 16.6 Investigations in suspected myeloma.

Screening test	Tests to establish diagnosis	Tests to assess prognosis and tumour burden	Tests to assess organ impairment
EPH of serum and urine Urea, Na, K Ca, creatinine (eGFR), albumin, FBC and ESR	Immunofixation of any monoclonal band Bone marrow with plasma cell phenotyping *SFLC	Quantification of monoclonal protein in serum and urine by densitometry β_2-microglobulin, albumin, total immunoglobulin, SFLC Skeletal survey	Urea, albumin, Ca albumin, creatinine (eGFR), plasma viscosity

*Serum free light chains (SFLC) should be measured where there is a strong suspicion of myeloma but EPH shows no abnormal band.

Table 16.7 Further investigations when myeloma has been diagnosed.

Non-paraprotein Ig – to assess the likelihood of immune paresis

Serum β_2-microglobulin – provides a prognostic index. Values >5.5 mg/L indicate a poor prognosis

Serum creatinine and eGFR to assess renal function

Serum calcium – this may be raised due to increased release of calcium from bone

Serum albumin – used for staging

Haemoglobin and full blood count – anaemia is quite common

Serum free light chains – for diagnosis and monitoring (particularly light-chain disease and MGUS)

 CASE 16.2

A 70-year-old man complained to his doctor of back pain that he had had for several months, and of feeling generally unwell. He appeared pale and he was tender over the lumbar spine. His urine contained protein (1 g/L) and his ESR was very high (90 mm in the first hour). The following abnormalities were reported.

How would you interpret these results, and what further chemical investigations would you request in this patient?

Serum	Result	Reference range
Albumin	32	35–50 g/L
Calcium	2.72	2.2–2.6 mmol/L
ALP	90	40–125 U/L
Creatinine	180	64–111 µmol/L
eGFR	35	>60 mL/min/1.73 m²
Total protein	84	60–80 g/L
IgA	<0.4	0.8–4.5 g/L
IgG	37	6–15 g/L
IgM	<0.2	0.35–2.90 g/L

Comment: Serum and urine protein electrophoresis would both be indicated. The serum pattern showed a discrete band in the γ-globulin region, with marked reduction of the other Igs, and urine electrophoresis revealed the presence of Bence Jones protein, subsequently identified as of the λ type. The diagnosis of multiple myeloma was confirmed on X-ray examination (which demonstrated osteolytic lesions in the skull, vertebral column, ribs and pelvis) and by the finding of atypical plasma cells in the bone marrow.

Hypercalcaemia is present in about 30% of patients with multiple myeloma, and about 50% show some evidence of impaired renal function at the time of presentation; this is associated with a poor prognosis. Serum paraproteins are not accurately quantitated using the usual immunological methods, and cannot distinguish between monoclonal and polyclonal Ig. Serum electrophoresis is thus required for screening for paraproteinaemia in symptomatic patients.

---

rapidly by the kidney. If Bence Jones protein is detected, the monoclonal nature of the light chains can be confirmed by immunofixation. In multiple myeloma, the light chains are nearly always dimers of type κ *or* type λ, but not a mixture of the two. Most cases of myeloma and many cases of macroglobulinaemia have Bence Jones proteinuria. In light-chain disease there is Bence Jones proteinuria but usually no serum paraprotein component.

Monoclonal gammopathy of unknown significance (MGUS)

On finding a paraprotein, the most important diagnostic decision is whether the condition is MGUS,

asymptomatic or symptomatic myeloma (Table 16.8). Often a paraprotein is found on electrophoresis in patients who have no symptoms and it may be unclear if this is due to early malignant disease or a benign disorder. MGUS is present in approximately 2% of individuals over 50 years of age and 3% of patients over 70. It is defined by a low concentration of paraprotein (<30 g/L), less than 10% of clonal bone marrow plasma cells and the absence of myeloma-related organ or tissue damage (Table 16.9). Serial measurement of both paraprotein concentration and serum free light chains is useful for risk stratification. In MGUS the overall rate of progression to myeloma is in the order of 1% per year; long-term follow-up is thus required.

Table 16.8 Diagnostic criteria for MGUS, asymptomatic and symptomatic myeloma.

	MGUS	Asymptomatic myeloma	Symptomatic myeloma
Monoclonal protein	In serum <30g/L	In serum >30g/L	In serum >30g/L and/or in urine*
Bone marrow	Clonal plasma cells <10%	Clonal plasma cells >10%	Clonal plasma cells >10% or plasmacytoma
Evidence of organ/tissue impairment	No evidence of organ impairment including bone lesions	No myeloma-related organ/tissue impairment	Any myeloma-related organ/tissue impairment

*Prognosis will depend on both the type of monoclonal protein and the concentration; IgA/IgM/or IgD paraproteinaemias usually indicate higher relative risk than IgG paraproteinaemias.

Table 16.9 Definition of myeloma-related tissue impairment.

Clinical effect due to myeloma	Definition
Increased calcium	Corrected serum calcium >0.25mmol/L above upper reference limit or >2.75mmol/L
Renal insufficiency	Creatinine >170µmol/L
Anaemia	Haemoglobin <100g/L
Others	Symptomatic hyperviscosity, amyloidosis, recurrent bacterial infection (2 episodes in 12 months)

Amyloidosis

Amyloidosis occurs when various proteins (amyloid) accumulate in a range of organs including the heart, kidneys, intestines, nervous system and liver, leading to tissue damage and organ dysfunction.

- Primary amyloidosis (AL) occurs in patients with multiple myeloma due to accumulation of aggregates of light chains in tissues.
- Secondary amyloidosis (AA) occurs in patients with chronic infection or inflammatory disease and in this situation a protein 'amyloid A' accumulates.
- Familial amyloidosis (ATTR) is a rare autosomal dominant condition in which transthyretin accumulates in tissues.
- β_2-Microglobulin amyloidosis occurs in patients undergoing renal dialysis where the protein accumulates in joints.

 CASE 16.3

A 66-year-old woman attended her GP with a history of fatigue. She had a previous history of type 2 diabetes and hypertension with CKD 3, and on investigation was found to have a mild normocytic anaemia. As a part of investigation into anaemia, a blood and urine sample was sent to the laboratory for serum electrophoresis and urine Bence Jones protein, respectively.

Serum	Result	Reference range
Creatinine	135	50–98µmol/L
eGFR	36	>60mL/min/1.73m²
Albumin	38	35–50g/L
Calcium	2.52	2.2–2.6mmol/L
Total protein	68	60–80g/L
IgA	4.3*	0.8–4.5g/L
IgG	13	6–15g/L
IgM	2.8	0.35–2.90g/L
Serum EPH	*A monoclonal band was detected in the γ-globulin region. Band: IgAκ; 3.8g/L	

Urine	Result
Urine total protein (spot)	0.09g/L
Urine Bence Jones protein	Bence Jones protein type kappa detected Band: 0.03g/L

On the basis of these results the GP referred the patient to the haematology clinic for further investigation, where a bone marrow biopsy and skeletal survey were undertaken. Bone marrow biopsy demonstrated a small clonal population of plasma cells (approximately 5%), which stained for kappa on immunohistochemistry. Erythropoiesis appeared within normal limits. There were no lytic lesions apparent on skeletal survey.

How would you interpret these results?

Comment: This patient has MGUS. This is supported by the relatively small monoclonal band in the serum and urine, the findings in the bone marrow biopsy, and by the lack of clear evidence of myeloma-related tissue damage. Although the patient has a degree of renal impairment, this was thought more likely to be a consequence of her diabetes and hypertension. Patients with MGUS require long-term monitoring as approximately 1% per year will progress to multiple myeloma. Analysis of serum free light chains can also provide a useful means of follow-up. This patient was reviewed after 6 months and found to be stable. Annual monitoring was arranged thereafter.

Cryoglobulins and cryoglobulinaemia

Cryoglobulinaemia is a syndrome caused by the presence of immunoglobulins that precipitate in the cold (4 °C) and redissolve when warmed to 37 °C. The most common symptoms in patients with cryoglobulinaemia are Raynaud's, weakness, arthralgia and purpura – symptoms that are particularly prevalent in cold weather; most people with cryoglobulins in their serum have no symptoms. Precipitates that form in plasma only, but not serum, are termed cryofibrinogen; such precipitates are usually composed of fibrinogen and fibrin breakdown products, although some are also associated with immunoglobulin.

Cryoglobulins occur in a number of diseases, including those associated with both diffuse and discrete hypergammaglobulinaemia, and are also found in many patients with hepatitis C.

Cryoglobulinaemia may be classified according to the type of Ig that is present:

- *Type I cryoglobulinaemia, 10% of cases:* Due to monoclonal Ig, usually IgM, or light chains, secondary to lymphoproliferative disorders such as myeloma and Waldenström macroglobulinaemia.
- *Types II and III cryoglobulinaemia* are characterised by rheumatoid factors (RFs), which are usually IgM (monoclonal for type II and polyclonal for type III) and are associated with inflammatory conditions such as systemic lupus erythematosus, viral infection and Sjögren syndrome. These RFs form complexes with the Fc portion of polyclonal IgG. Types II and III cryoglobulinaemia represent around 60% and 30% respectively of all cryoglobulinaemias.

If cryoglobulin determinations are to be performed, blood needs to be collected into warmed syringes (with and without anti-coagulant), and maintained at 37 °C until the plasma and serum have been separated from the cells.

17

Malignancy and tumour markers

Learning objectives

To understand:

✔ the clinical circumstances in which to request tumour markers;

✔ the routine tumour markers and the limitations of such measurements.

Introduction

Tumours may secrete a wide range of substances into blood, including hormones, enzymes and tumour antigens, which are collectively referred to as tumour markers. Tumour marker measurements can contribute to patient management in a number of ways (Tables 17.1 and 17.2).

When interpreting the results of serum tumour markers it is essential to remember the following:

- Concentrations within the reference range do not exclude malignancy.
- A rise in concentration within the reference range should raise the suspicion of tumour recurrence in previously diagnosed patients.
- Nonmalignant conditions may increase the concentration of some tumour markers.

Care must be exercised when requesting tumour markers, as inappropriate requesting can lead to unnecessary further investigations, with the potential risk of harm (e.g. biopsy) and considerable patient anxiety. The screening of nonspecifically unwell patients with panels of tumour markers should be discouraged, as their diagnostic sensitivity and specificity is low under such circumstances. Examples of some of the most commonly used tumour markers in clinical practice are discussed. The measurement of paraprotein concentration as a tumour marker for myeloma is discussed in Chapter 16 (Monoclonal hypergammaglobulinaemia).

Tumour markers commonly used in clinical practice

Carcinoembryonic antigen (CEA)

CEA is a high molecular weight glycoprotein and its measurement remains the most widely used marker as an aid to prognosis, surveillance and monitoring in patients with colorectal cancer. CEA measurements appear to define a subgroup of node-negative patients of Dukes B colon cancer patients that have poor prognosis and could benefit from adjuvant chemotherapy. CEA levels should return to normal post-operatively following successful surgical resection. Failure to do so suggests residual or metastatic disease. Serial monitoring with CEA can detect recurrent disease with a sensitivity of approximately 80% and specificity

Clinical Biochemistry Lecture Notes, Tenth Edition. Peter Rae, Mike Crane and Rebecca Pattenden.
© 2018 John Wiley & Sons Ltd. Published 2018 by John Wiley & Sons Ltd.
Companion website: www.lecturenoteseries.com/clinicalbiochemistry

of approximately 70%, and provides an average lead-time of about 5 months. Patients monitored frequently with CEA have an improved 5-year survival rate, and CEA testing is often carried out every 2–3 months for at least 3 years after the initial diagnosis. Monitoring the response to chemotherapy using CEA is also desirable, with measurements being taken every 2–3 months of active treatment. A clinically significant rise in CEA can be regarded as an increase of 30% over the previous value and such a rise should prompt a repeat measurement within

1 month. Smaller but persistent incremental rises in CEA should also prompt further investigation. It should be remembered that CEA is also increased in a variety of non-GI malignancies (including breast, lung and haematological cancers), as well as in non-malignant conditions (Table 17.3).

CEA is raised in only 30–50% of patients at the time of diagnosis and is thus not recommended for screening; only about 3% of patients with early colorectal cancer (Dukes A) have elevated CEA. In the UK, the faecal occult blood test or the more sensitive faecal immunochemical test is used as a screening test for colorectal cancer in asymptomatic subjects.

Figure 17.1 illustrates how CEA can be an effective aid in monitoring the management of a patient with colorectal cancer.

Table 17.1 Uses for tumour marker measurements.

1 *Monitoring treatment and detecting recurrence of disease* These are their most useful roles.
2 *Diagnosis* Tumour markers provide an aid to diagnosis, but only when used in conjunction with clinical and radiological evidence. Not all patients with a malignancy may exhibit increased concentrations of the tumour marker. Tumour marker concentrations may also be increased in clinical conditions not associated with malignancy.
3 *Screening* With a few exceptions (Table 17.2), tumour markers are of little value in screening for asymptomatic disease, but in some specific instances may be used to screen high-risk groups.
4 *Prognosis* Tumour markers can only be used for prognosis on the few occasions when the plasma concentration correlates with tumour mass (Table 17.2).

CA-125

CA-125 is a high molecular weight glycoprotein that has a well-defined role in the screening and monitoring of ovarian carcinoma. The majority (around 90%) of ovarian cancers are diagnosed in women >45 years, with the highest rates being found in the 60–64 year age group. The CA-125 antigen is found on the endothelium of the fallopian tubes, endocervix and endometrium and also in the normal ovary and the mesothelial cells of the pleura, pericardium and peritoneum. Serum CA-125 is elevated when there is vascular invasion, tissue destruction and

Table 17.2 Malignant disease where tumour markers are used in clinical practice.

Malignancy	Marker	Follow-up	Diagnosis	Prognosis with other factors	Screening
Breast	CA 15.3	*Yes	No	No	No
Choriocarcinoma	hCG	Yes	Yes	Yes	Yes
Colorectal	CEA	Yes	No	Yes	No
Germ cell	hCG	Yes	Yes	Yes	No
Germ cell	AFP	Yes	Yes	Yes	No
Hepatocellular carcinoma	AFP	Yes	Yes	Yes	**Yes
Myeloma	Paraprotein	Yes	Yes	Yes	No
Ovarian	CA-125	Yes	Yes	Yes	Yes
Pancreatic	CA 19-9	Yes	Yes	Yes	No
Prostatic	PSA	Yes	Yes	Yes	No
Thyroid, medullary	Calcitonin	Yes	Yes	Yes	***Yes
Thyroid, follicular, papillary	Thyroglobulin	Yes	No	No	No

* Only when disease cannot be evaluated by other means.
** Subjects at high risk, e.g. chronic hepatitis B and C or cirrhosis.
*** Screening relatives of diagnosed patients.

inflammation associated with malignancy. It is increased in over 90% of women with advanced ovarian cancer disease and in 40% of patients with advanced intra-abdominal malignancy. However, serum CA-125 can also be increased during menstruation and pregnancy and in other nonmalignant conditions such as endometriosis, peritonitis and cirrhosis. Values in patients with ascites can be particularly high, regardless of whether malignancy is present or not.

Guidelines issued by the National Institute for Health and Excellence (NICE) in the UK recommend that primary care physicians should measure serum CA-125 in all women who present with *persistent* symptoms suggestive of ovarian cancer as listed in Table 17.4. If the CA-125 concentration is >35 kU/L, ultrasound of the pelvis and abdomen should be performed and the 'risk of malignancy index' (RMI) calculated. Patients who have a score >250 should be referred for specialist investigation.

There are many causes of a raised CA-125 other than ovarian cancer, particularly in pre-menopausal women (see Table 17.3). Moreover, up to a third of patients with ovarian cancer will not demonstrate elevated CA-125.

Important points:

- In stage 1 ovarian cancer, CA-125 is only elevated in 50% of cases.
- A result within the reference range should never be used to exclude ovarian cancer.
- There are many causes of a raised CA-125 other than malignancy, particularly in pre-menopausal women.
- The likelihood of a raised CA-125 being caused by an ovarian malignancy increases with age.
- CA-125 is a relatively reliable marker of response to treatment and disease progression.

Table 17.3 Examples of nonmalignant conditions that may cause increases in serum tumour markers.

CA-125
- Liver disease
- Pancreatitis
- Acute urinary retention
- Rheumatoid arthritis
- Renal failure
- Colitis
- Congestive heart failure
- Cystic fibrosis
- Diabetes
- Diverticulitis
- Endometriosis
- Irritable bowel syndrome (IBS)
- Menstruation
- Ascites
- Peritoneal inflammation
- Respiratory disease
- Lupus
- Pregnancy Surgery

CEA
- Liver disease
- Renal failure
- Colitis
- IBS
- Respiratory disease
- Smoking

PSA
- Prostatitis
- Benign prostatic disease
- Urinary tract infection
- Digital rectal examination

AFP
- Hepatitis
- Liver repair/regeneration
- Pregnancy
- Physiological in neonates/infants

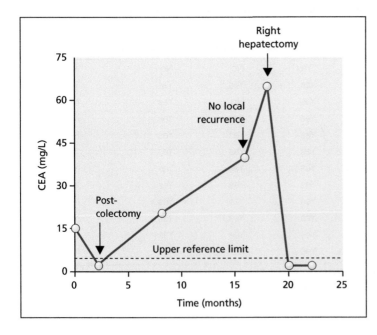

Figure 17.1 Carcinoembryonic antigen (CEA) levels in a 68-year-old man who presented with a colonic tumour.

Table 17.4 Summary of the investigation of suspected ovarian cancer. *See NICE guidelines for full details of assessment.*

Persistent or frequent (>12 times per month) symptoms requiring investigation with CA-125
- Abdominal bloating/distension
- Pelvic pain
- Unexplained weight loss
- Fatigue
- Loss of appetite or early satiety
- Increased urinary urgency or frequency.
- 50 years of age or over with IBS–like symptoms

If CA-125 is >35 kU/L, calculate the risk of malignancy index (RMI)
- RMI = U × M × CA-125
- U is the ultrasound score (0–5)
- M is menopausal status score: 1 = pre-menopausal; 3 = post-menopausal
- CA-125 is serum concentration in kU/L

If RMI >250, refer patient for specialist investigation

 CASE 17.1

Mrs PA, 32 years old, presented to her GP complaining of feeling bloated after eating; this had been going on for a couple of months. Her mother had died of ovarian cancer. Examination found no evidence of an abdominal or pelvic mass.

The CA-125 was found to be 45 IU/L (reference range <35 IU/L).

An ultrasound of the abdomen and pelvis was carried out and found to be entirely normal. What should be done now?

Comment: Given the normal ultrasound and age of the patient, ovarian malignancy is unlikely despite the increased CA-125. Further clinical assessment and investigations should be carried out and any alternative diagnosis considered. It may be worth repeating the CA-125, ensuring the sample is not taken during menstruation. This case illustrates the problem of screening using CA-125, i.e. abnormal CA-125 levels may be found in many women who do not have ovarian cancer (Table 17.3).

Prostate-specific antigen (PSA)

PSA is a glycoprotein used as a tumour marker to aid diagnosis and to monitor patients with prostatic cancer. PSA is detectable in the serum of healthy men and the concentration rises with age; thus age-related reference ranges are useful (Table 17.5). Most PSA circulates in plasma bound to α_1-antichymotrypsin, but

Table 17.5 Age-specific PSA reference ranges.

Age (years)	PSA reference range (µg/L)
<50	≤2.5
50–60	≤3.0
60–70	≤4.0
≥70	≤5.0

a small fraction circulates unbound to any protein (free PSA). Patients with prostatic cancer appear to have a higher ratio between bound and free PSA than patients with benign hypertrophy, however the assessment of free PSA is not widely available. Like most tumour markers, PSA is also increased in a number of nonmalignant conditions (Table 17.3).

Important points:

- Approximately 50% of men with prostatic cancer who have a PSA between 4 and 10 µg/L will have disease outwith the prostate capsule.
- Approximately 15% of patients diagnosed with prostatic malignancy will have a PSA between 3 and 4 µg/L
- Bone metastases are unlikely in patients with a PSA below 4 µg/L.

The value of screening asymptomatic patients remains controversial and, if performed, screening should only be done after appropriate counselling. Recent large-scale studies indicate that the 10-year survival rates for males with early-stage prostate cancer detected by PSA testing do not differ between those given treatment (surgery/radiotherapy) and those that undergo active monitoring.

 CASE 17.2

A 73-year-old man presented to his doctor, complaining of back pain and increasing problems with passing urine. The following results from chemical tests were obtained:

Serum	Result	Reference range
Prostate-specific antigen	70	<5 µg/L
Albumin	38	35–50 g/L
ALP activity	200	40–125 U/L
ALT activity	35	10–50 U/L
Bilirubin total	10	2–21 µmol/L
GGT activity	35	10–55 U/L

What is the likely diagnosis?

Comments: The man is likely to have metastatic prostatic cancer. Although there is overlap in the levels of PSA seen in men with benign prostatic hypertrophy and those with prostatic cancer, the high levels of PSA found in this patient are usually seen only in patients with metastatic disease.

The elevated ALP in the presence of normal GGT and other liver function tests also suggests metastatic spread to bone.

Examination of the prostate per rectum disclosed an enlarged and hard prostate, and tissue obtained during a transurethral resection demonstrated the presence of tumour.

α-Foetoprotein (AFP)

Patients with cirrhosis, haemochromatosis and persistent infection with hepatitis B and C are at high risk of developing hepatocellular carcinoma. Measurement of serum AFP on a regular basis (every 6–12 months) appears to be of value to allow early detection of tumour. Serum AFP is increased in many patients with cirrhosis, but a concentration in excess of 400 kU/L is almost diagnostic of malignancy; those with a concentration greater than 40 kU/L require close investigation. In such circumstances serum AFP is of value both for monitoring response to treatment and potential recurrence.

Measurement of serum AFP is also important in the investigation of patients presenting with potential germ-cell tumours. If raised due to secretion by the tumour, AFP provides an effective means to monitor treatment. Approximately 50–70% of non-seminomatous germ-cell tumours secrete AFP. Care should be exercised in interpreting values during pregnancy, or in neonates and infants, where AFP concentrations are greatly increased; values in premature neonates may be as much as 10^5-fold normal adult values.

 CASE 17.3

A 50-year-old male lecturer presented to his doctor, complaining of tiredness, abdominal discomfort and poor appetite. He had worked in Africa in the past, where he had contracted hepatitis B and had become a carrier. On examination, he was jaundiced and his liver was enlarged. Urine was positive for both bilirubin and urobilinogen.

The following results were found:

Serum	Result	Reference range
Albumin	34	35–50 g/L
ALP activity	420	40–125 U/L
ALT	146	10–50 U/L
Bilirubin total	60	2–21 μmol/L
GGT activity	164	10–55 U/L
AFP	3130	5 kU/L

What is the likely diagnosis?

Comments: The patient has a primary hepatocellular carcinoma. This is a relatively uncommon malignancy in the developed world, but common in China, South-East Asia and parts of Africa as a result of the high incidence of hepatitis B in these regions. Chronic carriers of the virus have an increased risk of developing the malignancy. The liver function tests show a mixed pattern of cholestasis, probably arising from the tumour, and hepatitis, arising from the chronic hepatitis. The very high concentration of AFP is highly suggestive of hepatocellular carcinoma, but levels of up to ~500 kU/L can be found in some patients with nonmalignant hepatobiliary disease.

Human chorionic gonadotrophin (hCG)

Patients presenting with a lump in the testes or malignancy of unknown origin should have hCG measured alongside AFP. The presence of hCG denotes the presence of trophoblastic tissue. When hCG testing is combined with that for AFP, approximately 75% of patients with non-seminomatous germ-cell tumours demonstrate elevated tumour marker levels. A small proportion of patients with seminomas (or dysgerminomas) will also secrete hCG as a tumour product; such tumours do not secrete AFP. Due to the existence of multiple forms of hCG in serum (intact, free β-subunit, nicked and hyperglycosylated), it is important that the laboratory hCG assay used for oncological purposes detects all possible forms of hCG.

One of the best defined applications of tumour marker screening is the measurement of hCG in patients with gestational trophoblastic disease. Approximately 8% of patients who have experienced a molar pregnancy will subsequently develop choriocarcinoma; screening urinary hCG in such patients is a highly effective means to detect occurrence (sensitivity and specificity ~99%). Measurement of hCG is also used to assess prognosis and response to treatment in these patients.

CA 19-9

Measurement of CA 19-9 is primarily indicated in the post-operative monitoring of patients with pancreatic tumours, although values can also be increased in patients with colorectal or other GI malignancies. However, the usefulness of CA 19-9 is limited by the fact that there are few effective treatments available for the disease.

Monitoring CA 19-9 may also be useful in patients with primary sclerosing cholangitis. Patients with this condition who subsequently develop cholangiocarcinoma often show a rapid rise in CA 19-9 concentration to greatly elevated values.

CA 15-3 and HER2/neu

CA 15-3 is a mucin glycoprotein of use in monitoring patients with breast cancer. Measurement of CA 15-3 provides prognostic information, and serial monitoring has the potential to detect recurrent disease and evaluate response to treatment. The marker may become more important when more effective treatments are developed to treat metastatic disease.

HER2/neu is a 185-kDa cell surface receptor protein which is a member of the epidermal growth factor receptor family. It is expressed in small amounts on the plasma membrane of normal cells. The protein appears to be involved in the growth and spread of breast cancer cells, and about 25% of patients have a high concentration of the protein. The presence of HER2/neu suggests an aggressive tumour and appears to provide a prognostic indicator. Patients with HER2/neu-positive tumours respond to treatment with monoclonal antibody therapy directed to the HER2/neu protein.

Inhibin A and B

Inhibin is a 32-kDa glycoprotein produced by the granulosa cells of the ovary and Sertoli cells of the testis (see Chapter 10). The primary use of inhibin measurements is for monitoring recurrence post-operatively in patients with granulosa or Sertoli-cell tumours. The concentration of inhibin in women varies markedly depending on the stage of the menstrual cycle and whether or not the patient is post-menopausal. Interpretation is therefore also dependent on whether unilateral or bilateral oophorectomy is performed.

Monitoring serum oestradiol post-operatively in patients with granulosa-cell tumours is also useful for detecting tumour recurrence; approximately 30% of such tumors also produce oestradiol.

Thyroglobulin

Patients with papillary or follicular thyroid cancer are usually treated by total thyroidectomy followed by ablative doses of radioiodine. Thyroxine is then prescribed at doses that suppress TSH to concentrations of <0.01 mU/L with a view to impairing the growth of any residual tumour. In patients with low-grade disease, complete suppression of TSH may not be required. Many of these tumours synthesise and secrete thyroglobulin, and the measurement of serum thyroglobulin is of value in monitoring progression of the disease and in assessing response to treatment. Measurement of thyroglobulin has no role in the diagnosis of thyroid cancer because elevated concentrations are found in many thyroid disorders other than malignancy. In patients who have been treated with total thyroidectomy and ^{131}I ablation, a serum thyroglobulin is usually undetectable. The finding of a detectable thyroglobulin is suggestive of residual or recurrent tumour, but could also indicate persistence of a remnant of normal thyroid tissue. The sensitivity of serum thyroglobulin measurements for detecting recurrence is enhanced by an elevated TSH concentration. Therefore, serum thyroglobulin should preferably be measured when the serum TSH is >30 mU/L; this can be achieved by either withdrawal of T4 or administering recombinant TSH. However, the introduction of high-sensitivity automated thyroglobulin assays that can measure thyroglobulin to <0.1 µg/L obviates the need for performing a recombinant TSH stimulation test in many circumstances.

Endogenous thyroglobulin antibodies are present in up to 20% of patients with thyroid cancer. These antibodies often interfere with the assays, leading to misdiagnosis. In the immunometric assays (used by most laboratories), antibody interference can lead to false-negative results whereas if radioimmunoassay is used the thyroglobulin antibodies may produce apparent increases in thyroglobulin. Therefore, thyroglobulin results should be interpreted with the knowledge of the thyroglobulin antibody status of the patient. Alternatively thyroglobulin should be measured by both immunometric assay and radioimmunoassay to identify discordant results.

Calcitonin

Medullary thyroid cancer (MTC) arises from the parafollicular, calcitonin-producing cells (C cells) of the thyroid gland, and accounts for about 10% of thyroid cancers. Sporadic cases account for 80% of all cases of MTC; a familial form of the disease occurs in conjunction with a syndrome known as multiple endocrine neoplasia (MEN). A description of MEN is given

Table 17.6 Characteristic tumours in the MEN syndromes.

MEN I	MEN IIa	MEN IIb
Hyperparathyroidism (95%)	Medullary carcinoma of the thyroid (100%)	Medullary carcinoma of the thyroid (100%)
Tumours secreting (50%) • Gastrin • Insulin • Glucagon • Vasoactive intestinal polypeptide (VIP) • Pancreatic polypeptide • Somatostatin	Phaeochromocytoma (30%) Hyperparathyroidism (50%)	Phaeochromocytoma (45%) Associated abnormalities: Mucosal neuroma (100%) Marfan habitus (65%) Megacolon
Carcinoid tumours (30%)		
Pituitary tumours (40%)		

Values in parentheses show the percentage of patients having the condition.

in Table 17.6. Developments in the molecular genetics of MTC that include *RET* proto-oncogene mutation testing have facilitated a rational framework for management and screening of affected family members. The use and interpretation of such molecular diagnostics requires careful application in individual patients and their families.

 CASE 17.4

A 54-year-old female shop assistant presented to the endocrine clinic for annual follow-up. She had been diagnosed 9 years earlier with a small focal papillary carcinoma of the thyroid that had been treated by partial thyroidectomy with no radioiodine ablation. She was taking thyroxine and had remained well with no evidence of recurrent disease.

At annual follow-up the following results were found:

Serum	Result	Reference range
TSH	4.0	0.2–4.5 mU/L
FT4	13	9–21 pmol/L
Thyroglobulin	5	µg/L

(Anti-thyroglobulin antibodies were negative.)

How would you interpret these results?

Comments: The patient has been taking inadequate doses of thyroxine. The aim of T4 therapy in patients with papillary carcinoma of the thyroid is to suppress TSH to undetectable concentrations; this has not been achieved in this patient. Compliance should be verified and the need for an increase in T4 dose ascertained. In patients who have undergone total thyroidectomy and in whom TSH is <0.01 mU/L, thyroglobulin should be undetectable. This patient has residual thyroid tissue (she only has had a partial thyroidectomy) and she has detectable circulating TSH that will stimulate thyroglobulin production from the thyroid remnant. It is thus impossible to determine from these results if the thyroglobulin is originating from the thyroid remnant or a recurrent tumour. Thyroglobulin was later found to be undetectable when the patient's TSH was <0.01 mU/L and no further action was required other than continued annual follow-up.

Plasma calcitonin is often greatly increased in patients with MTC, but plasma calcium is usually normal. Raised plasma calcitonin may occur in other conditions, including Hashimoto thyroiditis, chronic renal failure and diseases associated with transformed neuroendocrine cells (e.g. carcinoid tumours and phaeochromocytoma). It is important to obtain a baseline calcitonin measurement in patients in order that response to therapy (usually thyroidectomy and central node dissection) and follow-up can be assessed. Lifelong follow-up is recommended. The response to primary surgery can be assessed clinically, and by the measurement of serum calcitonin. The presence of an elevated but stable calcitonin level post-operatively may be managed conservatively. Progressively rising levels should trigger imaging for further staging. In the absence of recurrent symptoms, appropriate intervals are 6–12 months. The use of a pentagastrin-stimulated calcitonin test should be considered as a screening test where there is strong presumptive evidence of inherited disease but no mutation in the *RET* gene has been found. In patients with MTC, plasma calcitonin increases by 2–5 times above the basal level following combined calcium and pentagastrin administration, whereas normal subjects show little or no response.

18

Disorders of iron and porphyrin metabolism

Learning objectives

To understand:

✔ assessment of iron status;

✔ laboratory investigation of porphyria;

✔ abnormal derivatives of haemoglobin.

Introduction

Iron is an essential element present mainly in the porphyrin complex, haem, and in iron storage proteins, ferritin and haemosiderin. Haem, which is present in haemoglobin (Hb), myoglobin and cytochromes, is formed by the insertion of ferrous iron, Fe^{2+}, into protoporphyrin (Figure 18.1) which itself is synthesised by a complex chain of reactions (see Figure 18.3). In this chapter, we discuss the disorders of iron and porphyrin metabolism and consider some abnormal derivatives of haemoglobin.

Iron metabolism

The adult human possesses about 70 mmol (4 g) of iron. Iron balance is regulated by alterations in the intestinal absorption of iron. There is only a limited capacity to increase or decrease the rate of loss of iron.

Dietary iron and iron absorption

The normal intake of iron is about 0.2–0.4 mmol/day (10–20 mg/day). Good sources are liver, fish and meat. Normally, about 5–10% of dietary iron is absorbed by

an active transport process. Most absorption occurs in the duodenum. The rate of absorption is controlled by physiological and dietary factors:

- *State of iron stores in the body:* Absorption is increased in iron deficiency and decreased when there is iron overload. The mechanism is unclear.
- *Rate of erythropoiesis:* When this rate is increased, absorption may be increased even though the iron stores are adequate or overloaded.
- *Contents of diet:* Substances that form soluble complexes with iron (e.g. ascorbic acid) facilitate absorption. Substances that form insoluble complexes (e.g. phytate) inhibit absorption.
- *The chemical state of the iron:* Iron in the diet does not usually become available for absorption unless released during digestion. This depends, at least partly, on gastric acid production; Fe^{2+} is more readily absorbed than Fe^{3+}, and the presence of H^+ helps to keep iron in the Fe^{2+} form. Iron in haem (in meat products) can be absorbed while still contained in the haem molecule.

Iron transport, storage and utilisation

After being taken up by the intestinal mucosa, iron is either (1) incorporated into ferritin and retained by

Clinical Biochemistry Lecture Notes, Tenth Edition. Peter Rae, Mike Crane and Rebecca Pattenden.
© 2018 John Wiley & Sons Ltd. Published 2018 by John Wiley & Sons Ltd.
Companion website: www.lecturenoteseries.com/clinicalbiochemistry

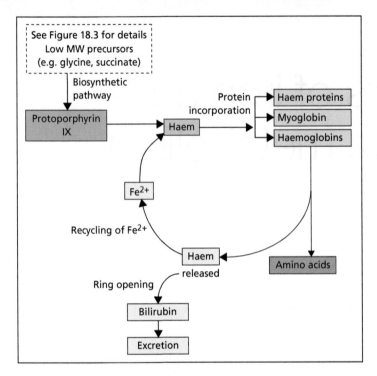

Figure 18.1 Schematic diagram illustrating the formation of haem, its incorporation into haem proteins and subsequent metabolism to bilirubin.

the mucosal cells, or (2) transported across the mucosal cells directly to the plasma, where it is carried mainly combined with *transferrin* (Figure 18.2). Iron retained by mucosal cells is lost from the body when the cells are sloughed. Mucosal cell retention is influenced by the body's iron status, being reduced in iron depletion and increased in states of iron overload.

The total iron circulating bound to transferrin is normally about 50–70 μmol (3–4 mg). Iron in plasma is taken up by cells and either incorporated into haem or stored as ferritin (or haemosiderin, probably formed by the condensation of several molecules of ferritin). Iron released by the breakdown of Hb, at the end of the erythrocyte's life, is normally efficiently conserved and later reused.

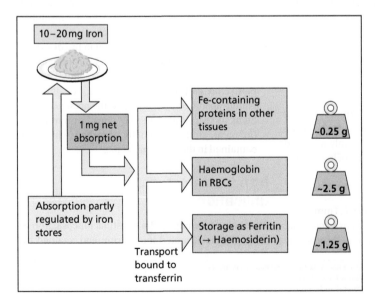

Figure 18.2 Summary of the absorption, transport and utilisation of iron. Total body iron stores (g) for the main iron-containing proteins are shown on the right side of the figure.

Iron excretion and sources of loss

Iron excreted in the faeces is principally exogenous, that is, dietary iron that has not been absorbed by the mucosal cells and transported into the circulation. In males, there is an average loss of endogenous iron of about 20 µmol/day (1 mg/day) in cells desquamated from the skin and the intestinal mucosa. Females may have additional losses due to menstruation or pregnancy. Urine contains negligible amounts of iron.

Laboratory assessment of iron status

This is necessary in the investigation of iron deficiency states and iron overload. The following tests are used (for reference ranges, see Table 18.1).

Serum iron

This is of limited diagnostic value because levels fluctuate widely in health. Much of this variation appears to be random, but some specific causes can be recognised:

1 *Diurnal variation*, with higher values in the morning.
2 *Menstrual cycle*, with low values just before and during the menstrual period.
3 *Oral contraceptives*, which cause increased serum iron.

4 *Pregnancy*, which tends to cause increased serum iron. However, it is often accompanied by iron deficiency so that serum iron falls.

Measurements of serum iron do *not* provide an adequate index of iron status. Although plasma iron is low in iron deficiency and is raised in iron overload, these changes occur relatively late when iron stores have already become either completely depleted or seriously overloaded. In addition, serum iron also alters in conditions not associated with changes in iron stores. Acute infections or trauma precipitate a rapid fall in serum iron. Chronic inflammatory disorders (e.g. rheumatoid arthritis) and malignant diseases are also associated with low levels.

Serum iron determination is only required for diagnostic purposes for a few conditions, for example in suspected cases of acute iron poisoning and in the assessment of individuals with an increased risk of haemochromatosis.

Serum ferritin

Serum ferritin is closely related to body iron stores, whether these are decreased, normal or increased, whereas serum iron becomes abnormal only in the presence of gross abnormalities of iron storage. A low, or low-normal serum ferritin indicates the presence of depleted iron stores. However, because ferritin is an acute-phase reactant, levels may be increased in patients with iron deficiency and concurrent

Table 18.1 Reference ranges for iron status.

	Iron (µmol/L)	Ferritin (µg/L)	TIBC (µmol/L)	TIBC saturation (%)
Reference ranges				
• Males	14–32	20–300*	45–72	20–50
• Females	10–28	15–200*	45–72	15–50
Physiological changes				
• Premenstrual	↓	N	N	↓
• Steroid contraceptives	↑	N	↑	N
• Pregnancy	Variable†	↓	↑	↓
Disease states				
• Iron deficiency	↓	↓	↑	Reduced
• Iron overload	↑	↑	N or ↓	up to 100
• Infections, neoplasms	↓	↑ or N	↓	N
• Hypoplastic anaemia	↑	↑ or N	N or ↓	>40

N = normal; ↑ = increased; ↓ = decreased.
*A serum ferritin below 20 µg/L suggests that the body's iron stores are depleted.
†See above.

inflammation, malignancy or hepatic disease, although at concentrations greater than 100 µg/L iron deficiency is almost certainly not present.

Increased serum ferritin is found in iron overload, irrespective of the cause, and in many patients with liver disease or cancer. A normal serum ferritin virtually excludes untreated iron overload. Determination of serum ferritin currently provides the most useful measure of iron status widely available on a routine basis.

Serum transferrin, total iron-binding capacity and iron saturation

Normally, nearly all the iron-binding capacity in serum is due to transferrin, and about 40% of the binding sites on transferrin are occupied by iron. Transferrin has a much longer half-life than iron, and serum transferrin shows fewer short-term fluctuations. Transferrin levels fall in PEM, during the acute-phase response, and with infections, neoplastic disease and chronic liver disease. Synthesis increases in iron deficiency.

Transferrin can be measured not only directly, but also indirectly as the ability of serum protein (largely transferrin) to bind iron, the so-called TIBC of serum. The ratio of serum iron to transferrin (or TIBC) then determines the transferrin (or TIBC) saturation.

In iron-deficiency anaemia, the low serum iron is typically associated with an increase in transferrin concentration (and TIBC). This leads to a low saturation of transferrin (and TIBC) with iron. Conversely, in iron overload, serum iron is high and transferrin is normal or low, that is, a high percentage saturation of TIBC (Table 18.1). This effect is particularly marked in haemochromatosis, in which saturation of the TIBC usually rises above 60% fairly early in the disorder.

As with serum iron, there is little place for determining serum transferrin or TIBC as a routine measure of iron status. However, in the detection of early or latent haemochromatosis, serum TIBC saturation should be measured. Also, in patients being treated with erythropoietin for the anaemia of chronic renal failure, the percentage saturation of TIBC provides a better index of available iron than serum ferritin, and it is also a better guide to the need to give iron treatment.

The serum transferrin (or TIBC) is also helpful in determining the significance of very high serum ferritin in patients with disordered liver function of unknown cause, in whom the differential diagnosis may be between haemochromatosis and malignancy. A high serum ferritin in the absence of an increased percentage saturation of TIBC indicates that cancer is more likely to be the diagnosis.

Serum transferrin receptor

A circulating form of the transferrin receptor, lacking the cytoplasmic and transmembrane domains of the intact receptor, has been identified in serum. Its concentration rises in iron deficiency following the depletion of iron stores and, because levels are unaffected by inflammation, its measurement has the potential to provide an indication of iron status in patients with anaemia associated with chronic disease. Assays for serum transferrin receptor are not yet widely available.

Iron deficiency

Worldwide, this is the most common single nutrient deficiency. The main causes (Table 18.2) are deficient intake (including reduced bioavailability due to dietary fibre, phytates, etc.), impaired absorption (e.g. intestinal malabsorptive disease, abdominal surgery) and excessive loss (e.g. menstrual, GI bleeding).

In patients who develop iron deficiency,

- serum ferritin falls, then
- serum transferrin and TIBC increase, after which
- serum iron falls, and finally
- anaemia becomes evident.

Table 18.2 Causes of iron deficiency and excess.

Iron deficiency	Iron overload
Decreased intake • Poor diet	Excessive intake • Over-supplementation with iron tablets
• Prolonged weaning (milk: poor iron source)	• Repeated blood transfusions
• Malabsorption	• Iron cooking utensils (especially with acid foodstuffs)
Increased requirements (in the presence of inadequate intake)	Excessive absorption • Haemochromatosis
• Adolescence	
• Pregnancy	
• Menstruating females	
Excessive iron losses • Menorrhagia	
• GI losses	
• Genito-urinary losses	
• Excessive blood donations	

A microcytic, hypochromic anaemia is characteristic, and storage iron is absent from macrophages in the bone marrow aspirate. In general, serum ferritin is the best diagnostic test for iron deficiency (renal failure is one of the few exceptions, see Chapter 18: Serum transferrin, total iron-binding capacity and iron saturation).

Biochemical tests may help to identify the underlying cause of iron deficiency anaemia. For example, practice guidelines recommend that where GI investigations are indicated, patients should be screened for coeliac disease (Chapter 14: Small intestine and colon/Serological tests for coeliac disease) as a possible cause of malabsorption. It should be noted that the traditionally widely used guaiac-based FOB tests are not sufficiently sensitive for excluding the possibility of GI blood loss in this setting and a negative result can give false reassurance and may delay diagnosis. However, there is potential for the use of quantitative faecal immunochemical tests (FITs) for haemoglobin to guide referral and further investigations in symptomatic patients presenting to primary care (Chapter 14: Small intestine and colon/Gastrointestinal inflammation).

 CASE 18.1

A 45-year-old woman presented with a flare-up of her inflammatory bowel disease and bloody stools. Her haemoglobin was 100g/L (reference interval 115–160) and her blood film revealed hypochromic and microcytic red blood cells.

Results of the iron studies investigations are shown below:

Serum	Result	Reference range
Ferritin	65	15–200g/L
Iron	4	10–28µmol/L
Transferrin	1.5	2.0–4.0g/L
Transferrin saturation	10	15–50%

How would you interpret the results?

Comments: The results are consistent with anaemia of chronic disease. However, the history of blood loss raises the possibility of iron deficiency in this patient. The low transferrin does not exclude iron deficiency, and iron deficiency may be associated with a normal ferritin in patients with inflammatory or chronic disease.

The patient responded well to treatment with oral iron supplements, confirming a diagnosis of iron deficiency.

Iron overload

This is much less common than iron deficiency (Table 18.2). Diagnosis is not usually difficult once the possibility has been considered. Increased serum iron with normal transferrin (or TIBC) often leads to 100% saturation of transferrin (or TIBC). Serum ferritin is increased, often to more than 1000µg/L. More common causes are as follows:

- Increased intake and absorption. Acute overdose, mainly occurring in children, may cause severe or even fatal symptoms, due to the toxic effects of free iron in plasma (see further on: iron poisoning). Chronic overload occurs when the diet contains excess absorbable iron (e.g. acid-containing food cooked in iron pots). Iron deposits form, for example, in the liver causing hepatic fibrosis and in the myocardium causing myocardial damage.
- Parenteral administration of iron, including repeated blood transfusions.
- Hereditary haemochromatosis.

Hereditary haemochromatosis

This autosomal recessive disorder is associated with a mutation of the *HFE* gene, which is located on chromosome 6. In 85–90% of cases, the mutation is due to a single base change that results in the substitution of tyrosine for cysteine at position 282 of the HFE protein (C282Y). Individuals homozygous for this mutation are predisposed to an unregulated increase in the intestinal absorption of dietary iron although the phenotypic expression is variable. At least 90% of symptomatic individuals are male, suggesting that iron losses in menstruation and pregnancy may protect females. Excessive iron deposits build up as haemosiderin in the liver, leading to a macronodular cirrhosis in untreated individuals. Fibrotic damage to the pancreas (with diabetes mellitus) and heart involvement are also described. Other clinical features include skin pigmentation ('bronzed diabetes'), endocrine organ involvement (testicular atrophy) and arthritis with chondrocalcinosis.

Hereditary haemochromatosis can be detected at the pre-clinical stage in affected members of a family in which an index case has occurred. In families at risk, apparently unaffected members with the susceptible genotype should have regular (e.g. annual) measurements of serum iron, ferritin and TIBC. The first abnormalities to appear in serum are increased ferritin and percentage saturation of TIBC; if either of these becomes abnormal, liver biopsy is indicated. Case finding for affected relatives is important, because treatment by phlebotomy can prevent the disease from progressing.

CASE 18.2

Two sisters, whose mother had recently received a diagnosis of haemochromatosis, were referred to a haematologist for assessment of their iron status and genetic testing. Both were well and asymptomatic. Initial biochemical findings were as follows:

Serum	Patient 1	Patient 2	Reference range
Ferritin	162	668	<150g/L
Iron	33	43	10–28µmol/L
Transferrin	1.7	2.1	2.0–4.0g/L
Transferrin saturation	74	78	15–50%

What would you consider to be the iron status of each sister?

Comments: Chromosomal analysis indicated that both sisters were homozygous for the C282Y mutation. The younger sister, aged 32 (patient 2), showed clear evidence of increased iron stores with an elevated serum ferritin, iron and transferrin saturation. She was subsequently treated by regular therapeutic phlebotomy. In contrast, the ferritin concentration suggested that the iron stores were only marginally increased in the elder sister, aged 40 (patient 1). Interestingly, this sister had been a regular blood donor for a number of years and had thereby protected herself from iron overload. No active treatment was necessary and she was subsequently reviewed on a regular basis.

Iron poisoning

This is potentially life threatening, particularly in children. Early clinical symptoms, which include epigastric pain, nausea and vomiting, often with haematemesis, may settle but be followed later by acute encephalopathy and circulatory failure. Acute liver and renal failure may also develop. Treatment involves giving desferrioxamine, an iron-chelating agent, which binds the iron in plasma, and the resulting complex is excreted in urine.

Serum iron values greater than 90µmol/L require treatment. An immediate IM injection of desferrioxamine is followed by gastric lavage, leaving desferrioxamine in the stomach.

Porphyrin metabolism

Porphyrins are tetrapyrroles, some of which are intermediates in the formation of haem. Haem itself is formed when Fe^{2+} combines with protoporphyrin IX (Figure 18.1). Most cells can synthesise haem, but liver cells and bone marrow are the most active. Inherited or acquired defects in the enzymes that are involved in haem formation can lead to overproduction of pathway intermediates, with different clinical consequences. These conditions, which are relatively rare, are collectively known as the porphyrias. Figure 18.3 summarises the haem biosynthetic pathway and the disorders that result from deficiency of specific enzymes, and indicates that the porphyrias may be classified according to their clinical presentation into acute, cutaneous and mixed forms. Only about 10–20% of patients with the enzyme defects of hereditary porphyria ever develop symptoms, but because of the protean manifestations of the porphyrias, the diagnosis is likely to be suspected more often than it presents.

Acute porphyrias

Enzyme deficiencies that lead to an accumulation of aminolaevulinic acid (ALA) and porphobilinogen (PBG) may be associated with potentially life-threatening acute attacks of severe abdominal pain often accompanied by neurological and psychiatric symptoms. Constipation, nausea, vomiting and hypertension are other common features. Acute attacks may be precipitated by a variety of factors including a wide range of commonly prescribed drugs, endogenous steroid hormones, fasting, substance abuse and stress. Skin lesions are absent in acute intermittent porphyria (AIP), the most common of the acute porphyrias, but they may accompany acute attacks in approximately half of patients with variegate porphyria (VP) and one third of patients with hereditary coproporphyria (HC). Cutaneous manifestations may be the sole presenting feature in VP and HC, but these patients are also at risk of acute attacks if exposed to acute precipitants. In between acute attacks, patients may be symptom free.

Laboratory diagnosis

The laboratory investigation of acute porphyria is summarised in Figure 18.4. With the exception of plumboporphyria, which is an exceedingly rare

CASE 18.3

A 35-year-old woman was admitted to a hospital with a history of abdominal pain and vomiting. She had been constipated for 5 days and also complained of numbness in the buttocks and aching at the tops of her legs. Her condition deteriorated rapidly and she was found on the floor hallucinating. A visiting aunt mentioned that there was a family history of porphyria.

Results of initial biochemical investigations were as follows:

Analyte	Result	Reference range
Serum		
Urea	7.8	2.5–6.6 mmol/L
Na	122	135–145 mmol/L
K+	3.4	3.6–5.0 mmol/L
Osmolality	256	280–295 mmol/kg
Urine		
Osmolality	556	

What do these results show? What further tests would be useful for investigating this patient for acute porphyria?

Comments: The initial biochemical results revealed marked hyponatraemia and a correspondingly low serum osmolality. The urine was relatively concentrated, suggesting inappropriate ADH secretion. A 30-fold elevation in the urinary concentration of PBG provided confirmation that the patient was experiencing an attack of one of the acute porphyrias. Faecal concentrations of porphyrin were not elevated, excluding the possibility of HC or VP. The activity of hydroxymethylbilane synthase in red cells was reduced, confirming the diagnosis of AIP. It was not possible to identify any specific precipitating factor in this case. Hyponatraemia and inappropriate ADH secretion are frequently observed in patients presenting with an acute attack of porphyria.

 CASE 18.4

A 27-year-old woman had become increasingly unwell over the previous 3 days and was admitted to hospital complaining of severe abdominal pains, nausea and vomiting. The diagnosis was uncertain but after 7 days her symptoms had largely resolved. Before discharge it was suggested that the patient may have experienced an attack of acute porphyia and therefore fresh samples of urine and faeces were tested for PBG and porphyrins. The following results were obtained:

Analyte	Result	Reference range
Urine		
PBG	1.4	<1.5 μmol/mmol creatinine
Porphyrin	34	<35 nmol/mmol creatinine
Faeces		
Coproporphyrin	201	<4 nmol/g
Protoporphyrin	725	<134 nmol/g

Comments: Because the urine PBG was within reference limits, the patient was not having an acute porphyria attack at the time the sample was collected. However, analysis of the faecal sample showed an accumulation of proto- and coproporphyrin that was consistent with a diagnosis of variegate porphyria. It was subsequently possible to retrieve an earlier urine sample that had been stored in the Microbiology Department since admission. Analysis showed an elevation of PBG, confirming that the patient had indeed experienced an acute porphyria attack around the time of admission.

This case demonstrates (1) the importance of obtaining urine samples for PBG analysis at the time of a suspected porphyria attack and (2) that in patients with variegate porphyria, PBG excretion may return to normal rapidly following an acute attack.

disorder that has not been reported in Britain, attacks of acute porphyria are invariably associated with an elevated urinary excretion of PBG. This relates to the reduced activity of hydroxymethylbilane synthase due to either an inherited deficiency in patients with AIP or the inhibitory effects of coproporphyrinogen III and protoporphyrinogen IX which accumulate in patients with HC and VP, respectively. Therefore, in the investigation of patients with a suspected attack of one of the acute porphyrias, a fresh random urine specimen, protected from light, should be sent to the laboratory for the quantitation of PBG (screening tests may be unreliable). A negative result excludes an acute porphyria provided the patient is symptomatic at the time of sample collection. In between acute attacks, the excretion of PBG may return to normal. This may occur within days in patients with HC and VP but take several months following an acute

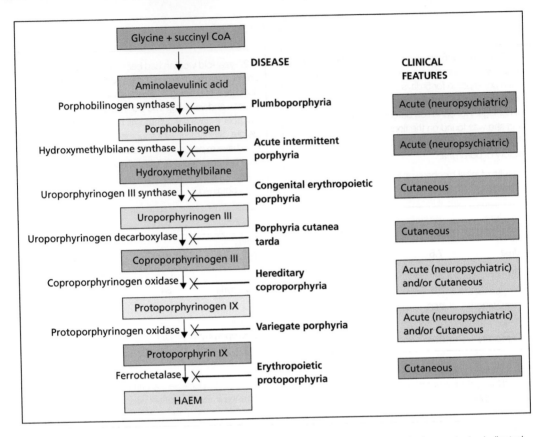

Figure 18.3 Haem synthesis. Enzyme deficiencies at various levels in the pathway result in the porphyrias indicated.

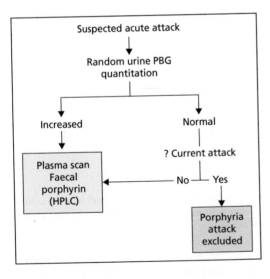

Figure 18.4 Laboratory investigation of the acute porphyrias. HPLC = high-performance liquid chromatography.

episode of AIP. The identification of asymptomatic patients who are in the latent phase of their disease can be particularly difficult (see Chapter 18: Family studies).

If PBG excretion is elevated, the acute porphyrias can be differentiated by the analysis of faecal porphyrins which are not usually elevated in AIP but show characteristic patterns in HC and VP. Initial screening tests involve the spectroscopic examination of an acid extract of faeces for porphyrins. Positive results should always be followed up by referral to a specialist laboratory for the identification of specific intermediates. Plasma porphyrin fluorescence scanning is particularly useful in the identification of VP when porphyrin is covalently bound to plasma protein.

The acute porphyrias are also associated with increased urinary ALA excretion, but it is only necessary to quantify ALA if plumboporphyria is suspected or, possibly, in the investigation of lead poisoning (Figure 18.4).

Family studies

It is most important to investigate relatives of patients with AIP, HC and VP so that gene carriers can be warned to avoid factors that may precipitate potentially fatal acute attacks. Unfortunately all of the standard biochemical investigations have limitations for identifying carrier status. PBG excretion is normal in virtually all children and in many adults with latent AIP. Although the measurement of red cell hydroxymethylbilane synthase activity may be helpful, because of overlap between normal subjects and patients with AIP unequivocal assignment of carrier status cannot be made. Similarly, urinary PBG and porphyrin excretion are usually unhelpful in identifying carriers of HC and VP. While an unambiguously positive pattern of faecal porphyrins or a characteristic VP porphyrin peak in plasma may identify carriers of HC and VP, negative results are inconclusive.

Genetic analysis is increasingly used in difficult cases. The gene locations of many of the porphyrias have now been identified and although a large number of mutations have been described, many are family specific and provide the opportunity for family studies.

Cutaneous porphyrias

The accumulation of porphyrins in the skin leads to photosensitivity which may present in two ways.

The cutaneous manifestations of erythropoietic protoporphyria (EPP) are present in childhood and include burning, itching and erythema occurring shortly after exposure to sunlight. In contrast, the skin lesions in porphyria cutanea tarda (PCT), HC, VP and congenital erythropoietic porphyria include fragile skin, subepidermal bullae, pigmentation and hypertrichosis. PCT is the most common of all the porphyrias and is usually sporadic (aetiological factors include alcohol, oestrogens, iron and chemicals), with only 10–20% of cases being familial.

Laboratory diagnosis

The laboratory investigation of the cutaneous porphyrias is summarised in Figure 18.5. The diagnosis of EPP is made by demonstrating excess free protoporphyrin (FPP) and zinc protoporphyrin (ZPP) in red cells. The examination of both urine and faeces for excess porphyrins is essential in the investigation of patients thought to have one of the remaining cutaneous porphyrias. Initial screening tests involve the spectroscopic examination of acidified urine or a plasma porphyrin fluorescence scan. Positive results should always be followed up by referral to a specialist laboratory for the identification of specific intermediates in urine and faeces. This is particularly important for the differentiation of patients with PCT from those with either HC or VP who may present

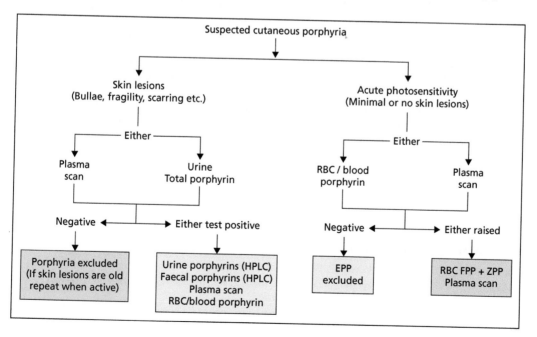

Figure 18.5 Laboratory investigation of the cutaneous porphyrias.

with skin lesions alone but still be at risk of life-threatening acute neurological attacks.

Lead poisoning

The accumulation of lead impairs the biosynthesis of haem through its inhibitory effects on the activity of PBG synthase, coproporphyrinogen oxidase and ferrochelatase. This results in an increase in:

- *Urinary ALA and coproporphyrin* which rise as the blood lead concentration increases.
- *Red cell zinc protoporphyrin* which, in the absence of iron deficiency, represents the average exposure of the erythrocyte to lead during its lifespan.

These tests are not sufficiently sensitive to detect reliably low levels of lead exposure, and the measurement of blood lead is the method of choice for investigating environmental or industrial exposure to lead.

Abnormal derivatives of haemoglobin

These all reduce the oxygen-carrying capacity of the blood (Table 18.3). The abnormal derivatives of Hb can all be identified by means of their characteristic absorption spectra, and it is possible to measure the various derivatives quantitatively if they are present in sufficient amounts.

Methaemoglobin

This is oxidised Hb, the Fe^{2+} normally present in haem being replaced by Fe^{3+}; the ability to act as an O_2 carrier is lost. The normal erythrocyte contains small amounts of methaemoglobin, formed by spontaneous oxidation of Hb. Methaemoglobin is normally reconverted to Hb by reducing systems in the red cells, the most important of which is NADH-methaemoglobin reductase. Excess methaemoglobin may be present in the blood because of increased production or diminished ability to convert it back to Hb. If there is more than $20\,g/L$ of methaemoglobin, cyanosis develops. Haemolysis sometimes occurs in cases of methaemoglobinaemia, and methaemoglobin then appears in the urine, giving it a brownish colour.

Both genetically determined and acquired conditions can cause methaemoglobinaemia; the acquired group is much more common.

- *Genetic causes of methaemoglobinaemia* include, first, a group of haemoglobinopathies, collectively termed Hb M, where an amino acid substitution stabilises Hb in the Fe^{3+} form. A second group has a deficiency in the enzyme system that reduces methaemoglobin. Reducing agents (such as ascorbic acid or methylene blue) work effectively in the second group, but are ineffective in the first group.
- *Acquired methaemoglobinaemia* usually arises following the ingestion of large amounts of drugs, for example phenacetin, the sulphonamides, excess of nitrites, or certain oxidising agents present in the diet. Treatment with reducing agents is also effective in reversing acquired methaemoglobinaemia.

Sulphaemoglobin

This is formed when Hb is acted on by the same substances as those that cause acquired methaemoglobinaemia, if they act in the presence of sulphur-containing compounds, such as hydrogen sulphide that may arise from bacterial action in the intestine. Sulphaemoglobin and methaemoglobin are often present at the same time in these patients. Sulphaemoglobin cannot act as an O_2 carrier, nor can it be converted back to Hb. Because of its spectroscopic characteristics, patients with even a mild degree of sulphaemoglobinaemia are cyanosed.

Table 18.3 **Abnormal forms of Hb.**

Hb derivative	Description
Methaemoglobin	Fe^{3+} replaces Fe^{2+}. Genetic or acquired causes
Haematin	Protoporphyrin containing Fe^{3+}, released from methaemoglobin. May combine with albumin to form methaemalbumin
Sulphaemoglobin	Produced by oxidation of Hb in the presence of SH-containing compounds. Often present with methaemoglobin
Carboxyhaemoglobin	Very stable compound where CO replaces O_2 in oxyhaemoglobin. Unable to transport O_2

Carboxyhaemoglobin (COHb)

Carbon monoxide is a colourless, odourless gas that avidly combines with the haem moiety in Hb and cytochrome enzymes. It combines at the same position in the Hb molecule as O_2, but with an affinity about 200 times greater than that of oxygen. As a result, even small quantities of CO in the inspired air cause the formation of relatively large amounts of COHb, with a corresponding reduction in the O_2-carrying capacity of the blood. This is due not only to the blocking effect of CO on O_2-binding sites, but also to a shift to the left of the oxygen dissociation curve (Figure 3.4) that occurs even when only one of the four O_2-binding sites on Hb is occupied by CO. As little as 1% CO in the inspired air can be fatal in minutes.

In general, nonsmokers have COHb values of less than 1%, except in some city dwellers. However, values of as much as 10% occur in heavy smokers. Acute poisoning (smoke inhalation, faulty heaters or flues, car exhaust fumes, attempted suicide) gives rise to nonspecific symptoms of lethargy, headache and nausea that may proceed to confusion, agitation and deep coma. When poisoning is suspected, COHb levels can be measured in the laboratory. Urgent treatment with 100% oxygen and, where necessary, cardiorespiratory resuscitation and treatment of cerebral oedema should be instituted. Hyperbaric oxygen is particularly helpful in the more serious cases, especially when COHb levels are 30% or more (concentrations >40% usually result in unconsciousness, and may be fatal).

19

Uric acid, gout and purine metabolism

Learning objectives

To understand:

✔ the origin and excretion of uric acid;
✔ the distinction between primary and secondary gout;
✔ the features of primary gout.

Introduction

The clinical importance of purines rests largely on the disorder termed gout, an inflammatory arthritis resulting from uric acid deposition in the joints. An increase in serum uric acid (as the anion, urate, at physiological pH) is the strongest risk factor for gout although gout may occur when serum urate levels are within the normal range. Descriptions of gout have been identified in ancient Egyptian writings but the earliest definitive report is ascribed to Sydenham, writing in the late 17th century. In man, urate is the end-product of purine metabolism such that urate accumulation may arise from:

- increased dietary purine intake or dietary factors affecting urate production;
- increased formation (either increased nucleic acid breakdown or increased *de novo* synthesis of purines);
- decreased renal excretion;
- a combination of the above.

Human beings and higher primates, unlike nonprimates, lack the enzyme called uricase that converts uric acid to the very soluble allantoin.

Primary (idiopathic) gout refers to the condition arising in the absence of clearly defined acquired or genetic conditions, although there may be a familial component to the problem. Associations of primary gout with obesity, alcohol excess, raised blood pressure and hypertriglyceridaemia are well described. Secondary gout refers to the condition in association with a specific acquired cause, such as renal failure, increased cell turnover or a drug-related cause (e.g. thiazide diuretic) or on the basis that the patient has a rare inborn error of one of the enzymes in purine metabolism. The classification is convenient but not always clear-cut because overlapping aetiologies are possible.

Understanding how urate is formed and then handled by the kidney aids our understanding of gout.

Purine metabolism and uric acid

Purines are simple, cyclic organic molecules that are essential constituents of the nucleic acids, both DNA and RNA. The purine bases adenine and guanine comprise the 'A' and 'G' of the DNA code. When a ribose

---

Clinical Biochemistry Lecture Notes, Tenth Edition. Peter Rae, Mike Crane and Rebecca Pattenden.
© 2018 John Wiley & Sons Ltd. Published 2018 by John Wiley & Sons Ltd.
Companion website: www.lecturenoteseries.com/clinicalbiochemistry

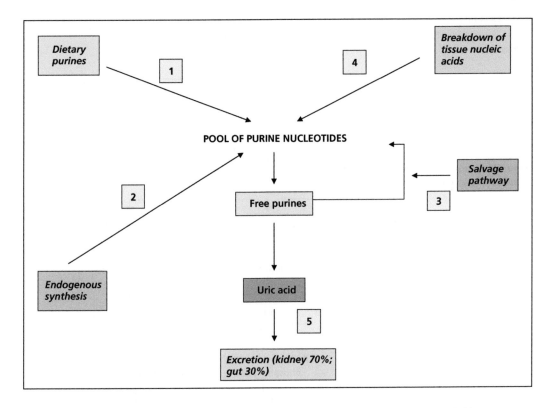

Figure 19.1 Routes to the formation of uric acid and examples: (1) purine-rich diet (meats, seafood); (2) 5-phosphoribosyl-1-pyrophosphate synthase overactivity; (3) hypoxanthine-guanine phosphoribosyltransferase deficiency; (4) tumour lysis syndrome; (5) renal failure.

sugar moiety is linked to the purine base a nucleoside is formed (e.g. adenosine, made up of the purine adenine linked to ribose). The addition of a phosphate group to the ribose ring generates the corresponding nucleotide (e.g. adenosine 5-monophosphate, AMP). As such the purines are essential constituents of metabolically important compounds such as ATP.

Figure 19.1 shows that uric acid is the end-product of breakdown of the purine bases. It emphasises that the source of the purines can be from the three routes of diet, nucleic acid breakdown or *de novo* purine synthesis. The liver is the main source of urate and, once formed, urate is predominantly excreted via the kidneys.

Figure 19.2 summarises the *de novo* synthetic route for purines from the simple activated ribose molecule, 5-phosphoribosyl-1-pyrophosphate (PRPP). The purine ring is built onto this sugar, and the nucleotide that is first formed (IMP; see Figure 19.2) can be converted to both AMP and GMP nucleotides. It also illustrates that the pathway to uric acid can be reversed at some points (converting the free purine bases to corresponding nucleotides), the so-called salvage

pathway. The nucleotides produced by the salvage pathway can be re-incorporated into nucleic acids.

Serum urate

A high serum urate, called hyperuricaemia, is a result of excessive formation, reduced excretion or a combination of both (Figure 19.1). Other factors that influence levels are as follows:

- *Sex:* Serum levels are higher in males (0.12–0.42 mmol/L) than in females (0.12–0.36 mmol/L).
- *Obesity:* Levels tend to be higher in the obese.
- *Social class:* The more affluent social classes tend to have a higher serum urate.
- *Diet:* Serum urate rises in individuals taking a high-protein diet (especially meat or seafood). High alcohol consumption and fructose-containing beverages are also associated with raised serum urate. Dairy foods and coffee drinking appear to lower urate when examined in epidemiological studies.
- *Genetic factors.*

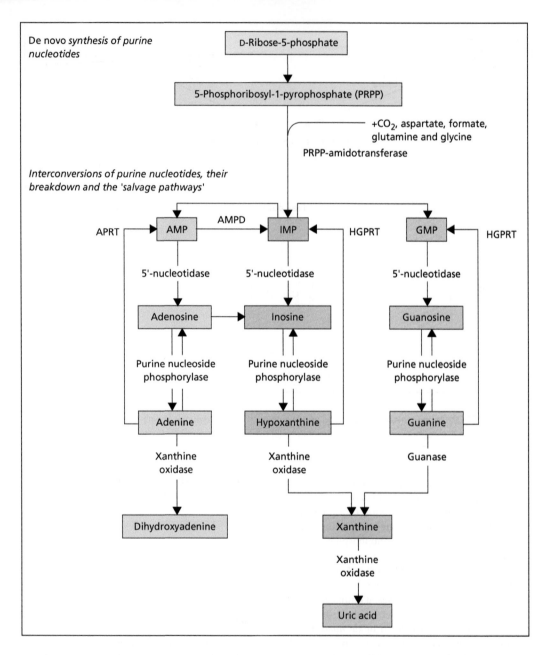

De novo *synthesis of purine nucleotides*

D-Ribose-5-phosphate

5-Phosphoribosyl-1-pyrophosphate (PRPP)

+CO$_2$, aspartate, formate, glutamine and glycine

PRPP-amidotransferase

Interconversions of purine nucleotides, their breakdown and the 'salvage pathways'

APRT   AMP   AMPD   IMP   HGPRT   GMP   HGPRT

5'-nucleotidase   5'-nucleotidase   5'-nucleotidase

Adenosine   Inosine   Guanosine

Purine nucleoside phosphorylase   Purine nucleoside phosphorylase   Purine nucleoside phosphorylase

Adenine   Hypoxanthine   Guanine

Xanthine oxidase   Xanthine oxidase   Guanase

Dihydroxyadenine   Xanthine

Xanthine oxidase

Uric acid

Figure 19.2 The upper part of this figure is a simplified representation of the synthetic pathway leading to the *de novo* synthesis of inosinic acid (IMP), a purine nucleotide that can then be converted to adenylic acid (AMP) and guanylic acid (GMP). The lower part of the figure shows the breakdown of AMP, IMP and GMP to the corresponding purines, and their further metabolism to uric acid (the main end-product of purine metabolism) and dihydroxyadenine. It also shows, with another set of curved arrows, the salvage pathways for re-forming AMP, IMP and GMP from their corresponding purine bases, by reactions catalysed by hypoxanthine-guanine phosphoribosyltransferase (HGPRT) and by adenosine phosphoribosyl transferase (APRT).

Hyperuricaemia

In addition to the deposition of sodium monourate crystals in affected joints (see Chapter 19: Gout) uric acid calculi in the kidneys may also form due to hyperuricaemia, and the lower pH values possible in urine can predispose to this problem.

As serum urate levels rise, the risk of precipitation of sodium urate increases, although the relationship between the presence and severity of hyperuricaemia and the development of arthritis or renal calculi is more complex than simple considerations of solubility might suggest.

Dietary factors

- *High-purine diets:* A high meat diet or one rich in seafood increases the purine load. The protein content per se does not appear to be responsible. For example, dairy foods have a relatively high protein content with low purine content and may actually lower serum urate, possibly as a consequence of a uricosuric effect of protein.
- *Alcohol excess:* Nutritional surveys have established a strong link between hyperuricaemia and alcohol intake. The mechanism is probably multi-factorial, including increased nucleotide breakdown, diuresis, dehydration and the influence of lactic acids and ketone bodies (arising from the effects of alcohol metabolism) in reducing urate excretion.
- *Fructose-containing beverages:* A possible mechanism is the consumption of ATP through the fructokinase reaction, with the ADP formed reconverted to ATP in the adenylate kinase reaction, generating AMP that serves as a precursor for uric acid (Figure 19.2).

Endogenous overproduction of urate

A number of mechanisms are possible. For example:

- Unspecified overactivity of the pathways of nucleotide metabolism, as opposed to nucleic acid synthesis, leading to urate formation ('endogenous overproduction').
- Decreased activity of the 'salvage' pathway so that purine bases are metabolised to urate rather than re-incorporated into nucleotides and nucleic acids.
- Increased nucleic acid breakdown when cell turnover or destruction is increased.

Defective elimination of urate

Renal excretion of urate is a complex process. Except for a small fraction bound to plasma proteins, urate is completely filtered at the glomerulus; this is then mostly reabsorbed in the proximal tubule. In the distal tubule, there is *both* active secretion *and* post-secretory reabsorption at a more distal site. These processes can all be affected by disease or drugs:

- *GFR:* When the GFR becomes reduced for any reason (Chapter 4: Tests of glomerular function), urate retention occurs.
- *Tubular reabsorption:* Around 90% of the filtered urate load is reabsorbed in the proximal nephron via specific anion transporters. The specific transport called URAT1 is a target for drugs such as probenecid that inhibit its activity and increase the excretion of urate.
- *Distal tubular secretion:* Urate excretion also depends upon distal tubular secretion. This process is competed for by other organic acid anions such as lactate and 3-hydroxybutyrate. Any condition that gives rise to lactic acidosis or ketosis tends to be associated with hyperuricaemia. Drugs may also compete with urate for this excretory mechanism (e.g. thiazide diuretics) and thereby increase serum urate concentration.

Salicylates and many other uricosuric agents have paradoxical and dose-dependent effects on the renal tubular handling of urate. *Low* doses of salicylates mainly reduce distal tubular secretion, tending to cause hyperuricaemia. The dominant effect of *high* doses is increased urate excretion through inhibition of urate reabsorption.

Gout

Hyperuricaemia is associated with *gout*, a condition characterised by recurrent attacks of monoarticular arthritis. Typically this involves the first metatarsophalangeal joint but the ankle, knee or other joints may be involved. Articular gout may be preceded by an asymptomatic phase of hyperuricaemia, followed by acute attacks with symptom-free periods and eventually leading to chronic, gouty arthritis. Patients with chronic, primary gout (see Case 19.1 and Table 19.1) often show deposition of urate as tophi in soft tissues. Some also develop renal stones, mainly composed of uric acid, increasing the risk of renal dysfunction. The incidence of renal stones varies widely, largely depending on the presence of other contributory factors such as dehydration or a low urinary pH. There appears to be a high prevalence of metabolic syndrome with increased cardiovascular risk, and an association of gout with hypertension is increasingly recognised. Cardiovascular disease, in particular, is an important cause of morbidity and mortality in patients with gout. The condition is more prevalent in men, rises with age and, in women, typically occurs after the menopause.

 CASE 19.1

A 48-year-old manager was admitted with severe colicky pain in his lower left lumbar region and an associated history of haematuria. He was overweight with a blood pressure of 165/105. Serum lipids on the admission sample showed triglyceride levels of 5.2 mmol/L, a total cholesterol of 7.2 mmol/L and an HDL cholesterol of 0.8 mmol/L. Serum calcium was normal but the urate was 0.75 mmol/L. Further questioning revealed an episode of severe pain in the first metatarsophalangeal joint of his left foot while holidaying in Spain. This was treated while abroad and resolved after a few days but he could not recollect what treatment had been given. What is the likely cause of this man's condition?

Comment: The clinical history here, together with the high serum urate level, all point towards the diagnosis of primary gout. The first metatarsophalangeal joint is the most common to be involved in first attacks of gout. The acute joint pain itself coincides with the time the patient was on holiday and possibly overindulging in alcohol and rich foods that may well have precipitated the initial episode. The high serum urate is likely to be longstanding and has led to the formation of renal stones. A history of severe lumbar pain, colicky in nature and associated with haematuria, is classical for renal colic. Where possible, examination of any stones passed or removed should be undertaken to confirm that these are composed of uric acid. There is a known association of gout with hyperlipidaemia, particularly a raised triglyceride. Associations with hypertension, obesity and IGT are also described.

A high serum urate does not always lead to gout, and the majority of patients with hyperuricaemia do not develop gout. A precipitating factor may be a sudden change in serum urate in either direction, perhaps as a result of a sudden dietary change or change in alcohol intake. For this reason, an acute attack of gout may not necessarily be accompanied by hyperuricaemia.

It is usual to subdivide gout into primary (Table 19.1) and secondary (Table 19.2) causes.

- Primary gout, by definition, occurs in the absence of acquired or monogenetic conditions although there is no doubt that genetic factors contribute, with about 60% of variability in serum urate genetically determined. The present evidence is that differences in urate excretion rates contribute principally to urate levels, overproduction being a less important factor. The association with hyperlipidaemia, ischaemic heart disease and metabolic syndrome may also reflect a familial component, although it is sometimes difficult to

---

Table 19.1 Features of primary gout.

- No obvious secondary cause (see Table 19.2)
- High serum urate (not always evident in an acute attack)
- Presents usually with an acute monoarthritis
- Asymptomatic periods with recurrent acute arthritis leading to chronic joint damage if untreated
- Tophi, renal stones, renal dysfunction may develop in chronic gout
- Associations with obesity, metabolic syndrome, hypertension
- Increased risk of cardiovascular disease

Table 19.2 Secondary causes of hyperuricaemia and gout.

Increased production
- Myeloproliferative disorders
- Malignancy
- Tumour lysis syndrome
- Psoriasis
- Alcohol (nucleotide breakdown)
- Fructose-containing beverages (increases AMP formation and purine breakdown)

Decreased elimination
- Renal failure (acute or chronic)
- Lactate or ketoacid excess (metabolic acidosis) with reduced secretion of urate
- Drugs, e.g. thiazide diuretics, low-dose salicylate with reduced secretion of urate
- Alcohol (increases lactate and ketoacid formation)

Excessive intake of purines
- Purine-rich diet (high meat and seafood diet)

Enzyme defects on urate pathway (rare)
- PRPP synthase overactivity
- PRPP amidotransferase overactivity
- HGPRT deficiency (salvage pathway)

disentangle the genetic and environmental factors. There are rare forms of gout that arise from clearly defined and inherited metabolic enzyme defects which increase uric acid formation. It is convenient to categorise these enzymatic defects as secondary gout to distinguish them from the common primary gout.

- Secondary gout describes the condition in association with other disorders that secondarily increase urate formation (e.g. increased cell death in myeloproliferative disorder) or decrease excretion (e.g. renal failure). The group also includes the rare metabolic causes of overproduction. Table 19.2 summarises these secondary causes.

In practice, both primary and secondary factors may contribute. For example, the patient may have a primary predisposition to hyperuricaemia which is then compounded by alcohol excess.

Primary gout

Diagnosis and pathogenesis

The diagnosis is often made clinically on the basis of the distribution of the joint involvement, a past history of similar episodes (especially if responsive to colchicine) and the presence of a raised serum urate. By definition, secondary causes of gout should have been excluded. Not all cases are typical clinically, and it should be remembered that:

- a high serum urate makes the diagnosis of gout probable, but not certain;
- a significant minority of patients (up to a third) with gout have a normal serum urate at the time of an attack.

For the definitive diagnosis of gout, it is necessary to aspirate joint fluid during an acute attack. This is then examined microscopically, and the finding of needle-shaped urate crystals that show negative birefringence establishes the diagnosis. Table 19.1 lists the features of primary gout.

The acute symptoms of gout are probably due to trauma or local metabolic changes causing crystals of monosodium urate to be shed into the joint cavity. The crystals are phagocytosed by leucocytes and macrophages and trigger a pro-inflammatory response with evidence that interleukin-1β is a key mediator of the inflammatory reaction to the monosodium urate crystals. Because the solubility of uric acid decreases with falling temperature, it is speculated that this may explain the predilection of gout to affect peripheral 'colder' joints such as the first metatarsophalangeal joint.

Treatment

- In an acute attack, anti-inflammatory drugs (e.g. indometacin) are usually prescribed. Low-dose colchicine is also effective during an acute attack and has a useful prophylactic effect. Steroids may also be helpful.
- Uricosuric drugs and allopurinol should be avoided at this stage.

Long-term treatment aims to reduce serum urate. Current European guidelines advocate levels less than 0.36 mmol/L and British guidelines recommend even lower levels at 0.3 mmol/L. The approaches to achieve this are:

- *Weight reduction:* This is encouraged (if appropriate). High-purine diets and certain drugs (e.g. thiazide diuretics) should be avoided. Alcohol restriction is encouraged.
- *Uricosuric drugs and inhibitors of urate synthesis (e.g. allopurinol):* These are often required. The first-line treatment is with allopurinol with the uricosuric drugs as second-line. Because acute changes in serum urate (increases or decreases) can precipitate attacks of gout, the uricosuric drugs and allopurinol should be avoided within several weeks of an acute attack. To prevent acute flare-up of joint problems the anti-inflammatory treatment should be continued while these drugs are introduced.
- *Allopurinol:* This isomer of hypoxanthine inhibits xanthine oxidase, thereby causing a fall in serum urate and in urinary urate excretion. Levels of the more water-soluble xanthine increase. More recently the xanthine oxidase inhibitor febuxostat has become available..
- In patients in whom urate stones seem likely to form, a high fluid intake and alkalinisation of the urine reduce the likelihood of stone formation.

Hypouricaemia

Low serum urate may arise as follows (Table 19.3):

- Dilutional states such as SIADH or pregnancy.
- Decreased production. This can be found in severe liver disease. Another example is the condition called xanthinuria arising from an inherited deficiency of the enzyme xanthine oxidase (which normally converts xanthine to urate). Xanthine crystals can form in the urinary tract.
- Increased excretion. This is usually in association with defective proximal tubular reabsorption (Fanconi syndrome).

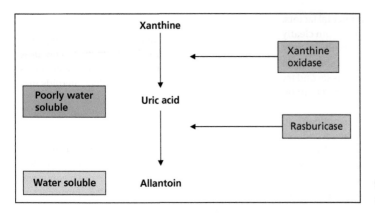

Figure 19.3 Formation of allantoin using rasburicase.

- Rasburicase (Figure 19.3). This is a genetically engineered enzyme that is a urate oxidase. It converts uric acid to the water-soluble allantoin. It is especially helpful in preventing the renal and other complications of excessive urate formation in the tumour lysis syndrome (massive cell lysis such as is found during treatment of haematological malignancies). It has a short half-life but can effectively reduce serum urate to very low levels. Modifications of rasburicase to increase its half-life are starting to find a place in the treatment of gout.

 CASE 19.2

While authorising clinical results prior to release to the wards, the clinical biochemist on duty was surprised to find a serum urate level that was extremely low (undetectable on the laboratory analyser). Initially, she felt that this must have been an analytical error and asked for the result to be repeated. Again, the serum urate was undetectable. She rang up the haematology ward to discuss this result with the Specialist Registrar. Can you suggest a likely explanation for this finding?

Comment: It turned out that the patient had an acute lymphoblastic leukaemia which was being actively treated. In anticipation of possible problems arising from the excessive formation of urate (as a consequence of massive cell lysis), the patient was on treatment with rasburicase. This is a genetically engineered urate oxidase which converts uric acid to the water-soluble allantoin. It is so effective as to reduce the serum urate to virtually undetectable levels, hence the laboratory finding which was a correct analytical result!

Table 19.3 **Causes of a low serum urate.**

Plasma dilution
- SIADH (Chapter 2: Hyponatraemia with normal ECF volume)
- Pregnancy

Decreased formation
- Xanthine oxidase deficiency
- Severe liver disease
- Rasburicase treatment

Increased excretion
- Uricosuric drugs (e.g. allopurinol)
- Fanconi syndrome

A low serum urate has not usually been regarded as pathological in its own right. However, uric acid has anti-oxidant properties that may be more important than have hitherto been realised. For example, there is a literature that reports associations between low serum urate and a variety of neurological disorders such as multiple sclerosis and Parkinson disease. It is speculated that urate may help prevent damage to nervous tissue from oxidants such as peroxynitrite, although it is unclear if the low urate is a causal factor or consequence of the neurological problem.

 FURTHER READING

Richette, P. and Bardin, T. (2010) Gout. *Lancet* **375**, 318–28.

20

Central nervous system and cerebrospinal fluid

Learning objectives

To understand:

✔ composition, appearance and identification of CSF;

✔ CSF spectroscopy in the investigation of suspected subarachnoid haemorrhage;

✔ examination of CSF for oligoclonal bands in the investigation of demyelinating disease.

Introduction

Many neurological disorders have a biochemical basis, or are associated with disturbances of metabolism. However, neurochemistry is a specialised subject that is beyond the scope of this book. Many generalised disorders of metabolism affect the CNS, for example Hartnup's disease, Wilson's disease and PKU, and these are considered elsewhere. In this chapter, we discuss the information to be gained from examining the CSF.

CSF composition

The CSF approximates to an ultrafiltrate of plasma. There are, however, differences between the relative concentrations in plasma and CSF of both low molecular mass and high molecular mass substances.

1 Low molecular mass substances
  - Differential rates of diffusion: Dissolved CO_2 diffuses into CSF more rapidly than HCO_3^-, so CSF H^+ (which depends on the $HCO_3^-:H_2CO_3$ ratio) may be significantly different from plasma H^+.
  - Effects of ultrafiltration: Bilirubin is nearly all protein bound in plasma, and normally very little crosses the blood–brain barrier. Calcium is only partly protein bound, and Ca^{2+} readily crosses into the CSF.

2 High molecular mass substances
  - Differential rates of diffusion: 80% of CSF protein is derived from plasma proteins by passive diffusion across the blood–brain barrier, and the total concentration of CSF protein is approximately 200 times less than that of plasma. The concentration of individual proteins depends both on the permeability of the barrier and on their plasma concentrations. All plasma proteins commonly measured are present in CSF and, in general, their relative concentrations are proportional to those in plasma.
  - Secretion of proteins: pre-albumin is synthesised by the choroidal epithelium and is present at concentrations greater than can be achieved by passive diffusion.

Clinical Biochemistry Lecture Notes, Tenth Edition. Peter Rae, Mike Crane and Rebecca Pattenden.
© 2018 John Wiley & Sons Ltd. Published 2018 by John Wiley & Sons Ltd.
Companion website: www.lecturenoteseries.com/clinicalbiochemistry

- Receptor-mediated transfer: desialylated transferrin (also known as β_2-transferrin or Tau protein) arises during receptor-mediated transfer of transferrin from plasma. It accumulates in CSF because the asialoreceptors of the reticuloendothelial system, which normally remove desialylated transferrin from the circulation, are not expressed in the central nervous system.

Examination of CSF

Appearance

CSF is normally clear and colourless. Turbidity is usually due to leucocytes, but it may be due to microorganisms. Blood-stained CSF may indicate recent haemorrhage, or damage to a blood vessel during specimen collection. Xanthochromia (yellow colour) is most often due to previous haemorrhage into the CSF, but it may indicate that CSF protein is very high. The CSF may be yellow in jaundiced patients.

CSF bilirubin

Patients investigated for suspected subarachnoid haemorrhage (SAH) initially undergo a CT scan. In experienced hands, this will be positive for subarachnoid blood in 98% of patients presenting within 12 h of SAH. In patients presenting later, the blood load may have cleared and the diagnostic sensitivity of the CT scan is reduced to 50% after 1 week. However, as erythrocytes in CSF undergo lysis and phagocytosis, oxyhaemoglobin is released and is converted into bilirubin in a time-dependent manner. In CT-negative patients, the identification of bilirubin in CSF may be helpful in establishing the diagnosis.

Specimen requirements

- CSF specimens should be obtained at least 12 h after the suspected SAH.
- The specimen should be protected from light.
- The specimen should be delivered to the laboratory immediately after collection for centrifugation and spectrophotometric examination.
- A simultaneous blood sample for bilirubin and total protein analysis should be taken as an aid to the interpretation of the CSF results. This information can be used to account for the elevation in CSF bilirubin that may result from an increase in serum bilirubin.

Because oxyhaemoglobin can interfere with the detection of bilirubin, *in vitro* lysis of any red cells present in the CSF specimen should be avoided. Therefore:

- The least blood-stained fraction of CSF (usually the last) should be taken for spectrophotometric examination.
- CSF should not be transported by pneumatic tube in order to minimise *in vitro* haemolysis of any contaminating red cells.

Spectrophotometric examination

Visual inspection for xanthochromia is unreliable, and it is essential that a spectrophotometric scan of the CSF supernatant be performed. The presence of an increased level of bilirubin is consistent with a recent bleed into the CSF. Available evidence suggests that bilirubin may be present for up to 2 weeks following SAH. However, this can vary greatly, especially in the case of small bleeds, therefore a negative bilirubin result cannot completely exclude SAH.

A spectral band characteristic of oxyhaemoglobin is usually present in CSF obtained from patients with SAH, especially within the first few days of the event. However, because oxyhaemoglobin may also be released following *in vitro* haemolysis of red cells introduced during collection, its predictive value for SAH is poor and the presence of oxyhaemoglobin alone is inconclusive.

CSF glucose

Lumbar CSF glucose is normally 0.5–1.0 mmol/L lower than plasma glucose, whereas CSF glucose in specimens obtained from the cerebral ventricles and from the cisterna magna normally differs little from plasma glucose.

Interpretation of CSF glucose requires a matching plasma glucose obtained at the same time as the lumbar puncture. The CSF to plasma glucose ratio is approximately 0.6 in normal individuals. In hypoglycaemia, CSF glucose may be very low; it is raised when there is hyperglycaemia.

CSF glucose may be low or undetectable in patients with acute bacterial, cryptococcal, tubercular or carcinomatous meningitis, or in cerebral abscess, probably due to consumption of glucose by leucocytes or other rapidly metabolising cells. In meningitis or encephalitis due to viral infections, it is usually normal.

CASE 20.1

A 38-year-old woman was referred to the neurologists by her GP. She had complained of a severe headache that had started suddenly 3 days earlier. The possibility of an SAH was considered but a CT scan did not reveal any evidence of subarachnoid blood. A lumbar puncture was performed and a sample of CSF was sent to the laboratory for spectroscopic examination. The CSF was blood-stained with a large RBC pellet and a protein concentration of 6 g/L. The serum bilirubin was within reference limits at 6 μmol/L.

The scan shown in Figure 20.1 was obtained:

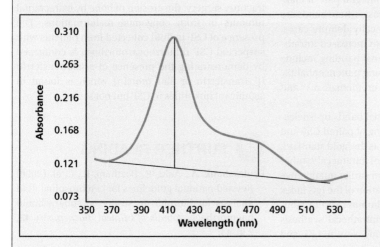

Figure 20.1
Spectrophotometric scan of CSF.

Comments: This scan showed an oxyhaemoglobin peak with a maximum absorbance of 0.19 AU at 414 nm. Adjacent to this peak was a shoulder demonstrating that bilirubin was also present. The net bilirubin absorbance (NBA) measured at 476 nm was elevated at 0.05 AU (NBA in unaffected patients is <0.007 AU). The elevation in CSF bilirubin was the key spectrophotometric finding. As the serum bilirubin was not elevated it was concluded that the increases in CSF bilirubin and oxyhaemoglobin were consistent with SAH.

CT angiography subsequently identified an aneurysm in the right posterior communicating artery. This was successfully coiled and the patient made a good recovery.

CSF total protein

Lumbar CSF protein (reference range 100–400 mg/L) is normally almost all albumin. Ventricular and cisternal CSF protein is lower than lumbar CSF protein. Much higher CSF protein may have no pathological significance in the neonatal period; for example, lumbar CSF protein may then be as much as 900 mg/L.

CSF protein is increased in a large number of pathological conditions. Whenever it is increased, organic disease of the CNS is probably present. In acute inflammatory conditions of the CNS, the increase may be very marked due to increased capillary permeability. CSF protein can be falsely elevated due to the presence of red blood cells from a traumatic tap or SAH.

In the demyelinating disorders, there is often a moderate increase in CSF protein, usually in the range 500–1000 mg/L. Primary and secondary neoplasms involving the brain or the meninges can cause very large increases in lumbar CSF protein if spinal block occurs. Values over 5000 mg/L may be observed. These specimens may be xanthochromic because of the high protein content, and a protein clot may form on storage after a few hours.

CSF oligoclonal bands

CSF normally contains small amounts of IgG (reference range 8–64 mg/L), a trace of IgA and minute amounts of IgM. An increase in CSF immunoglobulin

(Ig), particularly IgG, can either result from intrathecal synthesis or it can be secondary to an increase in plasma Igs and/or impairment of the blood–CSF barrier. Increased intrathecal synthesis of Ig results from the expansion of a limited number of clones of plasma cells and is associated with discrete oligoclonal bands that are present in CSF but not a paired serum.

Examination of CSF for oligoclonal bands is an essential laboratory test in the investigation of demyelinating disease. It is an integral part of making a diagnosis of multiple sclerosis where bands are seen in more than 95% of clinically definite cases. Other conditions associated with increased intrathecal IgG synthesis and oligoclonal banding include neurosyphilis, subacute sclerosing panencephalitis, polyneuritis, systemic lupus erythematosus and sarcoidosis.

The identification of oligoclonal bands by isoelectric focusing and immunoblotting of paired CSF and serum samples is now regarded as the 'gold standard' laboratory test for the detection of intrathecal synthesis of IgG. It is more sensitive than earlier quantitative approaches involving the calculation of the IgG index (CSF IgG : serum IgG ÷ CSF albumin : serum albumin). This attempts to detect intrathecal synthesis against a background of varying serum IgG and impaired CSF–blood barrier function, but at best is positive only in approximately 75% of patients who turn out to be oligoclonal band positive.

CSF rhinorrhoea and otorrhoea

Leakage of CSF into the subarachnoid space may result in a life-threatening infection of the central nervous system. It may arise as a result of traumatic fracture, surgery, the erosion of bone by extracranial tumours or from congenital malformations. The presence of CSF in fluid collected from patients with suspected CSF rhinorrhoea/otorrhoea is confirmed by demonstrating the presence of asialotransferrin (β_2-transferrin or Tau protein) which is found in significant quantities in CSF but not serum.

 FURTHER READING

Cruickshank, A., Auld, P., Beetham, R., et al. (2008) Revised national guidelines for cerebrospinal fluid analysis for bilirubin in suspected subarachnoid haemorrhage. *Annals of Clinical Biochemistry* **45**, 238–44.

21

Therapeutic drug monitoring and chemical toxicology

Learning objectives

To understand:

✔ when there is clinical benefit in therapeutic drug monitoring (TDM);

✔ when blood samples should be taken in relation to the last dose of the drug;

✔ the advantages and disadvantages of drug measurements in urine;

✔ the drugs that are most commonly measured for TDM;

✔ the concept of pharmacogenomics, giving clinical examples of its importance;

✔ the principal substances that give rise to hospital admissions for poisoning and what laboratory measurements can be helpful;

✔ the concepts that govern when N-acetyl cysteine is given to patients with suspected paracetamol overdose;

✔ the importance of determining the anion gap and osmolar gap in patients presenting with suspected methanol or ethylene glycol poisoning;

✔ when it is appropriate to screen patients for drugs of abuse.

Introduction

Poisoning is one of the most common causes of emergency admission to hospitals. Of the numerous potentially fatal chemicals and drugs, only a limited number are encountered in practice. It may be important to know the nature and blood levels of the poison, as this may help patient management and determine prognosis. Drug therapy is usually monitored on clinical grounds rather than on blood levels. However, for a few drugs, measurement of blood levels (and occasionally genotyping or phenotyping of a particular enzyme) is essential to ensure a therapeutic effect without toxicity.

Drug abuse is an increasing social and medical problem. Urinary or salivary drug measurements

---

Clinical Biochemistry Lecture Notes, Tenth Edition. Peter Rae, Mike Crane and Rebecca Pattenden.
© 2018 John Wiley & Sons Ltd. Published 2018 by John Wiley & Sons Ltd.
Companion website: www.lecturenoteseries.com/clinicalbiochemistry

have an important part to play in the management of a number of these individuals.

Therapeutic drug monitoring (TDM)

When is therapeutic drug monitoring required?

For many drugs, the dose given correlates well with a pharmacological effect, and the correct dosage can be satisfactorily determined by clinical assessment. For example, the pharmacological actions of anti-coagulants and of anti-hypertensive drugs can be assessed, and dosage adjusted, on the basis of pro-thrombin time and blood pressure measurements, respectively.

TDM is important in specific clinical circumstances, particularly if the actions and pharmacokinetics of the drug dictate that TDM will provide clinically useful information. These circumstances are given in Table 21.1.

Table 21.2 lists some common drugs for which the case for TDM has been clearly established. Regular monitoring of patients taking these drugs is not usually required once the patient has been stabilised on a dose of drug that has produced the desired clinical effect.

When should the blood sample be taken?

When a single dose of drug is taken for the first time, plasma levels will initially rise rapidly and then

Table 21.1 Situations where TDM may be useful.

- Establishing a dose regimen at the start of therapy, or when dose changes need to be made
- Failure to achieve therapeutic control, although dosage is apparently adequate
- Loss of control in a patient previously stabilised on treatment (e.g. check on compliance)
- When additional drugs are given or liver/renal dysfunction occurs that modify clearance
- Assess toxicity, especially if several drugs are being given
- Patients taking drugs which in overdose may produce symptoms that are similar to those of the disease being treated (e.g. phenytoin or ciclosporin)
- Drugs that have a narrow therapeutic range, for example lithium
- When there is a wide inter-individual variation in the therapeutic window
- When the drug may produce changes in hepatic or renal clearance
- When drug absorption may vary with dose or other circumstances

Table 21.2 Therapeutic drug monitoring; examples of drugs for which it is indicated.

Drug	Therapeutic range in plasma level	Units	Time to collect blood	Half-life (h)	Reason[†]
Amikacin	Peak 20–30 Trough <10	mg/L	30min to 1h after last dose / Just before next dose	2–3	b, c, d, e
Carbamazepine	4–12	mg/L	Just before next dose	8–24	c
Ciclosporin	110–270	µg/L	Just before next dose	6–24	c
Digoxin	0.5–2.0	µg/L	6–18h after last dose	36–48	a, b, c, d
Gentamicin	Peak 3–5 Trough <1	mg/L	30min to 1h after last dose / Just before next dose	2–3	b, c, d, e
Lithium	0.4–1.0	mmol/L	12–18h after last dose	10–35	a, b, e
Phenytoin	10–20	mg/L	Long half-life – not critical	20–40	a, c
Tacrolimus	5–15	mg/L	Just before next dose	12	a, b, c, e
Theophylline	10–20	mg/L	Not critical[‡]	3–13	a, b, c, d
Vancomycin	Trough 10–15	mg/L	Just before next dose	4–6	b, c, d, e

[†]Key to the reasons for performing therapeutic drug monitoring: (a) wide inter-individual variation; (b) low therapeutic index; (c) therapeutic effect or signs of toxicity difficult to recognise; (d) administration of a potentially toxic drug to a seriously ill patient; (e) very toxic in overdose.
[‡]Timing of peak levels will depend on formulation, for example slow-acting preparations.

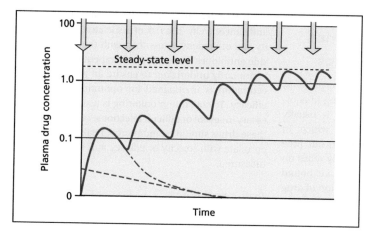

Figure 21.1 The effect on plasma drug concentration of giving repeated regular doses of a drug. As can be seen, after approximately five doses of the drug, a steady-state level is reached, with peak and trough values being found. The hatched line represents the elimination half-life and the hatched/dotted line shows the plasma drug concentration profile if a single dose of the drug had been given. Arrows show the time of each dose of the drug.

decline in a curvilinear manner similar to that shown in Figure 21.1. The characteristics of this curve provide essential details about the kinetics of the drug and the information needed to calculate the approximate dose and frequency of the drug for the desired therapeutic concentration in plasma. For any drug given at regular intervals, a steady-state relatively constant concentration in plasma is reached after about five half-lives (Figure 21.1). However, peak levels (achieved just after administration) and trough levels (achieved immediately prior to the next dose) may still be recognised. For most drugs, it is important that trough levels are adequate to achieve the desired therapeutic effect. Thus, blood samples are often withdrawn just before a dose of the drug is taken, but at any rate samples should usually be taken after the initial peak has subsided, unless toxicity is suspected. In all cases, the time of blood sampling in relation to the last dose of the drug must be known.

Interpretation of drug levels

Therapeutic ranges: If the blood has been taken at the appropriate time, the plasma level can be compared with published therapeutic ranges (Table 21.2). These published ranges indicate the range of plasma drug levels which in the majority of the population have been shown to provide the desired therapeutic effect without a high risk of toxicity. Published ranges offer little more than guidelines, because of inter-individual variation in the clinical response to drugs. Other important points to consider are given in Table 21.3.

Table 21.3 Important information that is required when interpreting drug levels.

Timing of sampling in relation to the dose
- If specimens are collected before a steady-state concentration of drug has been achieved, TDM results will be misleading.

Units in which concentrations are measured by the local laboratory.
- Concentrations may be expressed in mass or molar units of concentration. The Association for Clinical Biochemistry and Laboratory Medicine has recommended that drug concentrations should be reported in mass per litre with the exception of iron, lithium, methotrexate and thyroxine. The practice of referring to numerical values of drug measurements without stating the units is dangerous and can lead to fatal mistakes.

Drug metabolites
- If drug metabolites have a therapeutic action, assay methods that are specific for the native drug may give misleading information (see the importance of drug metabolites below).

Clinical information
- Therapeutic ranges assume normal rates of drug clearance and also do not take into account drug interactions.
- Patients with renal or liver impairment may eliminate drugs at a subnormal rate. In contrast, patients taking drugs that induce hepatic drug-metabolising enzymes will have enhanced clearance of other drugs. Drug metabolism may also be modified by polymorphisms in enzymes that metabolise drugs.

Other important issues in therapeutic drug monitoring

'Free' and protein-bound drugs

Most drugs circulate partly bound to plasma proteins, the bound and unbound (free) forms being in equilibrium. The pharmacological response is usually determined by the tissue concentration which, in turn, is related to the plasma [free drug] but [free drug] is difficult to measure. TDM usually relies on the measurements of plasma [total drug, i.e. bound and free]. For some drugs, the concentration of drug in saliva may reflect the concentration of [free drug] in plasma. Salivary drug measurements are now widely used in screening for drugs of abuse.

The importance of drug metabolites

Most drugs are metabolised to inactive products, although some are inactive when taken and are converted to active drug in the liver or GI tract. For example, primidone is converted to phenobarbitone. If primidone therapy is to be monitored, plasma phenobarbitone is the measurement required. A variety of analytical methods are used for measurement of drugs. Methods based on mass spectrometry are the most specific and accurate; unfortunately these methods may give rise to misleading results if they fail to measure metabolites that have pharmacological actions. Immunoassay and colorimetric methods are also used and may lack specificity; these less-specific methods may give rise to misleading results if there are high concentrations of inactive metabolites in plasma that cross-react in the assay.

Examples of drugs that often require TDM

Antibiotics

Aminoglycoside antibiotics (gentamicin, tobramycin, amikacin and netilmicin): These have a very short half-life of 2–3h if renal function is normal, but in patients with infection or renal impairment the half-life becomes prolonged (up to 100h). In addition, tissue pools of gentamicin may become saturated if treatment is for more than a week, and then plasma levels may start to rise sharply. Gentamicin and amikacin are *nephrotoxic* and *ototoxic*, therefore TDM is particularly important in patients with impaired renal function who receive the drug for more than 7 days, or those on high loading doses for serious infection. Peak and trough levels should be measured.

Glycopeptide antibiotics: These include teicoplanin and vancomycin. The risk of associated nephrotoxicity and ototoxicity is less than with the aminoglycoside antibiotics. Vancomycin therapeutic monitoring is primarily undertaken to ensure an adequate concentration is maintained for optimum therapeutic efficacy. Teicoplanin monitoring is usually only necessary in severe or difficult infections. Trough levels of these drugs should be monitored; peak levels do not correlate with toxicity or efficacy and should not be measured.

Anti-convulsants

Carbamazepine: Carbamazepine has fewer side effects, mainly neurotoxic, than phenytoin. Monitoring is of value in patients with poor control, because there is a variable relationship between dose and plasma concentration. The sample should be taken just before a dose.

Phenytoin: Phenytoin has a low therapeutic ratio and is subject to variable rates of hepatic metabolism, leading to a nonlinear relationship between dose and plasma concentration. Because of phenytoin's undesirable side effects, which include neurotoxicity and increased frequency of fits, TDM is required in new patients, where there is an unexpected loss in control, in pregnancy or when other drugs that interact with phenytoin are added or withdrawn.

Drugs that prevent graft rejection

Ciclosporin, tacrolimus and *sirolimus* are used to prevent graft rejection. TDM is recommended to ensure efficacy of each of these drugs because it is essential to achieve the correct level of drug in the blood to prevent rejection while minimising side effects such as nephrotoxicity. Blood is usually taken just before the next dose.

Digoxin

Digoxin has little clinical effect at plasma concentrations below 1 nmol/L, whereas toxicity (often manifest as cardiac arrhythmia and vomiting) is common when plasma levels rise above 3.8 nmol/L. Digoxin results should always be interpreted together with a plasma potassium concentration, because hypokalaemia potentiates the effect of digoxin. Thus, toxic effects of the drug may occur in a hypokalaemic patient who has a plasma digoxin within the therapeutic range. A similar effect may be seen in hypercalcaemia, hypomagnesaemia and hypothyroidism. Equilibration of digoxin within cardiac tissue takes some time, and thus blood should not be taken until at least 6–8h after the dose.

Lithium

Lithium is used for the treatment of depressive illness. It has a short half-life, and plasma levels should be determined 12 h after the last dose. TDM is essential because the drug is toxic, producing a range of symptoms including polyuria, hypothyroidism and, in severe cases, renal failure and coma. Patients with plasma lithium above 1.4 mmol/L are at risk of oliguria and acute renal failure. TDM may also be necessary in order to monitor compliance.

 CASE 21.1

A 25-year-old male was admitted with nausea, vomiting and diarrhoea following deliberate ingestion of a large quantity of lithium carbonate tablets earlier that day.

The following results were found:

Serum	Result
Lithium	5.2 mmol/L (therapeutic range 0.4–1.0)
Creatinine	131 μmol/L (reference range 64–111)

Comments: The patient has taken a large quantity of lithium and has the common GI symptoms of acute lithium ingestion. He has mild renal impairment; this requires close monitoring as deterioration could lead to neurotoxicity. Furthermore, as lithium excretion is dependent on renal function, correction of fluid balance and ongoing hydration with IV fluids is required.

Haemodialysis should be considered in those with impaired renal function or neurological features.

 CASE 21.2

A 65-year-old woman presented to her GP complaining of nausea. She had been treated with digoxin and diuretics for cardiac failure, and had tolerated the drugs well, with no previous evidence of poor compliance or poor therapeutic control. On examination, she was found to have bradycardia.

The following results were found (sampling at 14 h after last digoxin dose):

Serum	Result
Digoxin	1.9 (therapeutic range 0.5–2.0 μg/L)
Potassium	3.1 (reference range 3.6–5.0 nmol/L)

What is the most likely cause of the patient's symptoms?

Comments: The patient is likely to be suffering from digoxin toxicity. Although the plasma level of digoxin is within the therapeutic range, it is at the upper limit. However, more importantly, the patient has hypokalaemia, which will potentiate the pharmacological effect of digoxin. Plasma digoxin concentrations are a poor guide to toxicity if there is hypokalaemia. A common cause of digoxin toxicity is concurrent administration of diuretics, which cause potassium depletion. The patient was treated successfully by giving potassium supplements to restore her plasma potassium to normal.

Methotrexate

Methotrexate is a dihydrofolate inhibitor, and therefore reduces intracellular folate, which in turn inhibits DNA synthesis. The drug is cytotoxic; high-dose regimens are used in the treatment of some cancers, and lower-dose regimens are used for immunosuppression. TDM is of value in patients receiving high doses of methotrexate, to identify those at risk of toxic effects and to provide a guide to the dose and timing of leucovorin (a drug that restores the pool of reduced folate) rescue.

Theophylline

This drug is used to prevent or treat bronchoconstriction in some children or elderly patients who cannot use an inhaler easily. The drug commonly produces minor side effects such as nausea and headache, even at concentrations within the therapeutic range. Serious toxicity leading to cardiac arrhythmia can occur with plasma levels above 110 mmol/L. TDM is particularly valuable to optimise the dose, confirm toxicity or demonstrate poor compliance. Some believe that the metabolite caffeine should also be measured.

Anti-tumour necrosis factor (anti-TNF) drugs

Anti-TNF therapies (such as infliximab and adalimumab) are now established therapies for the treatment of chronic inflammatory conditions such as inflammatory bowel disease and rheumatoid arthritis. Despite evidence of their proven efficacy, there are patients who fail to respond to therapy or lose their response to therapy during maintenance treatment. Some patients also develop antibodies to these drugs, reducing their efficacy.

TDM of anti-TNF drug levels and their associated antibodies is becoming routine practice within certain clinical settings in the UK; it is used as a tool to optimise the prescription of these drugs and impact on patient care.

Pharmacogenomics

People may have markedly different responses to the same drug due to the presence of polymorphisms in the expression of phase 1 and phase 2 drug-metabolising systems. For example, it was recognised over 40 years ago that suxamethonium toxicity in some individuals was caused by impaired metabolism due to a genetic variant of cholinesterase (Table 21.4). There are now known to be marked variations in the ability of an individual to metabolise drugs catalysed by a wide range of phase 1 enzymes such as cytochrome P450 (CYP) 2D6 and the phase 2 enzyme thiopurine methyltransferase (TPMT). Knowledge of the specific enzyme polymorphisms expressed by a patient allows the therapeutic action of a drug to be maximised with a low possibility of an adverse drug reaction.

Suxamethonium (scoline) apnoea and choline esterase

There are two principal choline esterases (ChEs): *plasma BChE* (formerly known as pseudocholinesterase) is synthesised in the liver; *acetylcholinesterase* is present at nerve endings and in the erythrocytes, but not in plasma. Assessment of plasma BChE is of particular value in the investigation of patients with suxamethonium apnoea and organophosphorus insecticide poisoning.

Suxamethonium (succinylcholine or Scoline) apnoea is rare; it occurs when a patient has been given this muscle relaxant prior to surgery but only slowly metabolises the drug due to a polymorphism in BChE. Such patients may remain paralysed and unable to breathe for several hours after the surgery.

Phenotypes with impaired ability to metabolise scoline are AA, AS, AF, FF, FS, SS and to a variable degree UA. The pharmacological action of the drug may be increased from 30 min to several hours over this range of phenotypes.

Most individuals with abnormal variants have low plasma ChE activity, but the only reliable way of demonstrating the variants is by means of inhibitor studies using dibucaine and fluoride or by carrying out genotyping. It is important to recognise these abnormalities of plasma ChE so that affected relatives can be traced and anaesthetists warned not to administer Scoline to them.

Azathioprine and thiopurine methyltransferase (TPMT)

Azathioprine is widely used in the treatment of rheumatic disorders, hepatobiliary disease, skin disorders and following renal transplant. Azathioprine is metabolised by a number of pathways through 6-mercaptopurine (6-MP) eventually to form the therapeutically active 6-thioguanine nucleotides (TGNs). The TGNs are cytotoxic, being eventually incorporated into DNA as a false base, and cause cell death by a mismatch repair pathway. The 6-MP can also be methylated by TPMT and oxidised by xanthine oxidase (XO) to produce inactive metabolites. Variations in the extensive metabolism of 6-MP play a role in the toxicity and efficacy of azathioprine. TPMT has been extensively studied with respect to its variation in specific patient groups. The expression of TPMT in tissue is controlled by a genetic polymorphism inherited as an autosomal co-dominant trait. Patients with low expression of TPMT develop profound bone marrow toxicity, a consequence of the intracellular accumulation of grossly elevated cytotoxic TGN concentrations (Figure 21.2). Around 28 variant alleles have been identified that are associated with decreased levels of TPMT activity but only a few cause clinical problems. The wild type is usually designated TPMT*1 and the mutated genes assigned as TPMT*2-*8, etc. (with TPMT*3 having three forms: 3A, 3B, 3C). The alleles TPMT*3A and TPMT*3C account for 80–95% of intermediate or low enzyme activity, with TPMT*3A being the most common allele in Caucasian populations (5% of the population) and TPMT*3C the most common (2%) in African and South East Asian populations.

Patients who express intermediate or low activities of TPMT can accumulate high concentrations of toxic 6-thioguanine metabolites when given azathioprine, which puts them at increased risk of fatal bone marrow toxicity. Conversely, patients who express high activities of TPMT may not receive the maximum benefit from standard doses of the drug because of increased clearance. Genotyping or phenotyping for *TPMT* is thus advisable before initiating therapy with azathioprine. During azathioprine therapy, therapeutic drug monitoring of the thiopurine metabolites 6-MP and TGNs is indicated in patients with low TPMT activity and those who fail to respond to treatment.

Table 21.4 Genotypes of choline esterase.

Alleles of choline esterase

U – usual form, present in >95% of the UK population

A – resistant to inhibition by dibucaine.

F – resistant to inhibition by fluoride.

S – silent protein little or no ChE activity.

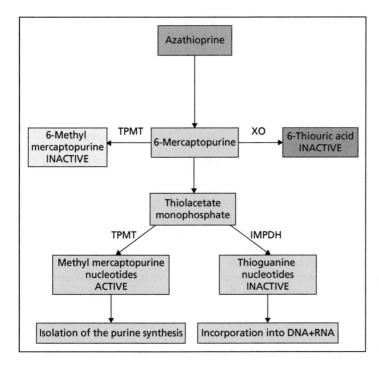

Figure 21.2 Azathioprine metabolism. TPMT=thiopurine S-methyltransferase; XO=xanthine oxidase; IMPDH=inosine monophosphate dehydrogenase. If TPMT activity is low, then more of the toxic thioguanine nucleotides will form.

Acute poisoning

The acutely poisoned patient accounts for around 5–10% of an emergency department's workload. Serious clinical sequelae occur in less than 5% of such patients and most can be treated with supportive care. There are up-to-date information services (e.g. the National Poisons Information Service (NPIS) and its online database TOXBASE®) that provide valuable advice and information on available toxicology tests and the clinical management of patients. The most common drugs that are taken in overdose are listed in Table 21.6 but paracetamol represents more than 50% of the intentional self-poisoning presentations in the UK. Over-the-counter medications (e.g. herbal remedies) and industrial chemicals (heavy metals, solvents etc.) can also give rise to severe toxicity in some cases.

Investigations in the poisoned patient (Table 21.5)

If the patient is conscious and presents with specific signs and symptoms of toxicity, then a reliable history, with the clinical examination, will often suggest which drug or drugs have been taken. This can be

Table 21.5 Investigation of patients with suspected poisoning.

History and examination
- Temperature, heart rate, blood pressure, respiratory rate

Laboratory investigations that are often helpful
- Urea and electrolytes
- Liver function tests
- Blood glucose
- Blood gases.(and acid–base status)
- Paracetamol
- Calcium (hypocalcaemia in ethylene glycol poisoning)
- Full blood count
- Prothombin time (PT)
- International normalised ratio (INR)

Laboratory investigations less frequently required
- Salicylate (unless clinical features are suggestive of salicylate poisoning)
- Bedside urine drug tests
- Toxicology screens (may be required for medico-legal reasons or in suspected child abuse)
- Plasma drug concentrations (helpful only in specific circumstances)
- Serum osmolality and osmolar gap
- Anion gap

confirmed by laboratory investigations if needs be. Unfortunately, few of the drugs commonly taken in overdose have specific clinical signs. It is quite common for a combination of drugs to have been taken, sometimes with large amounts of alcohol. Problems arise when the patient is unconscious and the history is unavailable or likely to be inaccurate.

In a few circumstances, the laboratory may be asked to perform a drug screen to identify which drugs and poisons may have been taken. Unfortunately the results of such toxicology screens are often not available for some time after admission and often do not impact on the immediate treatment.

Treatment

A few drugs have a specific antidote (Table 21.6), but some antidotes may themselves have unpleasant side effects. For the majority of poisons, there is no antidote available, and the patient is treated conservatively until the drug has been eliminated from the body. If there is poor renal or liver function, it may be necessary to use haemodialysis or haemoperfusion to eliminate the drug and, in such a case, measurement of plasma levels can be important.

Specific drugs and poisons

Paracetamol (acetaminophen)

Overdose with paracetamol is common. During the first few hours, there may be few symptoms, unless these arise from another drug that has been taken simultaneously. A very large overdose may produce symptoms of depressed consciousness and metabolic acidosis. In patients presenting after 20 h, biochemical evidence of liver dysfunction is often apparent.

Approximately 10% of paracetamol is converted in the liver by a P450 mixed function oxidase to a toxic metabolite, N-acetyl-p-benzoquinoneimine (NABQI), which is usually detoxified by conjugation

Table 21.6 The principal examples of substances that cause acute poisoning in the UK. Full details of management of poisoned patients can be found from the NPIS and web-based systems such as 'TOXBASE'® (www.toxbase.org).

Substance	Treatment or toxin
Drugs commonly taken as overdose	
• Benzodiazepines	Flumazenil (rarely required)
• Ethanol	No specific treatment available
• Paracetamol	N-Acetylcysteine
• Salicylates	Sodium bicarbonate, haemodialysis
• Tricyclic anti-depressants/SSRI	Sodium bicarbonate
Drugs less commonly taken as overdose	
• Carbamazepine	Repeated oral activated charcoal
• Digoxin	Anti-digoxin antibody
• Iron	Desferrioxamine
• Lithium	Saline
• Opiates	Naloxone
• Phenobarbitone	Repeated oral activated charcoal
• Phenytoin	Repeated oral activated charcoal
Toxic substances	
• Carbon monoxide	Oxygen
• Cyanide (nonfatal dose)	Cobalt edetate, hydroxocobalamin
• Ethylene glycol	Ethanol, haemodialysis, fomepizole
• Methanol	Ethanol, haemodialysis, fomepizole
• Heavy metals	EDTA, DMSA, DMPS
• Organophosphorus agents	Pralidoxime, atropine

DMSA = dimercaptosuccinic acid; DMPS = 2,3-Dimercapto-1-propanesulfonic acid.

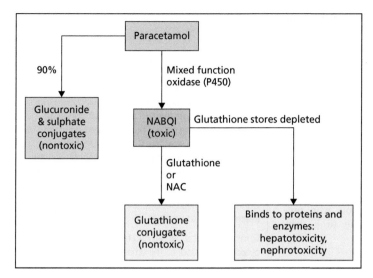

Figure 21.3 Metabolism of paracetamol. Around 10% is metabolised to toxic N-acetyl-p-benzoquinoneimine (NABQI). When glutathione stores are adequate, NABQI–glutathione conjugates are produced that are nontoxic. Glutathione stores can be replenished by giving intravenous N-acetylcysteine (NAC).

with glutathione. If large amounts of paracetamol are taken, the hepatic stores of glutathione become depleted, and NABQI binds irreversibly to proteins within the hepatocyte, producing centrilobular necrosis. In some cases, renal damage is also produced by a similar mechanism (Figure 21.3).

Increased production of NABQI occurs in patients with a chronic alcohol problem and in patients taking certain enzyme-inducing drugs such as phenytoin and phenobarbitone; these patients are at risk of hepatotoxicity at lower doses of paracetamol as are those with poor nutrition who may have low stores of glutathione.

If paracetamol overdose is diagnosed quickly, a specific treatment is available (IV N-acetylcysteine or oral methionine). The decision to treat is based on the plasma paracetamol concentration related to the time from overdose (Figure 21.4), *although 4 h should elapse from the time of ingestion to take into account drug absorption*. These treatments

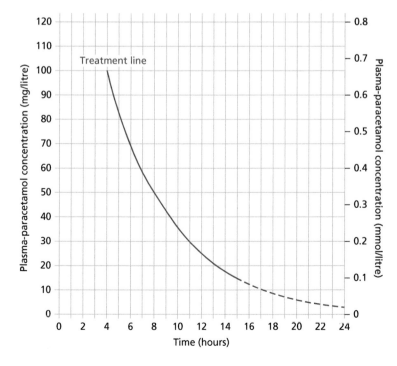

Figure 21.4 The decision to give N-acetylcysteine depends on the time since the overdose and on the plasma paracetamol concentration. Patients with a plasma paracetamol concentration that lies above the treatment line should be treated with N-acetylcysteine, as should those where the timing of the overdose is uncertain or staggered. The timing of specimen collection is important. At less than 4 h, the drug may not have been fully absorbed.

show most benefit if instituted within 12 h of the overdose, and are unlikely to be effective if used after 24 h. *When the time of the overdose is unknown or the overdose of paracetamol has been staggered, active intervention with N-acetylcysteine is advisable.* The prothrombin time is usually the first liver function test to become abnormal (after ~ 12 h) and is of value in assessing prognosis. Other liver function tests do not show an abnormality until at least 24–36 h after the overdose.

Paracetamol is taken commonly by patients who have taken an overdose either alone or in combination with other drugs. It is thus advisable to measure plasma paracetamol in most patients who present with suspected poisoning due to a drug overdose.

Salicylates

Patients often present with nausea, vomiting and increased rate of respiration. Dehydration, due to vomiting, is often severe. Acid–base disturbances are common – usually a mixed respiratory alkalosis and metabolic acidosis, but if vomiting is severe a metabolic alkalosis can develop.

The diagnosis and severity of poisoning are assessed using clinical and biochemical features and by measuring the plasma salicylate concentration. Plasma salicylate concentrations greater than 350 mg/L (2.5 mmol/L) are usually associated with poisoning. Most deaths in adults occur in patients whose concentrations exceed 700 mg/L (5.1 mmol/L). Concentrations of over 900 mg/L (6.4 mmol/L) are almost invariably associated with very severe toxicity and haemodialysis is almost always required in this situation.

Ethanol

The acute effects of overindulgence in ethanol sometimes lead to admission to hospitals. If the diagnosis is in doubt, or if help is required in assessing the severity of toxicity, blood ethanol should be measured. Blood concentrations of 3500 mg/L (76 mmol/L) are associated with stupor and coma. Concentrations of >4500 mg/L (98 mmol/L) are often fatal. Results should be used in combination with clinical symptoms to provide a more accurate guide. Patients taking a deliberate drug overdose frequently take alcohol with the drug. Some patients may have drunk methylated spirits rather than ethanol, and rapid identification of both methanol and ethanol is then needed.

 CASE 21.3

A 23-year-old woman was admitted to an A&E department after being found by a flatmate lying unconscious on her bed. Next to the patient was an empty bottle of vodka and on the bedside table there was a bottle of paracetamol tablets that appeared about half-full. The patient had appeared normal when seen by the flatmate 6 h earlier. On admission, the patient's breath smelt strongly of alcohol, and the plasma paracetamol level was found to be 105 mg/L. Liver function tests were normal, as was the PT.

Comment on these results, and also on what treatment should be given.

Comments: The patient had taken a paracetamol overdose with vodka. The time of the paracetamol overdose was not known accurately, and the patient was therefore treated with IV N-acetylcysteine.

No abnormalities were found in liver function tests on admission. Plasma ALT activity showed a transient increase over the next few days, with levels peaking at 400 U/L and then gradually falling back to reference values. These results indicate that some mild degree of liver damage had occurred.

 CASE 21.4

A 19-year-old student was admitted to an A&E department after calling his doctor to state that he had taken an overdose of aspirin 3 h previously. On admission, it was found that he had been vomiting and was now hyperventilating. The following results for blood tests were obtained:

Serum	Result	Reference range
Urea	7.3	2.5–6.6 mmol/L
Na	140	135–145 mmol/L
K⁺	3.3	3.6–5.0 mmol/L
Total CO₂	10	22–30 mmol/L
Salicylate	3.8	mmol/L
Paracetamol	Not detected	

Comment on these results.

Comments: The results and presenting features are consistent with a salicylate overdose. There is an acidosis, and salicylate is present in plasma.

Paracetamol was measured, as some preparations of salicylate also contain paracetamol. The patient was treated conservatively, and made a full recovery.

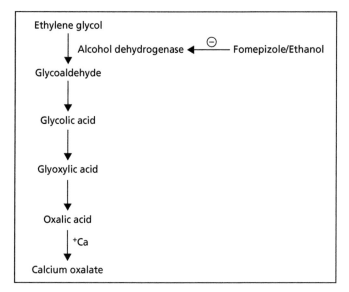

Figure 21.5 Metabolism of ethylene glycol. The formation of calcium oxalate results in the hypocalcaemia observed in patients following ethylene glycol ingestion.

Methanol and ethylene glycol

Methanol is metabolised to formaldehyde and formic acid, while ethylene glycol is metabolised to a number of products including glycoaldehyde, glyoxylic and oxalic acids. Many of these are toxic, and also give rise to metabolic acidosis. Severe methanol poisoning frequently leads to permanent visual impairment or complete blindness. Due to the formation of complexes with oxalic acid, hypocalcaemia occurs with ethylene glycol poisoning (Figure 21.5) As little as 10 mL of methanol can cause blindness. Lethal doses can be as little as 30 mL for methanol and 100 mL for ethylene glycol. After ingestion, there are latent phases of 8–36 h for methanol and 4–12 h for ethylene glycol.

Urgent measurement of plasma concentrations of these substances is required if poisoning is suspected, but it may be difficult to get such measurements performed out of normal laboratory hours. Measurement of the osmolar gap (i.e. the difference between the measured and calculated osmolality) and anion gap (Chapter 3: Anion gap) is useful in all suspected cases of methanol/ethylene glycol ingestion. An osmolar gap greater than 10 mos/kg is widely regarded as being indicative of an abnormality, but others have suggested that a value over 6 mos/kg should be regarded as abnormal. The osmolality must be measured using freezing point depression and not vapour pressure as the latter will produce falsely low results. A number of formulae have been published for the calculation of osmolality, for example $2 \times [Na^+ + K^+] + [urea] + [glucose]$.

The osmolar gap may only be present early in the poisoning, while a high anion gap may only occur late in the presentation when the ingested poisons have been metabolised to the acidic products.

Treatment consists of giving ethanol or fomepizole to inhibit the metabolism of the methanol or ethylene glycol to their toxic metabolites. The metabolic acidosis and hypocalcaemia must also be corrected. Severe poisoning with methanol or ethylene glycol should be treated by haemodialysis, which removes methanol, ethylene glycol and their metabolites in addition to correcting metabolic abnormalities.

 CASE 21.5

A 43-year-old woman was admitted to the A&E department after she had complained of abdominal cramps, vomiting, dizziness and blurred vision. She had drunk about a quarter of a bottle of cheap vodka, which she had bought at the local market, approximately 8 h previously. The following were found:

Serum	Result	Reference range
Urea	7.0	2.5–6.6 mmol/L
Na+	134	135–145 mmol/L
K+	5.0	3.6–5.0 mmol/L
Total CO₂	15	22–30 mmol/L
Chloride	100	95–107 mmol/L
Osmolar gap	11	<10 mos/kg

Calculate the anion gap and comment on the results. What treatment should be given?

Comments: The patient has a significant osmolar gap (>10 mos/kg) and an anion gap of 24 mmol/L. This, together with the low total CO_2 and presenting complaints, suggests a marked metabolic acidosis caused by ingestion of methanol or ethylene glycol. A blood methanol concentration of 550 mg/L (17 mmol/L was detected with no ethylene glycol. She was treated with an ethanol infusion, IV bicarbonate and haemodialysis. She made a full recovery. The vodka she had bought was found to contain some methanol.

Poisoning in children

Diagnosis is often more difficult than in the adult because the range of substances that may have been taken or administered is very large, symptoms may be atypical and often more severe, and the child may not be able to give useful information. The history obtained from parents may be vague or misleading, especially if one or both parents has been responsible for unauthorised drug administration. There are a number of urine drug-screening methods available which may, if necessary, be followed up by more accurate and specific methods such as mass spectrometry.

Drug abuse

The marked growth in drug misuse has resulted in increasingly frequent requests for the screening of urine specimens from patients suspected of being drug abusers, for the possible presence of opiates, cocaine, LSD, benzodiazepines, methadone, buprenorphine, amphetamines and amphetamine derivatives such as ecstasy, etc. Common reasons for requesting drugs of abuse screens are shown in Table 21.7.

Table 21.7 **Common reasons for screening for drugs of abuse.**

- Corroborate claims that drugs are being misused when patients request maintenance therapy
- Determine whether prescribed drugs (e.g. methadone) are being taken
- Determine whether drug abuse is continuing
- Monitor changing patterns of drug abuse
- Medicolegal reasons

Drug-screening procedures used to be performed mainly on urine specimens, but salivary and hair measurements are becoming more widely used. It is essential to ensure that the sample has not been tampered with by the patient, for example with the sample being diluted or exogenous drugs added. The preliminary drug screen may use immunoassays that are sensitive, but may lack specificity due to cross-reaction with related compounds. Confirmatory tests using specific chromatographic methods with mass spectrometry are required as a follow-up to positive results because of the possibly very serious implications for patients that can stem from being identified, correctly or incorrectly, as abusers of drugs.

Industrial and occupational hazards

Metal poisons

Arsenic, cadmium, lead, mercury and thallium are all highly toxic to humans. Their effects depend partly on the type of compound involved, whether inorganic or organometallic, and partly on the route of absorption. In all cases, the kidney is liable to be severely damaged, and often the liver and the nervous system also. Whole blood and urine measurements of the metal are important to confirm diagnosis and assess the severity of the poisoning. Iron poisoning is particularly important in children who ingest iron tablets. Hair or nail analysis can sometimes be used.

Patients with chronic renal failure maintained on haemodialysis regimes are particularly at risk from poisoning by dialysis fluid constituents. Aluminium toxicity leading to *dialysis dementia* and to *metabolic bone disease* has been described. Prevention of toxicity requires periodic checks of aluminium content in the water supply and in the effluent from deionisers used with dialysers.

 CASE 21.6

A 48-year-old decorator went to his GP complaining of persistent lethargy, nausea and headache which had been going on for the past few weeks. It had started when he had been employed to do some renovation work on an old Victorian house. He wondered if it could be due to the fumes from all the paint-stripping he had been doing using a gas blow torch.

The GP wondered if he may have been exposed to lead in the old paintwork; blood lead was found to be 4.2 μmol/L.

What course of action should this blood lead level initiate?

Comments: The patient has been exposed to toxic levels of lead from the old paintwork that he had been removing. Paints produced more than 50 years ago contained high levels of lead and this would have been absorbed by the patient as both lead fumes from the paint stripping and ingestion from any sanding he had been doing. He was treated initially with intravenous sodium calcium edetate to mobilise lead from bone and tissues followed by a course of oral chelators (e.g. DMSA (Succimer)). In the UK if a blood concentration in excess of 2.4 μmol/L is reached following occupational exposure, the employer is required by the Health and Safety Executive to reduce exposure. If the blood lead concentration is in excess of 2.9 μmol/L, the worker has to be suspended from work. Erythrocyte zinc protoporphyrin is sometimes measured in lead poisoning and elevated levels provide an indication of over-exposure to lead over the previous 3 months.

Organic solvents

Many organic solvents used in industry are toxic (e.g. chlorinated hydrocarbons, ethylene glycol). Toxicity may be due to accidental exposure, or sometimes to solvent abuse. The toxic agent can usually be identified specifically (e.g. by gas chromatography). Other biochemical and haematological investigations may be needed, to assess hepatic and renal function.

Pesticides

Organophosphates (e.g. parathion, malathion) may cause poisoning among farm workers by inhibiting acetylcholinesterase; plasma BChE is also inhibited. Measurements of plasma BChE activity can help in the recognition of excessive exposure to organophosphates.

 ## FURTHER READING

Thompson, J.P., Watson, I.D., Thanacoody, H.K.R., et al. (2014) Guidelines for laboratory analyses for poisoned patients in the United Kingdom. *Annals of Clinical Biochemistry* **51(3)**, 312–25.

22

Clinical biochemistry in paediatrics and the elderly

Learning objectives

To understand:

✔ the range and types of biochemical problems that are found at the extremes of age;

✔ that biochemical values may differ at the extremes of age, as compared to adult values, and that different reference ranges may apply;

✔ the types of inherited and acquired metabolic problems that present in the neonatal period or early childhood;

✔ that multi-organ problems and multiple drug usage may contribute to biochemical abnormalities in the elderly;

✔ the importance of disease screening for certain disorders at the extremes of age.

Introduction

Disorders of *children*, particularly the neonate, often differ from those in the adult. In the neonate, there may be problems associated with immaturity, problems in adapting to the new external environment and, rarely, inherited metabolic disorders. In childhood, disorders of growth and failure to thrive require investigation.

In *old age*, the differences from general adult medicine are fewer. However, multiple pathology is common, and diagnosis is often made difficult by the fact that symptoms may be minimal, atypical or confounded by drug treatment. For this reason, more reliance may have to be placed on laboratory tests.

Paediatrics

In this section, we discuss the following areas of diagnosis:

1 Causes and diagnosis of biochemical disturbances commonly found in the neonate and in early childhood.
2 Inherited metabolic disorders.
3 Biochemical abnormalities associated with failure to thrive, malnutrition and short stature.

Clinical Biochemistry Lecture Notes, Tenth Edition. Peter Rae, Mike Crane and Rebecca Pattenden.
© 2018 John Wiley & Sons Ltd. Published 2018 by John Wiley & Sons Ltd.
Companion website: www.lecturenoteseries.com/clinicalbiochemistry

Specimen collection from neonates and children

This should be done expertly, and the amount of blood taken minimised. Capillary blood is used in neonatal units and for newborn screening. Blood specimens from babies are obtained using an automated neonatal device by heel-prick from the fleshy (lateral) parts of the heel. In older children, finger-prick capillary sampling is used to monitor diabetes.

Paediatric reference ranges

Age-related reference ranges must always be used where available. In neonates, particularly when premature or small for gestational age, interpretation of results is difficult and requires considerable experience.

Table 22.1 Infants at risk of developing hypoglycaemia.

Poor milk intake	Hormone imbalance
• Establishment of breastfeeding	• Hyperinsulinaemia
Decreased glycogen stores	• Growth hormone deficiency
• Prematurity	• Adrenal insufficiency
• Small for gestational age	• Hypopituitarism
• Some inborn errors of metabolism	
Increased demand	
• Sepsis	
• Hypoxia, hypothermia and pyrexia	
• Inborn errors of metabolism	

Causes and diagnosis of biochemical disturbances in the neonate and early childhood

Glucose

Neonates

The foetus utilises maternal glucose and any excess is stored as hepatic glycogen. Fat is also stored in foetal adipose tissue during the last trimester. After birth the baby has to maintain its own blood glucose between feeds by fat and glycogen catabolism and gluconeogenesis. In some babies these mechanisms are insufficient to maintain blood glucose concentration, and hypoglycaemia occurs. In the neonate, there is no single cut-off for defining hypoglycaemia, although blood glucose below 2.6 mmol/L is often regarded as being an intervention threshold. The presence of clinical symptoms will also depend on the rate of fall in glucose. The principal causes of neonatal hypoglycaemia are as follows (see Table 22.1):

- Transient hypoglycaemia in healthy term infants is most commonly due to a low milk intake during establishment of breastfeeding. Premature infants, and infants that are small for gestational age, are particularly at risk from hypoglycaemia due to their lack of glycogen and fat stores.
- Hypoglycaemia may also become evident if there is an increased demand for glucose such as may occur in the septic, hypoxic, hypothermic or pyrexial infant.
- In rare cases the hypoglycaemia may be due to an inherited metabolic disorder or a deficiency or

imbalance in a range of hormones including GH and glucocorticoids.

Hyperinsulinaemia is the most common cause of persistent or recurrent neonatal hypoglycaemia after the first 24 h of life. There are a number of causes, including maternal hyperglycaemia due to poor diabetic control during pregnancy. Maternal hyperglycaemia induces hyperplasia of foetal islet cells, resulting in foetal hyperinsulinaemia that cannot be suppressed in the neonate, and hypoglycaemia results.

Rare genetic causes of *persistent* hyperinsulinism have been identified, including deficiencies of glucokinase or glutamate dehydrogenase, or recessive mutations of the genes for the sulphonylurea receptor (SUR 1) and the ATP-dependent potassium channel (KIR 6.2) in the plasma membrane of the pancreatic β-cells. The gene defects in SUR 1 and KIR 6.2 give rise to hyperplasia of insulin-producing cells in the pancreas (congenital hyperinsulinism). Sporadic causes of transient hyperinsulinism also occur in association with other disorders, such as the overgrowth disorder Beckwith–Wiedemann syndrome.

Neonates at risk of hypoglycaemia should have their blood glucose monitored regularly by POCT, with low readings (<2.5 mmol/L) confirmed by laboratory measurement; however treatment must not be delayed in the intervening period. Investigations to identify the cause of hypoglycaemia must be undertaken during the hypoglycaemic episode, otherwise the diagnostic opportunity may be missed.

Table 22.2 Investigations in the hypoglycaemic child.

Investigation	Interpretation and disorders
Glucose	Essential to confirm hypoglycaemia
Lactate	Present in tissue hypoxia and some inborn errors of metabolism (e.g. mitochondrial disorders, glycogen storage disease, etc.)
Ammonia	Elevated in some organic acid/fatty acid oxidation disorders
Insulin/C-peptide	Hyperinsulinism; exogenous insulin (only interpretable if glucose ≤2.5 mmol/L)
Free fatty acid/β-hydroxybutyrate (FFA/HOB)	Low in hyperinsulinism. Elevated FFA:HOB ratio occurs in fatty-acid oxidation disorders
Cortisol and GH	Lack of appropriate response may indicate pituitary or HPA axis disorder. Cut-offs are age-dependent
Amino acids	Amino acid disorders
Acylcarnitine profile	Disorders of long chain fatty-acid oxidation disorders and organic acidurias
Urine organic acid analysis	Organic acidurias and fatty acid oxidation disorders

During childhood

Recurrent hypoglycaemia of infancy and childhood may be due to any of the causes listed in Table 6.7 (Chapter 6: Hypoglycaemia) as well as several other inherited metabolic disorders (e.g. fatty acid oxidation disorders and mitochondrial disorders). Although islet cell hyperplasia usually presents in the first few days of life, symptoms may be delayed for up to 6 months. Table 22.2 indicates the biochemical investigations that should be performed in the hypoglycaemic child.

Calcium and magnesium

Plasma calcium falls, in normal full-term infants, by about 10–20% in the first 2–3 days of life. It then returns to normal (2.0–2.8 mmol/L) over the course of the next 3–4 days.

Neonatal hypocalcaemia within the first 48 h, sufficient to give rise to twitching, irritability and convulsions, occurs particularly in infants who are premature, those of diabetic mothers and those who have experienced birth asphyxia. Maternal vitamin D deficiency may be a factor (e.g. in Asian women). The mechanism is complex, but the hypocalcaemia tendency usually corrects spontaneously, although calcium gluconate may need to be given if convulsions occur, or if plasma calcium falls below 1.50 mmol/L. Rarely, hypocalcaemic convulsions in the neonate are associated with maternal hyperparathyroidism, which may produce temporary hypoparathyroidism in the neonate due to suppression of the foetal parathyroid glands by maternal hypercalcaemia.

Late neonatal hypocalcaemia, between the fourth and tenth days of life, may occur in full-term as well as in premature infants. Hyperexcitability of muscles is usually also present. This is liable to occur in infants whose mothers had a low intake of vitamin D during pregnancy; these infants may also have low plasma magnesium. Rarely, hypocalcaemia may be due to renal failure. Treatment with calcium, and often magnesium, may be required.

Neonatal rickets. Premature infants have increased requirements for calcium, phosphate and vitamin D for bone growth. The most sensitive indicator of inadequate intake is a rising plasma ALP, which precedes abnormalities in plasma calcium or phosphate.

Hypomagnesaemia is an occasional cause of neonatal convulsions. It can lead to hypocalcaemia by reducing PTH secretion. Plasma magnesium should be measured in all cases of hypocalcaemia.

Hypercalcaemia in the neonatal period is less common than hypocalcaemia. Inadequate phosphate supplements in rapidly growing preterm infants can lead to hypophosphataemia, bone resorption and thus hypercalcaemia. Oversupplementation may also lead to hypercalcaemia. Much rarer causes include malignancy, hyperparathyroidism, familial hypocalciuric hypercalcaemia, subcutaneous fat necrosis and Williams' syndrome.

Neonatal jaundice (Table 22.3)

Table 22.3 **Causes of jaundice in the neonatal period.**	
Early jaundice	**Prolonged jaundice**
Physiological	Breastfeeding
Haemolysis	Prematurity
Infection	Infection
Genetic defects of bilirubin metabolism	Biliary atresia
	Endocrine disorders
	Genetic disorders

Physiological unconjugated hyperbilirubinaemia

Approximately half of all infants develop hyperbilirubinaemia during the first week of life due to:

- Increased production from breakdown of red cells, which have a shortened lifespan in the neonate.
- Decreased excretion, because of immaturity of hepatic bilirubin uptake, conjugation and biliary excretion.
- Reabsorption from the intestine. Bilirubin is deconjugated by the intestinal enzyme β-glucuronidase. In adults it is further metabolised to urobilinogen by normal intestinal bacteria. The newborn's GI tract has not yet acquired these organisms, and some bilirubin is reabsorbed, a process which is stimulated by breast milk.

Pathological causes of unconjugated hyperbilirubinaemia

Babies may be at increased risk of severe hyperbilirubinaemia if they have one or more of the following, in addition to normal physiological factors:

CASE 22.1

A neonate born at 37 weeks was observed to be jaundiced about 48h after delivery. The bilirubin was found to be 172 μmol/L and this had risen to 220 mmol/L by 72h. Laboratory investigation confirmed that the bilirubin was largely unconjugated. The baby was administered phototherapy and the bilirubin started to fall such that within 7 days of delivery it had reduced to 28 μmol/L. The child was otherwise feeding well and showed no other LFT abnormalities or other problems.

Comment: This baby shows all the features of physiological jaundice of the newborn. The bilirubin is unconjugated and other LFTs are normal. The child is well and shows no other problems and the bilirubin responds to simple phototherapy which is required for only a short time. After a few days bilirubin levels return to normal. The problem reflects the relative immaturity of the glucuronyltransferase bilirubin conjugation system leading to a short-term unconjugated hyperbilirubinaemia.

- Dehydration, intercurrent infection, bruising, polycythaemia.
- Increased haemolysis.
- Lysis due to Rhesus incompatibility. This is now a rare occurrence; however, lysis may also result from ABO or other blood group incompatibility.
- Predisposition to lysis due to glucose-6-phosphate dehydrogenase deficiency or hereditary spherocytosis.
- Defective hepatic uptake or conjugation. This may occur in association with Gilbert's syndrome, mutations in anion transporters or rarely inherited disorders of bilirubin metabolism (Crigler–Najjar syndrome, Chapter 13: The congenital hyperbilirubinaemias).

In most infants, hyperbilirubinaemia is a self-limiting condition that requires no treatment. A tiny percentage of bilirubin exists free in the circulation, not bound to protein. Only free bilirubin can cross the blood–brain barrier, where high concentrations can cause bilirubin encephalopathy and kernicterus. The relationship between total plasma bilirubin and free brain bilirubin is complex because of:

- Variation in the concentration of circulating proteins (particularly albumin) that bind unconjugated bilirubin.
- Displacement of bilirubin from protein-binding sites by drugs (e.g. benzyl penicillin, phenobarbital, furosemide), free fatty acids (hypoglycaemic and ketotic infants) or hydrogen ions (acidotic infants).
- Impairment of the blood–brain barrier in premature and sick infants, allowing some albumin-bound bilirubin to penetrate the brain.

Total plasma bilirubin measurement is used routinely as a proxy for free bilirubin. First-line screening for healthy term babies is by visual assessment or transcutaneous bilirubin monitor. Confirmation requires laboratory measurement of total plasma bilirubin. Circulating unconjugated bilirubin is removed by phototherapy or, if concentrations are grossly elevated, by exchange transfusion. Action limits for treatment to prevent kernicterus are age related and are lower for pre-term or sick infants.

Prolonged jaundice is defined as jaundice persisting beyond 14 days of age. It is most commonly breast milk jaundice, mainly due to increased enterohepatic circulation, and caused by unconjugated bilirubin alone. It does not usually require treatment. All prolonged jaundice requires measurement of total and conjugated (or 'direct') bilirubin.

Conjugated hyperbilirubinaemia

Any increase in conjugated bilirubin always indicates pathology and requires identification and further investigation of its aetiology by appropriate biochemical and other tests.

Causes include infective, endocrine and genetic disorders (Table 22.4).

Biliary atresia: Extra-hepatic biliary atresia is a rapidly progressing condition where the bile ducts are rapidly obliterated. Diagnosis is confirmed by ultrasound scan to demonstrate absence of the gall bladder. Surgery before 60 days of age may be curative; otherwise the only treatment option is liver transplant. To identify potentially life-threatening but treatable causes, it is imperative to investigate all cases of prolonged jaundice without delay, by measurement of total and conjugated bilirubin, and LFTs in the first instance. Further tests such as thyroid function, galactosaemia screening and biliary tract imaging are carried out after clinical assessment of the infant.

Table 22.4 Causes of conjugated hyperbilirubinaemia in the neonate.

Biliary atresia	Cystic fibrosis
Sepsis or neonatal hepatitis (TORCH* infection)	Galactosaemia
Hypothyroidism	Tyrosinaemia
Hypopituitarism (± septo-optic dysplasia)	α_1-Antitrypsin deficiency

*TORCH includes toxoplasma, rubella, cytomegalovirus, herpes and others.

 CASE 22.2

A female baby born at 38 weeks by normal vaginal delivery was discharged breastfeeding after 24 h. She was re-admitted to the hospital after 5 days with marked jaundice (total bilirubin 390 μmol/L; direct bilirubin 75 μmol/L). She was given phototherapy but, despite this, after 6 weeks the jaundice persisted (total bilirubin was 190 μmol/L and direct bilirubin was 80 μmol/L). ALT was slightly raised at 60 U/L but GGT was markedly elevated at 600 U/L. What might be the differential diagnosis?

Comments: The baby has prolonged conjugated hyperbilirubinaemia. The differential diagnosis is between infection, inherited metabolic disorder and a biliary tree abnormality. Further investigations showed no evidence of infection. Galactosaemia screen was negative, as were urinary organic acids and amino acids. Thyroid function tests and serum cortisol were normal. Ultrasound of the liver demonstrated a small gallbladder. Further imaging, liver biopsy and laparotomy confirmed a diagnosis of extra-hepatic biliary atresia. The baby was treated surgically by Kasai hepatoportoenterostomy. Early diagnosis of this disease is very important. If surgery is performed before the baby is 2 months old, success is much more likely. For this reason, all infants who are jaundiced after the age of 4 weeks should be evaluated for biliary atresia if other causes cannot be found.

Inherited metabolic disorders

Inborn errors of metabolism usually present in infancy or childhood. They result from alteration in a single gene, leading to a protein product that has suboptimal function. Most of these rare conditions show autosomal recessive inheritance: heterozygotes do not manifest the disorder. The affected protein may be an enzyme, a structural or transport protein or an enzyme co-factor affecting the activity of several enzymes (Table 22.5).

The consequences of an inherited defect affecting a metabolic pathway include:

- accumulation of potentially toxic metabolites that occur in the pathway before the defect;
- deficiency of essential metabolites produced by the pathway after the defect;
- increased flux of potentially toxic metabolites through alternative metabolic pathways;
- storage of macromolecules in organs such as liver and spleen if the defect is in their breakdown pathway;
- failure of negative feedback inhibition of the pathway because production of the end-product is decreased.

Figures 22.1–22.3 illustrate these effects in PKU, defects in fatty acid oxidation and galactosaemia, respectively. The age at presentation depends on residual protein activity and is not constant for a given disorder.

Table 22.5 Examples of inherited metabolic disorders and diagnostic tests.

General disorders	Examples	Useful diagnostic test(s)
Amino acid metabolism	Phenylketonuria, tyrosinaemia	Plasma amino acids Urine organic acids
Organic acid metabolism	Methylmalonic aciduria	Urine organic acids
Fatty acid oxidation	Medium chain acyl-CoA dehydrogenase deficiency	Urine organic acids Acylcarnitine profile
Urea cycle defects	Ornithine transcarbamylase deficiency	Plasma ammonia/amino acids, urine organic acids
Carbohydrate disorders	Galactosaemia	Galactose-1-phosphate uridyl transferase bloodspot
Defects of intermediary metabolism	Mitochondrial respiratory chain defects	Enzyme activity in muscle biopsy
Steroid synthesis defects	21-Hydroxylase, 11-hydroxylase deficiencies	Plasma 17-hydroxyprogesterone, urine steroid profile
Macromolecule breakdown defects	Lysosomal storage disorders	Plasma lysosomal enzyme
Transport protein defects	Cystic fibrosis	Sweat chloride, mutation studies
Co-factor defects	Biotinidase deficiency	Plasma biotinidase activity
Organelle assembly or uptake	Peroxisomal defects	Plasma very-long chain fatty acids

In some cases addition or deletion of chromosomes or parts of chromosomes occurs, leading to clinically significant abnormalities (e.g. Down's syndrome, Turner's syndrome).

Diagnosis

The individual disorders are rare, but *collectively* they are not uncommon. The true incidence is unknown, except for those that are detected by screening programmes. Within the UK, bloodspot screening is performed on neonates at 5–8 days old using filter cards that are posted to national screening centres. This timing is not suitable for detecting all disorders (e.g. patients with galactosaemia will often have life-threatening symptoms before the sixth day of life.) In the UK, the panel of disorders screened has recently been expanded, as listed in Table 22.6.

Screening programmes require considerable organisation, and before embarking on them, several questions need to be considered:

1 What is the incidence of the disease?
2 Is the disease life threatening or liable to be severe?
3 Is there an asymptomatic period before irreversible damage occurs?
4 Is acceptable treatment available?
5 Is a suitable screening test available?
6 Are the costs acceptable?

Table 22.6 Newborn screening in the UK.

Disorder	Screening test
Congenital hypothyroidism	TSH
Cystic fibrosis	Immunoreactive trypsin
Sickle cell disease	Haemoglobin fractionation
Phenylketonuria	Phenylalanine/tyrosine
Medium chain acyl-CoA dehydrogenase deficiency	Octanoylcarnitine/decanoylcarnitine
Glutaric aciduria type 1	Glutarylcarnitine
Maple syrup urine disease	Leucine/isoleucine/alloisoleucine
Homocystinuria	Methionine/total homocysteine
Isovaleric aciduria	Isovalerylcarnitine

A screening programme should only be considered if all these criteria have been met.

For those disorders not detected by screening programmes, the clinical manifestations of patients with inborn errors of metabolism vary considerably. In acute neonatal presentations, an infant assessed as normal at birth typically develops reluctance to feed, vomiting and abnormal breathing. Without treatment the affected infants can rapidly progress to multiple organ failure, coma and death. In those disorders with a more chronic course, symptoms such as failure to thrive, progressive hepatomegaly or neurological deterioration may develop over months or years. Several inherited metabolic disorders that present less acutely may nevertheless carry a very poor prognosis. Only a minority present with a clearly defined clinical syndrome.

For the index case in a family, the recognition that there is a metabolic disease present, and its identification, can present complex diagnostic problems.

The index case

In an acutely ill infant, or one presenting with chronic signs and symptoms, the results of routine laboratory tests may provide a clue to a potential inborn error of metabolism. These include metabolic acidosis identified by blood gas analyser or calculated anion gap, hypoglycaemia, lactic acidaemia, or haematological abnormalities such as neutropenia, haemolytic anaemia, megaloblastic anaemia and coagulation defects. Suggestive clinical features include dysmorphia, hepato- or splenomegaly, cardiomyopathy, neurological disturbance (seizures/hypotonia), intractable feeding difficulties or onset of acute symptoms in response to fasting or weaning.

In sick children suspected of having an inherited metabolic disorder, the early measurement of plasma ammonia is particularly important; hyperammonaemia can lead to cerebral oedema with irreversible neurological damage, and immediate treatment is critical. The main causes of hyperammonaemia are listed in Table 22.7. Clinical signs associated with hyperammonaemia include encephalopathy, seizures and respiratory alkalosis associated with the presence of hyperventilation and/or grunting in neonates. Ammonia is inherently unstable in blood, and samples requiring analysis must be cooled and sent to the laboratory without delay; failure to do so can result in falsely elevated

values. Treatment of hyperammonaemia usually includes administration of 10% dextrose infusion and measures to directly reduce ammonia with L-arginine, sodium benzoate therapy, haemofiltration or dialysis. Ammonia is further discussed later in this chapter (Chapter 22: Urea cycle defects and hyperammonaemia).

If a child is suspected of having an inherited disorder of metabolism, samples may be referred to a regional paediatric laboratory for specialised tests, including:

- urine, plasma or CSF amino acids;
- urine organic acids;
- galactosaemia screening test (red cell galactose-1-phosphate uridylyltransferase, available as a bloodspot test);
- plasma or bloodspot acylcarnitines;
- mucopolysaccharide excretion;
- specific enzyme tests (to diagnose, for example, lysosomal storage disorders or mitochondrial respiratory chain defects).

For the correct interpretation of results it is essential to provide clinical details including fed/fasted status (fasting potentiates abnormalities in fatty acid oxidation and gluconeogenetic defects), transfusion history (any transfused red cells invalidate the galactosaemia screening test) and drug therapy (antibiotics mask amino acid abnormalities) at the time of specimen collection. In children who are acutely unwell, it is important to collect blood and urine samples during the acute episode, because in many cases the biochemical abnormalities are only apparent during this time.

Confirmation of the diagnosis

Diagnostic confirmation may require tissue biopsy (skin, muscle, liver) to demonstrate deficient enzyme activity or a pathological DNA mutation. Specific therapy (e.g. enzyme replacement therapy for Gaucher's disease, biotin supplements in biotinidase deficiency) is available for some disorders. Even if no such therapy is available, precise diagnosis is essential to allow genetic counselling for the family, including investigation of siblings and other relatives, genetic advice on recurrence rates and potential pre-natal diagnosis during future pregnancies.

Foetal tissue can be obtained by the technique of chorionic villus biopsy for the purpose of pre-natal enzyme testing, although nowadays genetic testing is used in the majority of cases. Heterozygote detection is not usually reliable by enzyme analysis, and is better performed by mutation studies. This is particularly

Table 22.7 **Causes of hyperammonaemia.**

- Organic acid disorders
- Urea cycle disorders
- Acute/severe hepatic failure
- Neonates (mild, physiological)
- Valproate therapy
- Post-ictal state

important for female relatives of boys diagnosed with an X-linked disorder (e.g. ornithine transcarbamylase deficiency or Fabry disease).

Examples of inherited metabolic disorders

Phenylketonuria (PKU)

This disease provides the best example of a treatable condition detected by neonatal screening. Screening for PKU has been performed for the past 50 years.

Phenylalanine is converted to tyrosine by hepatic phenylalanine hydroxylase (Figure 22.1). In classical PKU, phenylalanine hydroxylase activity is undetectable or very much reduced. However, a minority (1–2%) of patients with inherited abnormalities of phenylalanine metabolism have defects in tetrahydrobiopterin (a co-factor for phenylalanine hydroxylase) metabolism. A third group of patients demonstrate a milder increase in phenylalanine (Phe <400 μmol/L). These rare forms of PKU must be differentiated from the classical form,

as they require different treatment. Classical PKU illustrates many of the principles that underlie the diverse effects of inherited metabolic disorders.

1 *Accumulation of the substrate of the blocked reaction.* This occurs in the liver. Plasma phenylalanine is much increased, unless dietary phenylalanine is restricted.
2 *Reduced formation of product.* Tyrosine formation is severely affected in patients, but tyrosine deficiency is avoided by supplements.
3 *Alternative paths of metabolism of the precursor that accumulates.* There is increased formation and urinary excretion of phenyl-pyruvate, phenyl-lactate and phenyl-acetate, and of various *o*-hydroxyphenyl metabolites. Dietary phenylalanine restriction reduces the output of these metabolites.
4 *Effects on other reactions.* Accumulation of phenylalanine and its metabolites competes with transport of other amino acids into the brain, potentially causing cerebral deficiency of other essential amino acids.

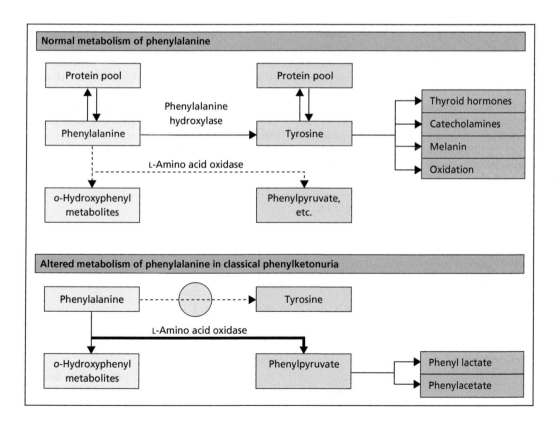

Figure 22.1 The metabolism of phenylalanine. In the classical form of PKU, the activity of phenylalanine hydroxylase is greatly reduced, and normally minor metabolites of phenylalanine are excreted in much increased amounts.

Elevated brain phenylalanine and concomitant deficiencies of other amino acids lead to cerebral damage in early life. This is prevented by restricting natural dietary protein to supply only the tiny amount of phenylalanine required for growth. Other essential amino acids, vitamins and minerals are given as supplements. Dietary protein is adjusted in response to frequently measured capillary phenylalanine. Even patients with classical PKU may show some fall in circulating phenylalanine in response to treatment with high doses of the biopterin co-factor. A commercial preparation of this is available. Each patient with PKU will require detailed assessment of its potential use, along with, or instead of, dietary treatment.

Medium chain acyl-CoA dehydrogenase (MCAD) deficiency

MCAD deficiency is the most common fatty acid oxidation defect in Europe, with an estimated incidence similar to PKU (1 in 10 000). The primary defect affects β-oxidation of fatty acids (Figure 22.2). Prior to the introduction of screening programmes, patients characteristically presented in the toddler age group, following a minor infection where vomiting induces a longer than normal fast. At this age, glycogen stores are rapidly exhausted and energy production depends on the defective fatty acid oxidation. Patients rapidly become hypoglycaemic and encephalopathic, due to toxic fatty acid-related compounds, and ammonia is often elevated. There is a relative lack of ketones; however, the presence of ketonaemia does not exclude the diagnosis. The child responds rapidly to dextrose infusion, which restores glucose concentra-tion, increases insulin secretion and thus suppresses fatty acid oxidation and production of the toxic fatty acids. Prolonged hypoglycaemia and encephalopathy can result in irreversible neurological damage and death.

Diagnosis is readily made when the patient presents in hypoglycaemic crisis, by identification of the characteristic pattern of urinary dicarboxylic acids and acyl-glycines identified by urine organic acid analysis, or by the abnormal acyl-carnitine pattern on tandem mass spectrometry. These two sensitive techniques are also capable of detecting small amounts of diagnostic compounds when the patient is well (Figure 22.2).

The clinical spectrum extends from fatal neonatal presentations to adults with no history of acute attack. Treatment consists of avoidance of prolonged fasting. If there is evidence of decompensation, dextrose infusion is urgently required.

When the patient has been diagnosed, episodes of decompensation can be readily prevented by the avoidance of fasting.

Galactosaemia

Galactose is metabolised by the liver. Three rare defects have been described: deficiency of galactose-1-phosphate uridylyltransferase (Gal-1-PUT), galactokinase or UDP-galactose epimerase (Figure 22.3). They all prevent normal metabolism of galactose, causing a rise in plasma and urine galactose. Galactose gives positive results if urinary tests for reducing substances are performed, and infants who have positive tests for reducing substances

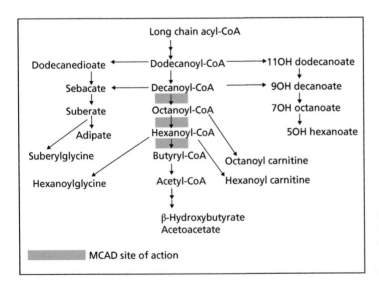

Figure 22.2 Pathways for fatty acid oxidation. In MCAD deficiency, fatty acid intermediates are metabolised by alternative β-oxidation pathways or excreted as glycine or carnitine conjugates.

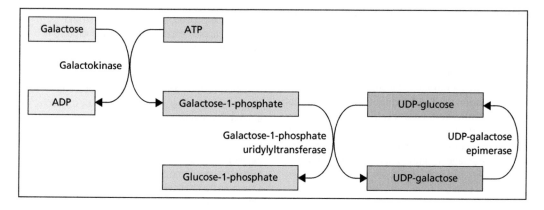

Figure 22.3 The enzymatic conversion of galactose to glucose. Galactosaemia may be caused by deficiency of any of these three enzymes, but the most common cause is deficiency of galactose-1-phosphate uridylyltransferase.

in urine should have the diagnosis excluded by enzyme or metabolite tests.

Galactosaemia is rare (1–2 per 100 000 live births). The most common and most severe enzymatic defect is Gal-1-PUT deficiency. This manifests itself in the neonatal period after feeding with galactose-containing milk, giving rise to vomiting, jaundice and abnormal LFTs, and sometimes hypoglycaemia. A bloodspot test for Gal-1-PUT is available and considered the first-line test for galactosaemia screening. Treatment is by galactose-free diet.

In babies that exhibit a classic picture of galactosaemia, hereditary fructose intolerance and tyrosinaemia type 1 should also be considered as part of the differential diagnosis.

Urea cycle defects and hyperammonaemia (Figure 22.4)

The urea cycle is the means by which metabolically generated ammonia is detoxicated and excess

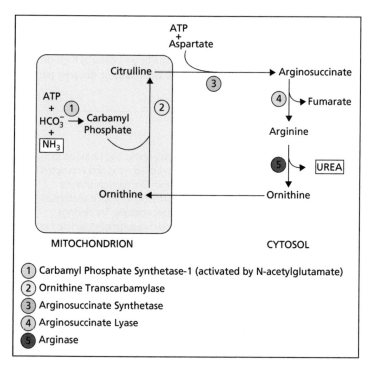

① Carbamyl Phosphate Synthetase-1 (activated by N-acetylglutamate)
② Ornithine Transcarbamylase
③ Arginosuccinate Synthetase
④ Arginosuccinate Lyase
⑤ Arginase

Figure 22.4 The urea cycle (in liver).

nitrogen present in the amine group of amino acids is removed; it also serves as a means to generate the amino acid, arginine. The full cycle only operates in the liver and comprises three intra-mitochondrial and three cytosolic steps. The substrates for urea formation are ammonia, bicarbonate and aspartate with utilisation and subsequent regeneration of ornithine. Inherited urea cycle enzyme defects interfere with the detoxification of ammonia that then accumulates with the potential for severe neurological damage (Figure 22.4). For this reason,

---

CASE 22.3

A previously well 11-month-old boy was admitted to a hospital with a 1-day history of vomiting and diarrhoea, pyrexia and a red macular rash. On the ward he fed poorly, vomited three times overnight and the following morning suddenly became drowsy and floppy, with unrecordable glucose on BM sticks. At that time, selected biochemistry results were:

Plasma	Result	Age-corrected reference range
Glucose	<0.5	2.2–6.4 mmol/L
Urea	10.8	1.4–6.6 mmol/L
Cortisol	2137	100–610 (6 am to 10 am) nmol/L
Urine qualitative analysis		Ketones – moderate

What causes of hypoglycaemia can be ruled out from these results?

What further tests should be requested?

Comments: It is important to confirm hypoglycaemia by laboratory measurement, and to collect sufficient samples for additional analyses to test the response to the provocation of falling plasma glucose. The cortisol response indicates an intact HPA axis and rules out adrenal failure and panhypopituitarism. The ketonuria rules out hyperinsulinism. The elevated urea reflects dehydration caused by vomiting and diarrhoea.

The remaining urine sample was analysed for organic acids. The pattern showed large peaks of fatty acid oxidation intermediates (adipate, suberate, sebacate, and their hydroxylated derivatives, with a relative lack of acetoacetate and β-hydroxybutyrate). Hexanoyl-, suberyl- and phenylprioninyl-glycine peaks were present. This pattern is diagnostic of MCAD deficiency presenting in crisis (see Figure 22.2).

The child responded rapidly to IV glucose and carnitine supplementation. He was discharged after the parents had been taught home glucose monitoring and given advice on the importance of avoiding fasting and of bringing him to the hospital should he develop another vomiting illness. The diagnosis was subsequently confirmed by mutation studies. The identified mutations, along with organic acid analysis, were used to rule out the diagnosis in two siblings born subsequently. The patient had one further precautionary hospital admission at 15 months following a low home glucose measurement. Otherwise he has been well and developed normally. Once patients reach school age, their increased hepatic glycogen stores make them less vulnerable to decompensation following common childhood illnesses.

---

immediate recognition of hyperammonaemia and its treatment are imperative.

Defects in all the urea cycle enzymes have been described but the commonest is X-linked ornithine transcarbamylase deficiency; this is a mitochondrial enzyme catalysing combination of carbamyl phosphate with ornithine to form citrulline (Figure 22.4). Severe, neonatal onset is seen in males with null defects and the prognosis is then poor. Identification of the problem in a severely affected male is important in allowing the possibility of ante-natal screening in subsequent pregnancies. Some males may have a mild disorder that may present later in life. A small proportion of female carriers may also have symptoms later in life that can be provoked by high-protein diets, drugs (such as valproate) or the post-partum

---

CASE 22.4

A 2-week-old boy was investigated for failure to thrive. He had a history of vomiting and was noted to be increasingly lethargic. Biochemical analysis revealed a low urea with mild LFT abnormalities. There was no significant acidosis. The findings prompted an ammonia measurement that was high at 520 μmol/L (normally <70 μmol/L). What condition do you suspect?

Comment: The high ammonia, in the absence of a metabolic acidosis, raises the possibility of an inherited urea cycle defect. The commonest cause is an X-linked disorder due to a deficiency in the enzyme ornithine transcarbamylase (OTC). Initial diagnosis requires assessment of the amino acid profile on plasma; this showed high levels of glutamine, alanine and orotic acid. Deficiency of OTC leads to an accumulation of carbamyl phosphate within the mitochondria in the liver prior to the block. This leaks into the cytoplasm where it can be used to synthesise carbamyl aspartate, the first intermediate on the pathway of pyrimidine biosynthesis. The excess orotic acid arises as this is a precursor in the formation of the pyrimidine, uracil. Confirmatory diagnosis requires mutation studies or demonstration of low levels of OTC on a liver biopsy. The prognosis is poor in severely affected males, although recognition allows for the possibility of ante-natal diagnosis in subsequent pregnancies.

period (in association with the extensive protein breakdown associated with the post-partum period).

Tyrosinaemia type 1

This is due to a deficiency of fumarylacetoacetate hydrolase. In severe cases it presents with acute liver failure, hepatomegaly and renal Fanconi syndrome; those with a more chronic form often demonstrate failure to thrive, irritability, jaundice and progressive neuropathy with neurological sequelae. Radiologically, there are signs of vitamin D-resistant rickets and renal stones. As liver disease from any cause gives rise to increased plasma tyrosine, the diagnosis of tyrosinaemia type 1 is signalled by the presence of succinylacetone, succinylacetoacetate and hydroxy-oxo-heptanoate in urinary organic acid analysis; biochemical confirmation requires the measurement of fumarylacetoacetate hydrolase activity in cultured skin fibroblasts or leucocytes. Tyrosinaemia type 1 is treated by the drug NTBC, which inhibits an earlier step in the affected pathway and reduces the accumulation of toxic metabolites. This disorder can also be detected as a result of screening for PKU; the severe liver damage usually results in elevated bloodspot phenylalanine and tyrosine, and screening protocols are often adapted to identify these patients.

Miscellaneous childhood disorders

Congenital hypothyroidism

The incidence of congenital primary hypothyroidism is about 1 in 4000. Bloodspot TSH is used as the new-born screening test. This condition is due to a defect in the development of the thyroid gland. It is amenable to treatment with thyroxine, particularly if started early, but it can be difficult to diagnose clinically.

Congenital adrenal hyperplasia (CAH)

Striking anatomical changes take place in the adrenal cortex immediately after birth; these are associated with marked alterations in the pattern of steroid output. There is a period of transition during the first 6 months of an infant's life in which the pattern of foetal steroid metabolism changes to the normal childhood pattern, which closely resembles the adult pattern. A number of enzyme deficiencies have been identified that are associated with abnormal steroid secretion or action. Figure 22.5 shows a simplified steroid biosynthetic pathway and some of the known sites of enzyme defect.

21-Hydroxylase deficiency (Figure 22.5)

This is an autosomal recessive condition (about 1 in 10000 live births in Caucasians) that may impair synthesis of cortisol and aldosterone. It accounts for approximately 95% of all cases of CAH. The low cortisol promotes ACTH secretion, so that the adrenal gland becomes hyperplastic. Severe cases show evidence of mineralocorticoid deficiency, with salt and water loss and neonatal adrenal crisis. Steroids accumulate before the enzyme block, and are diverted to moderately strong androgens (e.g. androstenedione, which is metabolised to testosterone in peripheral tissues). This causes virilisation of the female foetus and precocious sexual development in boys if the latter are not diagnosed in the neonatal period. Late presentation (in adult life) is also possible in less severe cases.

The diagnosis can be established by finding a raised concentration of 17-hydroxyprogesterone in a plasma sample taken at least 2 days after birth. Earlier samples may contain maternally derived 17-hydroxyprogesterone, which complicates the interpretation of the results. Measurement of other steroids that accumulate before the block and gene probing for 21-hydroxylase can also be helpful. Treatment with glucocorticoids (e.g. hydrocortisone) suppresses the excessive output of ACTH and limits the excessive androgen production. It may also be necessary to administer a mineralocorticoid. Monitoring of treatment requires measurement of serum 17-hydroxyprogesterone.

11β-Hydroxylase deficiency (Figure 22.5)

Inherited deficiencies in this enzyme affect the production of cortisol, corticosterone and aldosterone. Increased androgen production also gives

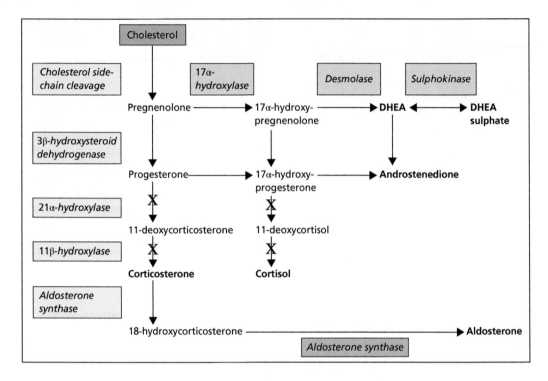

Figure 22.5 Defects in the steroid biosynthetic pathways leading to CAH. 21α-Hydroxylase deficiency leads to overproduction of androstenedione and 17α-hydroxyprogesterone. In 11β-hydroxylase deficiency, high concentrations of 11-deoxycortisol are found. The conversion of corticosterone to aldosterone is restricted to the zona glomerulosa. X indicates sites of enzyme defect.

rise to virilisation in the female. High concentrations of 11-deoxycorticosterone are produced; this steroid has mineralocorticoid activity. Diagnosis requires demonstration of a high serum concentration of 11-deoxycortisol or its urinary metabolites. Treatment involves giving cortisol alone, because the excess 11-deoxycorticosterone provides adequate mineralocorticoid action even if aldosterone synthesis is impaired.

17-Hydroxylase, 18-hydroxylase and 3β-hydroxysteroid dehydrogenase deficiency are extremely rare causes of CAH.

Failure to thrive in childhood

Poor nutrition is by far the most common cause of failure to thrive; however, it is important to exclude chronic disease, including renal disease, coeliac disease and cystic fibrosis.

Malnutrition in children

PEM, in its severest forms, includes kwashiorkor and marasmus; there is a range of less severe clinical pres-

entations. There may be other important factors, for example deficiency of essential fatty acids, or the consequences of immune defence mechanisms being impaired by malnutrition.

Plasma albumin is a widely used, though insensitive, test for malnutrition. A concentration below 30 g/L should be regarded as abnormally low; values below 25 g/L are associated with increasing degrees of oedema. Parallel changes in plasma pre-albumin and transferrin also occur.

Malnutrition severe enough to cause hypoglycaemia is encountered in children with kwashiorkor and in starvation (e.g. due to gross parental neglect). If malnutrition is severe enough to cause liver failure to develop, many other biochemical tests become abnormal.

Vitamin deficiency diseases make up a potentially important group of nutritional causes of failure to thrive, bcause the growing child has relatively greater requirements for vitamins than the mature adult. Rickets (Chapter 5: Rickets and osteomalacia) due to inadequate nutrition or lack of sunlight continues to occur, even in developed countries.

Cystic fibrosis

This autosomal recessive disorder is the most common inherited metabolic disease in Caucasians, occurring in about 1 in 2000 live births. Abnormalities of the cystic fibrosis transmembrane conductance protein, expressed in all epithelial cells, result in failure of cyclic adenosine monophosphate (cAMP)-regulated chloride transport across the cell membranes. The most common disease-causing mutation, DF_{508}, is found in about 70% of cystic fibrosis chromosomes in Northern Europe. Alterations in the ion concentrations in the secreted fluid lead to abnormally thick mucus in the lung, which predisposes to chronic infection and the development of obstructive airway disease. It also produces exocrine pancreatic insufficiency and high concentrations of chloride and sodium in secreted sweat. Biochemical investigations used as part of the diagnostic process include sweat testing and measurement of stool elastase.

Newborn screening for cystic fibrosis uses measurement of immunoreactive trypsin, which is greatly increased in blood specimens collected from infants with cystic fibrosis only in the first month of life. If this is elevated, cascade testing is by a panel of DNA mutations targeted to the population. Further tests, including a sweat test, are often required to help establish the presence of atypical forms of cystic fibrosis or act as a prognostic indicator.

Sweat test

This is used to confirm the diagnosis following newborn screening, and to investigate older children presenting with suggestive symptoms. Chloride or conductivity is measured in sweat obtained by iontophoresis from a small area of skin using standardised conditions; sweating is induced by applying pilocarpine to the skin under a low electric current. The test demands close attention to detail if reliable results are to be obtained, and should only be carried out by staff that are experienced in performing it.

In healthy children and adults, the pilocarpine-stimulated sweat chloride is normally below 40 mmol/L (or 30 mmol/L in neonates). In patients with classical cystic fibrosis, the concentration is nearly always above 60 mmol/L. Variant forms may give intermediate results between 40 and 60 mmol/L.

Short stature

Table 22.8 lists the principal categories of disordered growth, with examples. In this section, we shall only consider in detail the investigation of children for possible GH deficiency and for coeliac disease.

Table 22.8 **Disorders of growth.**

Growth abnormality and category	Examples
Short stature	
• Genetic	Familial short stature, delayed development
• Intrauterine	Small for gestational age infants
• Nutritional	Inadequate food supply, malabsorption, coeliac disease, infections
• Systemic disease	Chronic renal disease, congenital heart disease
• Endocrine disease	GHD, hypothyroidism, corticosteroid excess
Tall stature	
• Genetic	Familial tall stature, advanced development
• Endocrine disease	Growth hormone excess, hyperthyroidism, precocious puberty
• Miscellaneous	Klinefelter (XXY) syndrome, XYY anomaly

Growth hormone deficiency (GHD)

This may be an isolated defect, partial or complete, or it may be a component of panhypopituitarism. GH is released into the circulation in pulses, mainly at night. Random plasma GH in daytime specimens from normal children is often therefore undetectable. The investigation of suspected GHD requires provocation tests to test the function of the hypothalamic–pituitary–GH release axis. Hypothyroidism, chronic disease, Turner's syndrome and poor nutrition should be excluded before these tests are performed.

GH provocation tests

In suspected isolated GHD, two GH provocation tests (sequential or on separate days) are recommended. However, in those with defined CNS pathology, history of irradiation, multiple pituitary hormone deficiency or a genetic defect, one GH test may suffice. The second test is only required if there is an inadequate response in the first test. Other tests of pituitary function may also be required if indicated clinically, for example a GnRH test. Provocative agents used include clonidine, arginine and insulin. The insulin hypoglycaemia test is only safe in children if it is performed under close supervision by experienced staff who regularly perform this test. It has the advantage of superior sensitivity and specificity. If a second test is required it should employ a provocative agent other than that used in the first test.

In the *clonidine test*, clonidine is given orally to stimulate GH release; blood specimens are collected before giving clonidine ($0.15\,mg/m^2$ body surface area) and at 30-min intervals for 2.5 h afterwards.

Arginine ($0.5\,g/kg$ body weight, maximum 30 g) can be infused IV (10% arginine in 0.9% saline) at a constant rate over 30 min and samples taken before the infusion and at 30-min intervals for 2.5 h. Arginine provocation should not be used in patients with electrolyte disturbances, uraemia, diabetes or liver disease, and anti-histamine and adrenaline should be available for treatment of anaphylaxis.

The *insulin hypoglycaemia test* uses a procedure modified slightly from the test as used in adults (Chapter 7: Dynamic function tests – insulin hypoglycaemia test) and the local laboratory should be consulted before performing the test. Specimens are taken before an IV injection of soluble insulin (0.075–0.10 U/kg) and at 20, 30, 45, 60 and 90 min after the injection. Plasma GH and glucose are measured in all specimens, alongside cortisol to help establish if panhypopituitarism is present. The test may also be combined with a GnRH test if a combined pituitary function test is to be performed. For each of the above stimulation tests a post-stimulated GH below $5\,\mu g/L$ supports the diagnosis.

Coeliac disease

This is a common cause of growth restriction. The first-line investigation is measurement of serum anti-tTG IgA antibodies, which are elevated in untreated coeliac disease. The definitive method of diagnosis is made by demonstrating abnormal villi in a duodenal biopsy collected by endoscopy. Other diagnostic features include the improvement that is brought about by a gluten-free diet, both physically and in the severity of diarrhoea and the relapse that follows dietary relaxation. Compliance with treatment with a gluten-free diet is monitored by measurement of anti-tTG IgA antibodies.

Childhood malignancy: neuroblastoma and ganglioneuroma

Neuroblastoma and related tumours, although rare, account for approximately one-third of childhood deaths from malignant disease. Most produce catecholamines. Marked pharmacological effects are uncommon, because the catecholamines are largely metabolised by the tumour tissue to form inactive metabolites. Only occasionally is there hypertension. Measurements of catecholamine metabolites are made in urine (4-hydroxy-3-methoxymandelic acid, homovanillic acid or 4-hydroxy-3-methoxyphenylacetic acid and dopamine) and are related to urinary creatinine because it is difficult to obtain complete 24-h urine collections in children. Age-related reference ranges are used. Elevated results may also occur in phaeochromocytoma, although this is uncommon in children.

The elderly

The additional diagnostic biochemical problems in the elderly arise mainly from the increased frequency of multi-organ disease, polypharmacy and the tendency for symptoms to be absent or atypical. There are a few aspects that merit emphasis.

Reference ranges in the elderly

The concentrations of certain analytes show clear changes in the elderly, even when monitored in apparently healthy individuals. For the most part these changes merely represent the extension of changes that have been gradually occurring throughout adult life, and include a gradual increase in cholesterol, glucose, ALP, PSA and urate, with decreases in total protein and albumin. Ideally laboratories should provide age-related reference ranges for the elderly, but in practice few do.

Screening for disease in elderly patients

Because of the masking of clinical symptoms and signs, it is common practice to perform an admission biochemical screen on patients admitted to assessment units for the elderly. Table 22.9 lists some of the tests that are commonly used.

Renal function, fluid and electrolyte balance

The GFR falls with age, as does the ability of the renal tubules to reabsorb and secrete various substances. There is also a progressive loss of nephrons that starts in middle age. The consequence of these changes is that creatinine clearance tends to fall and the concentration of creatinine and urea rises slightly. The reduction in muscle mass and the smaller dietary intake of protein that tend to occur in older people may offset these effects to some extent in some

Table 22.9 Admission screening of elderly patients with biochemical tests.

Examination	Abnormalities commonly detected
Measurements on blood specimens	
• Albumin, total protein	Evidence of poor nutrition
• Creatinine, urea	Renal disease, post-renal uraemia
• Glucose	Diabetes mellitus
• Calcium	Hypocalcaemia (osteomalacia)
	Hypercalcaemia (hyperparathyroidism or malignancy)
• ALP	Increased in Paget's disease, malignancy and osteomalacia
• Potassium	Hypokalaemia (often due to diuretic therapy)
	Hyperkalaemia (poor renal function and K^+-sparing diuretics)
• Thyroid function tests	Hypothyroidism or hyperthyroidism
• C-reactive protein (or ESR)	Nonspecific indicator of the presence of organic disease
Point of care tests	
• Urine	Glucosuria, proteinuria

patients. The use of formulae to estimate GFR (which take into account age) can negate some of the interpretative problems in this age group.

The regulatory mechanisms that control water and electrolyte balance become less efficient in the elderly. The renal response to vasopressin is reduced and, in addition, the sensation of thirst is impaired which makes water conservation less efficient. Renin and aldosterone levels decrease with age, leading to problems with sodium conservation. The elderly also have an impaired ability to adapt to volume expansion because the secretion of ANP in response to hypervolaemia and the renal response to this hormone may both be diminished. In addition many elderly patients are on long-term diuretic treatment that, in turn, can produce hypovolaemia, postural hypotension, hyponatraemia, hypokalaemia and hyperuricaemia. Some patients taking diuretics may increase their water intake to an extent that it induces hyponatraemia. The maximum rate of secretion of hydrogen ions in response to an acid load is also impaired in the elderly.

These changes make the elderly patient particularly susceptible to disorders of fluid and electrolyte balance, and a full assessment of fluid and electrolyte balance is an essential component of the evaluation of an elderly patient who is ill.

 CASE 22.5

A 73-year-old retired schoolteacher had been admitted to a hospital with exacerbation of her chronic asthma. She gave a history of having moderately severe hypertension, which her GP had been treating with a combined preparation of atenolol and chlorthalidone for the previous 2 years. She was treated with an increase in the dose of oral glucocorticoid that she was already taking and discharged home. Two weeks later, she was seen by her GP because her ankles had begun to swell, and he prescribed furosemide. However, her ankle swelling persisted, and she began to complain of feeling very weak. She was readmitted to the hospital, where examination of a blood specimen gave the following results:

Serum	Result	Reference range
Urea	5.0	2.5–6.6 mmol/L
Na^+	148	135–145 mmol/L
K^+	2.7	3.6–5.0 mmol/L
Total CO_2	30	22–30 mmol/L

Comment on the likely causes of this patient's hypokalaemia.

Comments: There are several drug-related reasons as to why this patient had developed marked hypokalaemia:

1 Chlorthalidone is a thiazide diuretic. It can cause modest K^+ depletion, although this is not usually sufficient by itself to require potassium supplements.
2 High doses of glucocorticoid cause potassium loss.
3 Furosemide causes K^+ loss. When using it for the treatment of oedema, it would be normal practice to use it in combination with a K^+-sparing diuretic.

The drug treatment of this patient was changed in the light of these analytical results.

Bone disease

The incidence of bone disease rises markedly in old age.

• *Osteoporosis* is the most common cause, particularly in women.
• *Paget's disease* is very common. It is one of the first diagnoses to be considered when increased serum

ALP activity is found as an isolated abnormality in an elderly patient. It is occasionally necessary to determine whether the increased total enzymatic activity is due to the bone isoenzyme, as would be the case in Paget's disease, or to the liver isoenzyme (e.g. due to secondary deposits of carcinoma in the liver).

- *Osteomalacia* may contribute to fractures and falls in the elderly, and should be considered in a patient who has been housebound or who has a low dietary vitamin D intake. Often in such patients a lack of exposure to sunlight, combined with nutritional deficiency, is the cause. Serum calcium and phosphate may both be reduced and ALP activity increased in many cases. Serum 25-hydroxycholecalciferol is often borderline low, owing to inadequate intake of vitamin D or lack of endogenous synthesis (Chapter 5: Vitamin D deficiency). It has been suggested that even minor vitamin D deficiency during the winter at higher latitudes can give rise to a PTH-driven negative bone balance and there are those who advocate the use of vitamin D supplements of 400–600 U/day during such periods.

The endocrine system

Although there is a small decline in the efficiency of a wide range of endocrine systems with ageing, there is no convincing evidence as yet to support the use of hormone supplements in the elderly. Despite this lack of evidence, there are still those who advocate that testosterone (in men), GH and DHEA replacement therapy may be of benefit to the elderly.

Some endocrine disorders are more common in the elderly than in other age groups.

Thyroid disease

Many assessment units for the elderly have reported that screening for thyroid dysfunction is worthwhile, and hitherto unsuspected thyroid disorders are said to have been detected in 2–6% of patients. Classical features of hypothyroidism and hyperthyroidism are less common in the elderly. The elderly patient with hypothyroidism is more likely to present with a general decline in health, with depression being a common feature. The hyperthyroid patient may present with weight loss, GI or cardiovascular problems; in a small group of patients apathy and inactivity may dominate the clinical picture (apathetic hyperthyroidism).

Screening in the elderly frequently produces abnormal thyroid function test results in patients who subsequently are found not to have a thyroid disorder.

For example, up to 3% of patients admitted to units for the elderly may have an undetectable serum TSH without there necessarily being clinical or other biochemical evidence of thyroid disease. These abnormalities in thyroid function tests are often due to the effects of NTIs and drugs (see Chapter 8: Situations in which thyroid function test results may be misleading).

Thyroid function tests must be interpreted with caution in the elderly.

Measurement of serum TSH provides the best screening test. The following conclusions can be drawn from its results:

1 A normal result excludes primary thyroid disease.
2 If, at the time the test is performed, the patient is not recovering from a recent NTI, a serum TSH above 10 mU/L indicates that the patient has hypothyroidism and may require treatment with thyroxine.
3 If the serum TSH is undetectable, serum FT4 and FT3 should be measured. If the results for either the T4 or T3 measurements are raised, the patient should be referred for specialist advice, as treatment for hyperthyroidism may be required. If, however, the results for the T4 and T3 measurements are normal or low, this suggests that the cause of the low serum TSH is NTI, subclinical hyperthyroidism or, rarely, secondary hypothyroidism.

 CASE 22.6

A 78-year-old retired civil servant was admitted to an assessment unit for the elderly with a recent history of rapidly progressing dementia. Point of care tests and the results of admission screening investigations were all normal, apart from the results of thyroid function tests, which were as follows:

Serum	Result	Reference range
TSH	<0.1	0.2–4.5 mU/L
FT4	19	9–21 pmol/L
FT3	3.0	2.6–6.2 pmol/L

How would you interpret these results?

Comments: Undetectable serum TSH is reported in 1–3% of patients admitted to assessment units for the elderly if thyroid function tests are performed as part of a routine admission screening of all patients. Although undetectable serum TSH is found in hyperthyroidism and in secondary hypothyroidism, in these elderly patients NTI and the effects of drug therapy are much more frequent reasons for this finding.

In this patient, the normal serum FT4 and the low-normal serum FT3 excluded overt hyperthyroidism and secondary hypothyroidism and suggest that the suppressed TSH was due to NTI. The final diagnosis was multiple cerebral infarctions caused by extensive atheromatous disease of the cerebral vessels, detected by CT scanning.

Diabetes mellitus

The diagnosis of diabetes in the elderly is often made as the result of routine testing during a concurrent illness or because of the development of peripheral vascular disease or cataracts. Few patients present with classical symptoms such as weight loss and polyuria. The presence of diabetes mellitus may not be detected by point of care testing of urine for glucose, as the renal threshold for glucose tends to rise with age; thus plasma glucose measurements may be needed (Chapter 6: Diabetes mellitus). Management of elderly diabetic patients may need to depend on the help of relatives.

Inadequate nutrition

Old people living alone are particularly at risk of having an inadequate diet, particularly if they are poor or unable to feed themselves properly. Although serum albumin may be low, its diagnostic value is limited.

Index

Page numbers in *italic* refer to figures or cases.
Page numbers in **bold** refer to tables.

abetalipoproteinaemia, 181
accuracy of tests, 4, *5*
acetaminophen, 270–272
acetoacetate, 85
acetylcholinesterase, 268
acid–base balance, 30–41, *see also specific disorders*
  chronic renal disease, 55
  diabetic ketoacidosis, 86
  indications for full assessment, 42
acidification tests, urine, 50–51
acidosis, *see also* metabolic acidosis; respiratory acidosis
  on calcium levels, 64
  potassium and, 26, 27
acrodermatitis enteropathica, **211**, *212*
acromegaly, 95–96
ACTH *see* adrenocorticotrophic hormone
activin, 140–141, 147
acute intermittent porphyria (AIP), 246, 249
acute kidney injury, 52–54
acute liver failure, 192, *195*
acute-phase response, 225–227
Addison's disease, 27, 132–134
adenylic acid, *254*
ADH (vasopressin), 14, 19, 44, 104
adipose tissue, effects of insulin, **78**
adrenal cortex, 121–134, *see also* congenital adrenal hyperplasia
adrenaline
  on glucose metabolism, **78**
  hypokalaemia, 25
adrenal medulla, 121
adrenocorticotrophic hormone (ACTH), 93, 122
  Addison's disease, 132, 133
  Cushing's syndrome, 124–126
  ectopic production, 93, 129, 130, *131*
  hypopituitarism, *102*
  placental secretion mimicking, 159
  plasma levels, **101**, 128–129
agammaglobulinaemia, 229
age, effect on test results, 6

ageing, *see also* elderly patients
  plasma cholesterol, 176
  testosterone deficiency, 144
alanine aminotransferase (ALT), 186, *187*, **193**
  acute hepatitis, 191
  cholestasis, 192
  coefficient of variation, **6**
  liver fibrosis, 194
albumin, 225, 226
  ascites, 197
  on calcium levels, 64
  elderly patients, 293
  fluid balance disorders, 23
  glycated, 84
  kwashiorkor, 222
  liver disease, 186–187, **193**
  nutrition assessment, 216, 288
  pregnancy, 160
  urine, 56
  variants, on thyroid function tests, 119
albumin-bound testosterone, 141
alcohol
  γ-glutamyltransferase, 194
  on HDL cholesterol, 176
  on lipids, 180
  liver disease, 195–196, *201*
  magnesium deficiency, 76
  on measured osmolality, 13–14
  paracetamol poisoning, 271
  poisoning with, 272
  pseudo-Cushing syndrome, 128
  thiamin deficiency, *215*
  urate levels, 255
aldosterone, 15, 21, 25–26, 123–124, 135, *see also* primary hyperaldosteronism
aldosterone:renin ratio, 136, *137*
aldosteronism, 52, 135–136
alkaline phosphatase, 64, **291**
  acute hepatitis, 191
  cholestasis, 186, 192
  metabolic bone disease, **71**

Clinical Biochemistry Lecture Notes, Tenth Edition. Peter Rae, Mike Crane and Rebecca Pattenden.
© 2018 John Wiley & Sons Ltd. Published 2018 by John Wiley & Sons Ltd.
Companion website: www.lecturenoteseries.com/clinicalbiochemistry

alkaline phosphatase (*cont'd*)
  Paget's disease, 292
  pregnancy, 160
  steatosis, 196
  vitamin D deficiency, 70
alkalosis, *see also* metabolic alkalosis; respiratory
      alkalosis
  potassium and, 25, 26
allopurinol, 257
α_1-antitrypsin, **225**, 227, *228*
α_1-globulins, 225
α_2-globulins, 225
α_2-macroglobulin, **225**
α-foetoprotein, 165, 193–194, **225**, 238
α-melanocyte stimulating hormone, 223
α-subunit, TSHoma, 118
α-tocopherol, 214
aluminium toxicity, 274
amenorrhoea, 148–149, *150*, 152
amikacin, monitoring, 266
amino acids
  absorption, 201
  essential, 210
  phenylketonuria, 284
  TPN, 219
aminoacidurias, 51–52
aminoglycosides, monitoring, 266
aminolaevulinic acid (ALA), 248, 250
aminotransferases *see* alanine aminotransferase;
      aspartate aminotransferase
amiodarone, on thyroid function, 117
ammonia
  inborn errors of metabolism, 282, 285–287
  liver disease, 188
  urinary buffer, 32
ammonium chloride, 51
amylase, 7, **57**, 200
amyloidosis, 230, 232
anaemia
  chronic renal disease, 55
  multiple myeloma, **232**
  pernicious, 215
analbuminaemia, 226
analytical errors, 2
androgen-binding protein, 140
androgen insensitivity syndrome, 144
androgens, 124, 141, *see also* free androgen index;
      testosterone
  deficiency, 144
  21-hydroxylase deficiency, 287
  polycystic ovarian syndrome, 153–154
andropause, 144
angioplasty, on biomarkers, 168

angiotensinogen, 123
angiotensins, 15, 123–124, 135
anion gap, 40, 273, *274*
anorexia nervosa, 99–100
anterior pituitary disease, 100–103
anterior pituitary hormones, 92–99
antibiotics, monitoring, 266
antibodies, *see also* thyrotrophin receptor antibodies
  Helicobacter pylori, 198–199
  heterophilic, 118
  islet cells, 79
  liver disease, 187
  thyroglobulin, 239
  thyroid peroxidase, 113, *114*, 119
  tissue transglutaminase (tTG), 203, 204, 290
anticonvulsants, monitoring, 266
antidiuretic hormone (vasopressin), 14, 19, 44, 104
antidotes, 270
antigen-binding fragments, immunoglobulins, *228*
anti-mitochondrial antibodies, 187
anti-Mullerian hormone (AMH), 141, 150
antipsychotic drugs, hyperprolactinaemia, 97, 98, **99**
anti-thyroid peroxidase antibodies, 113, *114*, 119
anti-TNF drugs, monitoring, 267–268
apathetic hyperthyroidism, 292
apolipoproteins, 174–175, 178, 179, 181
appetite control, 223
arachidonic acid, 209
arginine, GH provocation test, 290
aromatase, 141, 153
artefacts, haemoglobin A_{1c}, 83
artefactual anion gap, 40
artefactual hyperkalaemia, 27
artefactual hyponatraemia, 21
arterial blood, 33, 41–42, 86
ascites, 187, 196–197
  CA-125, 236
ascorbic acid *see* vitamin C
asialotransferrin, 260, 262
aspartate aminotransferase (AST), 186, **193**
  acute hepatitis, 191
  cholestasis, 192
  coefficient of variation, **6**
  liver fibrosis, 194
aspirin, poisoning, 272
asthma, carbon dioxide, *41*
atherogenic lipid profiles, 177
ATP7B (copper transporter), gene, 194, 195
ATP-dependent potassium channel gene, 277
atrial natriuretic peptide (ANP), 16, 291
atrophic thyroiditis, 113
audit, clinical, 10–11
autoimmune Addison's disease, 134

autoimmune disorders, *see also* coeliac disease
  chronic hepatitis, 192
  premature ovarian failure, 155
autoimmunity, diabetes mellitus, 79
automation, 1
avidin, 216
azathioprine, 192, 268, *269*
azoospermia, 141, *143*

bacterial colonisation, small intestine, 202–203, 205
Bartter's syndrome, 26
basal hormone measurements, pituitary, **101**
BChE (choline esterase), 268, 275
Bence Jones protein, **57**, 230–231
benign proteinuria, 56
β_2-microglobulin, 58, **225**, **231**, 232
β_2-transferrin, 260, 262
β-globulins, 225
β-hydroxybutyrate, 85
β-lipotrophin, 93
bicarbonate, 30, 34, 35–36, *see also* sodium
      bicarbonate
  reabsorption, 31–32, 36, 50–51
  reference ranges, 37
  renal tubular acidosis, 51
  in total CO_2, 39
big ACTH, 93
bile acids, 164, 188, 202
biliary atresia, 280
biliary obstruction, 192–194, *see also* cholestasis
  bilirubin and urobilinogen, **189**
  vitamin D deficiency, 70
bilirubin, 184–185, **189**, **193**, *242*
  cerebrospinal fluid, 260, *261*
bilirubin UDP-glucuronyltransferase, 186, 190
binding proteins, *see also* sex hormone-binding
      globulin; transferrin
  androgen-binding protein, 140
  cortisol-binding globulin, *122*
  growth hormone, 94
  IGF-1, 94
  thyroid hormones, 107
  vitamin A, 213
bioavailable testosterone, 141
bioelectrical impedance, 216
bio-identical hormones, 157
biomarkers *see* markers; tumour markers
biopterin co-factor, 284
biotin, **212**, 216
bisalbuminaemia, 226
blindness, methanol poisoning, 273
blood glucose, 82, **83**
blood pressure, metabolic syndrome, 222

bloodspot screening, 281
blunders, 5
body mass index, **217**, 221
bone, 61
  alkaline phosphatase, 64
  chronic renal disease, 55
  elderly patients, 291–292
  metabolic disease, 71–73
  parathyroid hormone on, 63
  turnover markers, 71, **72**
breast cancer, tumour markers, 239
breast milk jaundice, 280
breath tests
  glucose–hydrogen, 203
  triglycerides, 202
  urea, 198
B-type natriuretic peptide, 16, 171–172
buffers, 30, 31–33

CA 15-3, 239
CA 19-9, 239
CA-125, 235–236, 237
caeruloplasmin, 194–195, **225**
calcitonin, 64, 239–240
calcitriol *see* 1,25-dihydroxycholecalciferol
calcium, 60–73
  balance, 60–61, *62*
  cerebrospinal fluid, 259
  chronic renal disease, 55
  functions, 61
  hypercalcaemia, 65–69
  malabsorption, 205
  metabolic bone disease, **71**
  metabolism, 62–64
  multiple myeloma, **231**, *231*, **232**
  paediatrics, 278
  pancreatitis, 200
  plasma, 62–63
  serum levels, 64
  TPN, **218**, 219, 220
  urine, 58–59
  vitamin D deficiency, 70
calculated osmolality, 13–14, 23
calculi *see* stones
calprotectin, 204
cancer *see* malignant disease
capillary blood
  arterialised, 33
  plasma glucose, 82, **83**
carbamazepine, monitoring, 266
carbamyl phosphate, *287*
carbimazole, *112*
carbohydrate-deficient transferrin, 196

carbohydrates, 209
^{14}C-triolein breath test, 202
carbonate dehydratase, 30
carbon dioxide, *see also* total CO_2
    alkalosis, 38
    asthma, *41*
    cerebrospinal fluid, 259
    diabetic ketoacidosis, 86
    excess with hypoxia, 42
    excretion, 30–31
    metabolic acidosis, 37
    normal H^+, 38
    reference ranges, 37
    respiratory acidosis, 34
    respiratory alkalosis, 35
carbonic acid, 30, 32–33
carbonic anhydrase, 30
carbon monoxide, 251
carboxyhaemoglobin, 251
carcinoembryonic antigen, 234–235, *236*
carcinoid tumours and syndrome, 206–207, 215
cardiac failure *see* congestive cardiac failure; heart
        failure
cardiovascular disorders, 167–182
    risk factors, 172–182
carriers
    acute intermittent porphyria, 249
    X-linked ornithine carbamoyltransferase
        deficiency, 286–287
case-finding programmes, 3
catecholamines, 137–138, 290
cell damage
    potassium balance, 27
    pseudohyperkalaemia, 27
central adiposity, 222
central hypothyroidism, 113, 115
central nervous system, 259–262
    hyponatraemia, **18**
central veins, liver, 183
cerebrospinal fluid, 259–262
chelators, for lead poisoning, *275*
children, 276–290
    poisoning, 274
    undernutrition, 221, 288
chloride, 40
    kidney, 43
    measurement, 23
    sweat test, 289
chlorpropamide, *89*
chlorthalidone, *291*
cholangiocarcinoma, CA 19-9, 239
cholecalciferol, 63, *see also* vitamin D
cholecalciferol 1α-hydroxylase, 55
cholecystokinin (CCK), **207**

cholestasis, 186, *187*, 190, 192–193, *see also* biliary
        obstruction
    lipoprotein X, 180
    obstetric, 163–164
    TPN, 220
cholesterol, 172, 176, 178, *179, see also*
        hypercholesterolaemia
    in lipoproteins, 173–174, 177
    metabolic syndrome, 222
    non-HDL, 177
    ratio to α-tocopherol, 214
    reduction, 182
    total, 176–177
choline esterases, 268, 275
choriocarcinoma, 158, 238
chorionic villus biopsy, 282
chromium, 210, 211
chronic obstructive airways disease, 42
chronic renal disease, 54–55, *56, see also* renal
        osteodystrophy
    hyperparathyroidism, 55, 75
    hypocalcaemia, *75*
    hyponatraemia, 21
    vitamin D deficiency, 70
chylomicrons, 173, 174–175
ciclosporin, monitoring, 266
cirrhosis, **193**, 194
    α$_1$-antitrypsin deficiency, 227
    primary biliary, *187*
11-*cis*-retinal, 213
clearance, 45, *see also* creatinine clearance
clinical audit, 10–11
clonidine
    GH provocation test, 290
    suppression testing, 138
clotting factors, liver disease, 187
clozapine, hyperprolactinaemia, 98
coagulation factors, liver disease, 187
cobalt, 210
Cockcroft–Gault equation, 45
coefficients of variation, **6**
coeliac disease, 203–204, 290
    iron status, 245
colchicine, 257
collecting ducts (renal), 44
colloid osmotic pressure, 13, 14
colorectal cancer
    carcinoembryonic antigen, 234–235, *236*
    faecal occult blood, 204
combined hyperlipoproteinaemia, familial, **178**, 179
combined oral contraceptives, 157
Combined Test, first trimester screening, 164
congenital adrenal hyperplasia (CAH), 134, 151,
        287–288

congenital hypothyroidism, 116, 287
congenital (inherited) metabolic disorders, 280–290
congestive cardiac failure, hyponatraemia, 21
conjugated hyperbilirubinaemia, neonate, 280
Conn's syndrome, 135, 136, *137*
contraceptives, 157
  menopause, 155, **156**
  for polycystic ovarian syndrome, 151
  T3 hyperthyroidism, *110*
copper
  liver disease, 194–195
  as trace element, 210, 211
coproporphyrinogen III, *247*
coproporphyrins
  congenital hyperbilirubinaemias, 191
  lead poisoning, 250
coronary syndromes
  acute, 167–182
  gout and, 256–257
corticotrophin-releasing hormone, 93
  stimulation test, 129
cortisol, 122
  Addison's disease, 132–133
  anorexia nervosa, 99–100
  diurnal variation, 122, *123*
  on glucose metabolism, **78**
  hypopituitarism, *102*
  insulin hypoglycaemia test, 103
  measurement, **101**, 126–128, 129
  pregnancy, 159
cortisol-binding globulin, *122*
cow's milk, acrodermatitis enteropathica, *212*
C peptide, 89
C-reactive protein, **225**, 226
  erythrocyte sedimentation rate *vs*, 227
  TPN monitoring, 219
  vascular disease risk, 181
  vitamin C measurement and, 214
creatine, 45
creatine kinase, *6*, 168, 170–171
creatinine
  acute kidney injury, 52
  chronic renal disease, 54
  multiple myeloma, **232**
  plasma concentrations, 46–47
  ratio to protein, 163
  undernutrition, 222
  water and sodium depletion, 23
creatinine clearance, 45, 46, 290
Crigler–Najjar syndrome, 190
Crohn's disease, *72*
crush injury, *see also* rhabdomyolysis
  acute kidney injury, *54*
  hyperkalaemia, *28*

cryofibrinogen, 233
cryoglobulins, 233
crystallisable fragment, immunoglobulins, *228*
Cushing's disease, 124, *125*, 128, *131*
Cushing's syndrome, 124–131
  carcinoid tumours, 206–207
  hypertension, **135**
  insulin hypoglycaemia test, 103
  potassium loss, 25
  pregnancy, 159
  treatment, 130–131
cutaneous porphyrias, 249
cut-off levels, 8, *10*
  faecal magnesium, *206*
  haemoglobin A_{1c}, 81
cyanocobalamin *see* vitamin B_{12}
cyclical Cushing's syndrome, 126
cyproterone acetate, 151
cystatin C, 48
cystic fibrosis, 289
cystinuria, 51, 201
cytosolic calcium, 61

daily oral intakes
  fats, 209
  sugar, 209
  trace elements, 210
  vitamins, **212**
dartboard analogy, *5*
DDAVP, test with, 49, 50
D-dimers, 172
1-deamino-8-D-arginine vasopressin, test with, 49, 50
deep vein thrombosis, 172
dehydration, 22–23, *76*, *88*
demyelinating disorders
  CSF protein, 261, 262
  osmotic demyelination syndrome, 18
11-deoxycorticosterone, 288
de Quervain thyroiditis, *111*
desferrioxamine, 246
desialylated transferrin, 260, 262
dexamethasone suppression tests, 126, 129
dextrose infusions, 16, **29**
  diabetic ketoacidosis, 86
  MCAD deficiency, 284
  TPN, **218**, 219
DF_{508} mutation, cystic fibrosis, 289
diabetes insipidus, 22, 50, 104
diabetes mellitus, 79–87
  acromegaly, *96*
  coeliac disease and, *204*
  diagnosis, 81–82, **83**
  elderly patients, 293

diabetes mellitus (*cont'd*)
   hyperglycaemia, *23*, 84, 86–87, *88*
   ketoacidosis (DKA), 74, 84–86, *87*
   on lipids, 180
   metabolic complications, 84–87
   monitoring treatment, 82–84
   nonalcoholic fatty liver disease and, 196
   potassium balance, 27
   pregnancy, 160–161
   secondary, 79
dialysis *see* haemodialysis
diarrhoea, factitious, 206
diet, *see also* nutrients
   effect on test results, 5
   gluten-free, 290
   plasma cholesterol, 176
   urate levels, 253, 255
digoxin
   monitoring, 266
   potassium balance, 27
   toxicity, *267*
5α-dihydrotestosterone, 141
1,25-dihydroxycholecalciferol, 63–64, 70
dilutional hyponatraemia *see* syndrome of
      inappropriate ADH secretion
dipeptidyl peptidase-4, 78
dipsticks *see* urine test sticks
disaccharidase deficiency, 201
discretionary testing, 2–3
distal convoluted tubules, 43
   parathyroid hormone on, 63
   potassium reabsorption, 24
   urate excretion, 255
distal renal tubular acidosis, 51
diuretic phase, acute kidney injury, 53
diuretics
   adverse effects, 291
   hyperaldosteronism, 135
   potassium loss, 26
   potassium-sparing, hyperkalaemia, 27
diurnal variation, 5
   cortisol, 122, *123*
   testosterone, 145
dopamine, on TSH release, 107
Down's syndrome, 164, *165*
drug abuse, 274
drug-induced liver injury, 192
drug-resistant hypertension, 134
drugs, *see also* poisoning; *specific drugs*
   monitoring, 263–269
Dubin–Johnson syndrome, 190–191
Duchenne muscular dystrophy, CK, 171
dysgerminomas, hCG, 238

ectopic ACTH production, 93, 129, 130, *131*
ectopic pregnancy, 160, *200*
EDTA, artefactual hyperkalaemia, 27
Edwards' syndrome, 164
eGFR *see* estimated GFR
egg white, 216
elastase, faecal, 200–201
elderly patients, 290–293, *see also* ageing
electrophoresis
   collection tubes for, **2**
   multiple myeloma, 230, *231*
   plasma proteins, 224, *225*
   urine, 55–56, 230–231
emphysema, pulmonary, 227, *228*
encephalopathy
   bilirubin, neonate, 279
   thiamin deficiency, 214
endocrinology, definition, 91
energy
   carbohydrates, 209
   fats, 209
   proteins, 210
   requirements, 217–218
   TPN, 219
enteral feeding, 217
enteroglucagon, **207**
enterohepatic circulation, 186, 202
enzymes, pharmacogenomics, 268
erectile dysfunction, 144
ergosterol, 63
errors, 2, 5
   artefactual hyponatraemia, 21
   urine collections, 46
erythrocytes
   lysis, neonate, 279
   mean cell volume, alcohol abuse, 195–196
   zinc protoporphyrin, 250, *275*
erythrocyte sedimentation rate, 227
erythropoietic protoporphyria, 249
erythropoietin
   chronic renal disease, 55
   therapy monitoring, 244
essential amino acids, 210, 219
essential free fatty acids, 209
essential trace elements, 210
estimated GFR
   chronic renal disease, 54
   MDRD equation, 48
ethanol *see* alcohol
ethinyloestradiol, 151, 157
ethnicity *see* race
ethylene glycol, poisoning, 273–274
European liver fibrosis panel, 194

exercise
  creatine kinase, *171*
  effect on test results, 5, *6*
  plasma cholesterol, 176
external balance, water and sodium, 12,
  14–16
extracellular fluid, 12, 13
  calcium, 61
  in hyponatraemia, 17, 19–21
  phosphate, 73–74
  potassium, 24
exudates, ascites, 197

Fab (antigen-binding fragments), *228*
factitious diarrhoea, 206
faecal calprotectin, 204
faecal elastase, 200–201
faecal fat test, 201
faecal occult blood, 204, 245
faecal osmotic gap, 206
failure to thrive, 288–290
familial benign hypocalciuric hypercalcaemia,
  67, 68–69
familial hypercholesterolaemia, 178, *179*
familial hypertriglyceridaemia, 178–179
Fanconi syndrome, 51–52, 71, 257
fasting
  lipids, 177
  MCAD deficiency, 284
  metabolism, 77
fasting hypoglycaemia, 87–90
fasting plasma glucose, 81, **83**
  metabolic syndrome, 222
fats, 209
  absorption, 202
  malabsorption, *201*, 202–203
  TPN, **218**, 219
fat-soluble vitamin K, 187
fat-soluble vitamins, 205, **212**, 213–214
fatty acids, 173, 209
  oxidation defects, 284, *286*
fatty liver *see* nonalcoholic fatty liver disease
febuxostat, 257
ferritin, 243–244, 245
  pregnancy, 160
fibrinogen, ESR, 227
fibrosis of liver, markers, 187, 194
first trimester screening, 164–165
flavin adenine dinucleotide, 214
fluid balance *see* water balance
fluid deprivation test, 49–50
fluid volume, TPN, 219
foetoplacental unit, 158–159

foetus
  chorionic villus biopsy, 282
  hypothyroidism, 161
  pre-natal diagnosis, 164–166
folic acid, 181, **212**, 215–216
follicle-stimulating hormone (FSH), 94
  anorexia nervosa, 99
  basal values, **101**
  fertility, 149
  menopause, 154, **155**, **156**
  menstrual cycle, *148*
  oral contraceptives and, 157
  polycystic ovarian syndrome, 152, 153
  premature ovarian failure, 155
  reference ranges, **148**
  on spermatogenesis, 140
48-hour dexamethasone suppression test, 126
Franklin disease, 230
free androgen index, 141, 143, 153
free β-hCG, *165*
free cortisol, urinary, 126
free drugs, 266
free fatty acids, 209
free protoporphyrin, 249
free PSA, 237
free T3, 107
  anorexia nervosa, 99
  elderly patients, 292
  hyperthyroidism, 110, 111, **113**
  hypothyroidism, 113
  measurement, 108
  pregnancy, 159–160, *163*
free T4, 107
  anorexia nervosa, 99
  basal values, **101**
  drugs affecting, 116–117
  elderly patients, 292
  hyperthyroidism, 109–110, 111, **113**
  hypothyroidism, 112–113
  measurement, 108, 109
  pregnancy, 159–160, 161, *163*
free testosterone, 143
Friedewald equation, 177
fructosamine, 84
fructose, on urate levels, 255
fructose intolerance, 201
fulminant hepatic failure, *195*
fumarylacetoacetate hydrolase deficiency, 287
functional proteinuria, 56
furosemide, *291*

Gal-1-PUT deficiency, 284, 285
galactorrhoea, *98*, *102*, 148–149

galactosaemia, 284–285
  screening test, 282
gallstones, *200*
γ-carboxyglutamate, 214
γ-globulins, 225, 229–230
γ-glutamyltransferase (GGT), 186, **193**
  alcohol abuse, 195–196
  cholestasis, 192
  cirrhosis, 194
  population distribution, *7*
  steatosis, 196
ganglioneuroma, 290
gastric outlet obstruction, *37, 40*
gastrin, 199, **207**
gastrinomas, 199
gastrointestinal hormones, 207
gastrointestinal tract, 198–207, *see also*
    malabsorption
  fluid balance, 12
  potassium balance, 26
Gaussian distribution, 4–5, *7*
G-cell hyperplasia, 199
gentamicin, monitoring, 266
germ cell tumours
  α-foetoprotein, 238
  human chorionic gonadotrophin, 238
gestational diabetes, 80, 160–161
gestational trophoblastic disease, hCG, 238
ghrelin, 94
gigantism, 95–96
Gilbert's syndrome, **189**, 190–191
glibenclamide, *89*
glomerular filtration rate (GFR), 43, 45, 48
  elderly patients, 291
  nephrotic syndrome, *57*
  pregnancy, 160
  sodium excretion, 15–16
  urate excretion, 255
glomerular proteinuria, 55, 56, **57**
glomeruli, 43
  function tests, 45–48
  potassium filtration, 24
  sodium filtration, 12
glomerulonephritis, 58
glucagon, on glucose metabolism, **78**
glucagon-like polypeptide-1, 78
glucocorticoids, 122
  deficiency, 21
  excess, 124–131
  therapy
    adrenocortical insufficiency after, 134
    Synacthen test and, 133
  on TSH release, 107
glucocorticoid-suppressible hyperaldosteronism, 135

glucokinase, mutation, 80
gluconeogenesis, 77
glucose, *see also* impaired glucose tolerance
  ascitic fluid, 197
  cerebrospinal fluid, 260
  homeostasis, 77–78
  metabolic syndrome, 222
  paediatrics, 277–278
  plasma, 81, 82, **83**
    hypoglycaemia, 87
    metabolic syndrome, 222
  TPN, **218**, 219, *221*
  undernutrition, 221
  urine, 81
glucose-dependent insulinotropic polypeptide,
    78, **207**
glucose hydrogen breath test, 203
glucose tolerance factor, 211
glucose tolerance test *see* oral glucose tolerance test
glucuronides, bilirubin, 186
glutamic acid decarboxylase, antibodies, 79
glutaminase, 32
glutathione peroxidase, **211**
gluten-free diet, 290
glycated haemoglobin, 81, 82–84
glycogen, 77, 209
glycogen synthase, 78
glycopeptides, monitoring, 266
glycosuria, 51
glyoxalate, urine, 59
gonadal function
  female, 147–157
  male, 140–147
gonadotrophin-releasing hormone (GnRH), 94, 140
  anorexia nervosa, 99
  deficiency, *144*
  on menstrual cycle, 147
gonadotrophins *see* follicle-stimulating hormone;
    human chorionic gonadotrophin; luteinising
    hormone
gout, 252, 255–257
Graafian follicles, 147
granulosa-cell tumours, 239
Graves' disease, 110
  pregnancy, 161, 162
  thyrotrophin receptor antibodies, 119
growth hormone, 94–96
  acromegaly, 95
  deficiency, 94–95, 289–290
  on glucose metabolism, **78**
  insulin hypoglycaemia test, 95, 103, 289, 290
  provocation tests, 289–290
  receptor, 94
  recombinant, NICE criteria, 95

regulation, *93*
  stimulation tests, 95
growth hormone-releasing hormone, 94–96
guaiac test, faecal occult blood, 204
guanylic acid, *254*
gynaecomastia, 146–147

haem, 241, *242*, 246, *248*
haematocrit, testosterone on, 146
haemochromatosis, 244, 245–246
haemodialysis
  on calcium metabolism, 73
  for methanol poisoning, 273
  toxicity, 274
haemoglobin, *see also* oxyhaemoglobin
  abnormal derivatives, 250–251
  as buffer, 30, 32
  oxygen saturation, 41, 42
  testosterone on, 146
  in urine, **57**
haemoglobin A$_{1c}$, 81, 82–84
haemolysis, *see also* HELLP syndrome
  bilirubin and urobilinogen, **189**
  Gilbert's syndrome *vs*, 190
  Wilson's disease, *195*
haemosiderin, 242
haptoglobin, **225**
Hartmann's solution, **29**
Hartnup disease, 201
Hashimoto's thyroiditis, 113, *114*, 119
Health and Safety Executive, on lead poisoning, *275*
heart failure, 171–172
  hyponatraemia, 21
heavy-chain disease, 230
heavy chains, immunoglobulins, 228
Helicobacter pylori, 198–199
HELLP syndrome, pre-eclampsia, 163
Henderson equation, 33
heparin, blood gases collection, 33
hepatic lipase, 174
hepatic nuclear factor 1 alpha, mutation, 80–81
hepatitis, **189**, 191–192
hepatitis B, hepatocellular carcinoma, *238*
hepatocellular carcinoma, 193–194
  α-foetoprotein, 238
hepatocellular hyperbilirubinaemia, 190
hepatocytes, 183–184
hepatolenticular degeneration, 194–195
HER2/neu, 239
hereditary coproporphyria (HC), 246, 247
hereditary haemochromatosis, 245–246
hereditary metabolic disorders, 280–290
heterophilic antibodies, 118
HFE gene, 245, *246*

high density lipoproteins (HDLs), **173**, 174, 176, 178, 222
high-dose dexamethasone suppression test, 129
hirsutism, 139, 150–154
home blood glucose monitoring, 82
homocysteine, 181, 215
homocystinuria, 181
hormone replacement therapy, 155–157
hsCRP assay, 181
human chorionic gonadotrophin (hCG), 158, *159*
  cross-reactivity with LH, 159
  ectopic pregnancy, 160
  free β-hCG, *165*
  on thyroid-stimulating hormone, 162, *163*
  as tumour marker, 238
hydatidiform mole, 158
hydrocortisone, after pituitary surgery, 103
hydrogen ions
  buffering, 32–33
  on calcium levels, 64
  cerebrospinal fluid, 259
  decreased, 38
  excretion, 31–32
  increased, 37
  metabolic acidosis, 35–36
  metabolic alkalosis, 36
  reference range, 37
  respiratory alkalosis, 35
  urine, 50–51
3-hydroxybutyrate, 85
25-hydroxycholecalciferol, 64, 70, 292
7α-hydroxy-cholestenone, 202
24-hydroxylase, 64
1α-hydroxylase deficiency, 70, *75*
11β-hydroxylase deficiency, 287–288
21-hydroxylase deficiency, 151, 287, *288*
1α-hydroxylation, 25-hydroxycholecalciferol, 64
4-hydroxy-3-methoxymandelic acid, 137
hydroxymethylbilane synthase, 247
17α-hydroxyprogesterone, 151
17-hydroxyprogesterone, 287
5-hydroxytryptamine, 206, 207
5-hydroxytryptophan, 206
hyperaldosteronism, 135–136
hyper-α-lipoproteinaemia, 179
hyperammonaemia, 282, 285–287
hyperbaric oxygen, CO poisoning, 251
hyperbilirubinaemia, 190–191, 279–280
hypercalcaemia, 65–69
  multiple myeloma, 68, *231*, **232**
  neonate, 278
hypercalciuria, 58–59
hypercholesterolaemia, 178, *179*, 180
hyperemesis gravidarum, 162

hypergammaglobulinaemia, 229–230
hyperglycaemia, 84, *88*
  hyperosmolar, *23*, 84, 86–87
  maternal, 277
hypergonadotrophic hypogonadism, 143
hyperinsulinemia, neonate, 277
hyperkalaemia, 26–28
  rhabdomyolysis, *28, 54*
hyperlipidaemia
  cholesterol reduction, 182
  gout and, 256–257
  secondary, 180
hyperlipoproteinaemias, 178–179
hypermagnesaemia, 76
hypernatraemia, 22–23, *88*
hyperosmolar hyperglycaemia, *23*, 84, 86–87
hyperosmolar hyponatraemia, 22
hyperoxaluria, primary, 59
hyperparathyroidism
  chronic renal disease, 55, *75*
  familial benign hypocalciuric hypercalcaemia
      vs, 69
  investigations, **71**
  maternal, 278
  primary, 65–68
  renal osteodystrophy, 73
  tertiary, 68
hyperphosphataemia, 74, *75*
hyperprolactinaemia, 97–99, *102*
  female, 149, *151*
  male, 143
  psychiatric patients, 98–100
hyperpyrexia (malignant), CK, 171
hypertension, 134–137
hyperthyroidism, 109–112, *see also* T3
      hyperthyroidism
  elderly patients, 292
  pregnancy, 161–162
  subclinical, 111
  thyroid function tests, **113**
  thyrotrophin receptor antibodies, 119–120
hypertonicity, potassium balance, 27
hypertriglyceridaemia, 178–179, 180
hyperuricaemia, 253–257
hyperventilation, 35, 36
hypoalbuminaemia, 226
hypobetalipoproteinaemia, 181
hypocalcaemia, 69–70, *76*
  chronic renal disease, *75*
  methanol poisoning, 273
  neonate, 278
  renal osteodystrophy, 73
  TPN, 220
hypogammaglobulinaemia, 229

hypoglycaemia, 87–90
  liver disease, 188
  malnutrition, 288
  MCAD deficiency, 284, *286*
  neonate, 277
  reactive, 89
hypogonadism, 141, 143–146
hypogonadotrophic hypogonadism, 143–144
hypokalaemia, 25–26
  diabetic ketoacidosis, 86
  digoxin and, 266, *267*
  elderly patients, *291*
  hyperaldosteronism, 135, *136–137*
  magnesium, 28
  renal tubular acidosis, 51
hypolipidaemia, secondary, 181
hypolipoproteinaemias, primary, 181
hypomagnesaemia, 75–76
  neonate, 278
  TPN, 220
hyponatraemia, 14, 17–22, *see also*
      pseudohyponatraemia
  acute kidney injury, 53
  acute porphyrias, *247*
  dilutional *see* syndrome of inappropriate ADH
      secretion
  elderly patients, 291
  post-operative patients, *20*
  TPN, *221*
  urine, 24
hypoparathyroidism, 70
  magnesium deficiency, *76*
hypophosphataemia, 74, *75*, 220
hypophosphataemic vitamin D-resistant rickets, 71
hypophosphatasia, 71–72
hypopituitarism, 100, 102–103, 134
hypoproteinaemia, 21, *57*
hypothalamic–anterior pituitary–adrenal axis,
      123, 159
hypothalamic–pituitary–gonadal axis, 139,
      143–144
hypothalamic–pituitary–ovarian axis, 147
hypothalamus, 91–93
hypothyroidism, 112–118, *180*, *see also* subclinical
      primary hypothyroidism
  congenital, 116, 287
  elderly patients, 292
  hypercholesterolaemia, 180
  neonate, 116
  pregnancy, 161
hypouricaemia, 257–258
hypovolaemia, effect on renal function, 44
hypoxia, 41, 42
hysterectomy, 155

IFCC assays, haemoglobin A$_{1c}$, 84
IgA deficiency, 204, 229
IgA immunoglobulins, 228, **229**
IgD immunoglobulins, 228–229
IgE immunoglobulins, 229
IgG immunoglobulins, 228, **229**
  cerebrospinal fluid, 262
IgM immunoglobulins, 228, **229**
  Waldenström macroglobulinaemia, 230
immune paresis, 230
immunoassay, plasma proteins, 224
immunochemical test, faecal occult blood, 204
immunoglobulins, 187, **225**, 228–233, *see also* IgA
    deficiency
  cerebrospinal fluid, 261–262
  deficiencies, 229
  liver disease, **193**
immunometric assays, parathyroid hormone,
    65–67
immunoreactive trypsin, 289
impaired fasting glucose, 82, **83**
impaired glucose tolerance, 82, **83**
  chronic renal disease, 55
  TPN, 220
  undernutrition, 222
impotence, 144
inborn errors of metabolism, 280–290
incretins, 78
index case, inborn errors of metabolism, 282
industrial hazards, poisoning, 274–275
infections
  acute phase response, 225–227
  CSF glucose, 260
  TORCH, **280**
  TPN, 220
infertility
  female, *97*, 149–150, *152*
  male, 141–147
inflammation, acute phase response, 225–227
inherited metabolic disorders, 280–290
inhibins, 140, 147, 239
inosinic acid, *254*
insulin, 78
  causes of excess, **88**
  for diabetic ketoacidosis, 86, *87*
  for hyperosmolar hyperglycaemia, 86–87
  hypokalaemia, 25
  polycystic ovarian syndrome, 153
  resistance
    polycystic ovarian syndrome, 152, 153
    undernutrition, 221
  TPN, 220
  for type 2 diabetes, 79
insulin hypoglycaemia test, 95, 103, 289, 290

insulin-like growth factor 1, 94, 95
insulin-like growth factor 2, paraneoplastic form, 90
insulinoma, 89
interferons, on thyroid function, 117
interleukin-1β, gout, 257
interleukins, on TSH release, 107
intermediate-density lipoproteins (IDLs), 173, 175
internal balance, water and sodium, 12
interstitial fluid, 12
intracellular fluid, 12, 13
  calcium, 61
  potassium, 24
intrathecal IgG synthesis, 262
intravenous infusions, *see also* dextrose infusions
  diabetic ketoacidosis, 86
  fluids for, 29
  specimens from sites, **2**
inulin, 45
iodide, thyroid hormone synthesis, 106
iodine, 210
  hyperthyroidism, **110**
  pregnancy, 159
  radioactive, 111
ionised calcium, 60, **71**
ion-sensitive electrodes, sodium measurement, 22
iron, 210
  coefficient of variation, **6**
  deficiency, 244–245
  malabsorption, 205
  metabolism, 241–246
  overload, **244**, 245–246
  poisoning, 246, 274
  pregnancy, 160
  saturation, **243**, 244
  serum, 243
islet-cell antibodies, 79
isoniazid, vitamin deficiencies, 215, 216
isotonic fluids, 16
  diabetic ketoacidosis, 86
  loss, 22
itching, pregnancy, 163–164

jaundice, 188–191, *see also* cholestasis
  neonate, 227, 279–280
joint fluid, gout, 257

Kallman's syndrome, *144*
Kayser–Fleischer rings, 195
kernicterus, 279
ketoacidosis, diabetic (DKA), 84–86, *87*
  hypophosphataemia, 74
ketone bodies, 84, 85–86
kidney *see entries beginning* renal...
KIR 6.2 (ATP-dependent K$^+$ channel gene), 277

Klinefelter syndrome, *143*
kwashiorkor, 222

labelling errors, 2
lactate dehydrogenase, ascites, 197
lactose intolerance, 201
lactulose, test for intestinal permeability, 201
late neonatal hypocalcaemia, 278
late night salivary cortisol, 126–128
latent autoimmune diabetes of adults, 79
late-onset hypogonadism, 144
laxative abuse, 206
lead poisoning, 250, *275*
lecithin cholesterol acyltransferase, 174
leptin, 223
leucovorin, 267
leukaemia, hyperkalaemia, *28*
Leydig cells, 140
light-chain disease, 230
light chains
   immunoglobulins, 228
   serum free, **230**, **231**
linoleic acid, 209
linolenic acid, 209
lipase, *see also* lipoprotein lipase
   hepatic, 174
   pancreatitis, 200
lipids, 172–182
   investigations, 176–181
   liver disease, 188
   metabolic syndrome, 222
   pregnancy, 160
lipoprotein lipase, 174
   deficiency, **178**, 179
lipoproteins, 173–176, *see also* low density
      lipoproteins
   cholesterol in, 173–174, 177
   high density (HDL), **173**, 174, 176, 178, 222
   very low density (VLDLs), 173, 175, 178–179
lipoprotein X, 180
lithium, *50*
   hypercalcaemia, 68
   monitoring, 267
   on thyroid function, 117
lithium-heparin anticoagulant, **2**
liver, 183–197
   α_1-antitrypsin deficiency, 227
   effects of insulin, 78
   failure, 192, *195*
   glucose metabolism, 77
   infiltrations, 193–194
   iron overload, 245
   serum electrophoresis, *225*
   structure, 183–184

liver biopsy
   copper, 195
   nonalcoholic fatty liver disease, 196
liver function tests, 184–188
   paracetamol poisoning, 272
   pregnancy, 160, 164
   TPN monitoring, 219, 220
log-Gaussian distribution, *7*
loops of Henle, 43
low density lipoproteins (LDLs), 173, 175–176
   plasma levels, 177
   receptors, 176
low-dose dexamethasone suppression test, 126
low-renin hyperaldosteronism, 135–136
Lp(a) (lipoprotein), 174, 179
luteinising hormone (LH), 94
   anorexia nervosa, 99
   basal values, **101**
   cross-reactivity with hCG, 159
   menstrual cycle, *148*
   oral contraceptives on, 157
   polycystic ovarian syndrome, 152, 153
   reference ranges, **148**
   spermatogenesis, 140
lysozyme, in urine, **57**, 58

macro-amylasaemia, 200
macroprolactin, 96, *97*
magnesium
   chronic renal disease, 55
   deficiency, 75–76
   familial benign hypocalciuric hypercalcaemia, 69
   hypokalaemia, 28
   laxatives, 206
   metabolism, 74–76
   paediatrics, 278
   TPN, **218**, 219, 220, *221*
malabsorption, 204–207, *see also* short bowel
      syndrome; steatorrhoea
   bacterial colonisation of small intestine, 202–203, 205
   iron status, 245
   tertiary hyperparathyroidism, 68
   vitamin D deficiency, 70
male sex differentiation, disorders, 144
malignant disease, *see also* multiple myeloma;
      tumour markers
   biliary obstruction, *193–194*
   children, 290
   choriocarcinoma, 158, 238
   colorectal cancer, 204, 234–235, *236*
   CSF protein, 261
   faecal occult blood, 204
   ferritin, 244
   gastrinomas, 199

hepatocellular carcinoma, 193–194, 238
hypercalcaemia, **65**, 68
hypoglycaemia, 90
hyponatraemia, 20–21
liver, **193**
parathyroid hormone, *66*
risk of malignancy index, 236, **237**
thyroid gland, 119
trophoblastic tumours, hCG secretion, 158
malignant hyperpyrexia, CK, 171
malnutrition, 208, 216, 288, *see also* undernutrition
elderly patients, 293
protein-energy malnutrition (PEM), 222, 288
vitamin D deficiency, 70
Malnutrition Universal Screening Tool, 216, **217**
maltose intolerance, 201
manganese, 210, 211
marasmus, 222
markers, *see also* tumour markers
bone turnover, 71, **72**
cirrhosis, 194
foetal abnormalities, 164, *165*
liver fibrosis, 187, 194
myocardial infarction, 167–168
maturity onset diabetes of the young, 80–81
MDRD equation, eGFR, 48
mean cell volume, erythrocytes, alcohol abuse,
195–196
medium chain acyl-CoA dehydrogenase deficiency,
284, *286*
medullary thyroid cancer, 239–240
melanin, 93
melanocortin-4 receptor, 223
α-melanocyte stimulating hormone, 93
menaquinone, 214
menopause, 154–155, 156
menstrual cycle, 5, 139, 147, *148*
6-mercaptopurine, 268
metabolic acidosis, 35–36, 37
anion gap, 40
chronic renal disease, 55
diabetic ketoacidosis, 85, 86
hyperparathyroidism, 65
methanol poisoning, 273, *274*
renal tubular acidosis, 41, 51
treatment, 41
for urine acidification test, 51
metabolic alkalosis, 36–37, 38, 41
metabolic bone disease, 71–73
metabolic disorders
acid–base balance, 33–34
inherited, 280–290
metabolic syndrome, 222
gout and, 256–257

metabolites, drug monitoring, 266
metadrenalines, 137–138
metals, poisoning, 274–275
methaemoglobin, 250
methanol poisoning, 273–274
methionine, 215, 271–272
methionine synthase, 215
methotrexate, monitoring, 267
metoclopramide, *98*
microadenomas, pituitary, 100
microalbumin, urine, 84
microbiology, malabsorption, 205
mid-arm muscle area, 216
migraine, drugs for, *98*
milk–alkali syndrome, 69
mineralocorticoids, *see also* aldosterone
deficiency, 27
mixed acid–base disturbances, 38–39
mobilising lipase, 174
molar pregnancy, hCG, 238
molybdenum, 210, 213
monoclonal gammopathy of unknown significance,
231–232, *233*
monoclonal hypergammaglobulinaemia,
229–230
motilin, **207**
Mullerian ducts, 141
multiple endocrine neoplasia syndromes, 68,
239–240
insulinoma, 89
multiple myeloma, 230–231, 232
hypercalcaemia, 68, *231*, **232**
serum electrophoresis, *225*
multiple sclerosis, CSF protein, 262
muscle
creatine kinase, 171
effects of insulin, **78**
muscle mass
on creatinine levels, 46
measurement, 216
muscular dystrophy, creatine kinase, 171
MUST score, 216, **217**
myeloma *see* multiple myeloma
myocardial infarction, 167–171
time course, 168
myoglobin
myocardial infarction, 168
in urine, **57**
myopathies, creatine kinase, 171

N-acetyl-*p*-benzoquinoneimine,
270–271
N-acetylcysteine, 271–272
NADH-methaemoglobin reductase, 250

natriuresis, 24
neonatal diabetes, 80
neonate
 cystic fibrosis, 289
 glucose, 277
 hypercalcaemia, 278
 hypocalcaemia, 278
 hypothyroidism, 116
 inborn errors of metabolism, 280–290
 jaundice, 227, 279–280
 specimens, 277
 thyrotrophin receptor antibodies, 120
nephrogenic diabetes insipidus, 50
nephropathy, microalbuminuria, 84
nephrotic syndrome, 56–57
 hypercholesterolaemia, 180
net bilirubin absorbance, CSF, *261*
netilmicin, monitoring, 266
neural tube defects, 165
 prevention, 215
neuroblastoma, 137, 290
niacin, **212**
 carcinoid syndrome, 206
 deficiency, 215
NICE criteria, recombinant GH treatment, 95
nicotinamide, 215
nitrogen
 nutritional requirements, 218
 TPN, **218**, 219
nonalcoholic fatty liver disease, 194, 196
 TPN, 220
nonalcoholic steatohepatitis, 196
non-HDL cholesterol, 177
noninvasive prenatal testing, 165
non-nutrients, 209
nonthyroidal illness (NTI), thyroid function tests,
 115–116
normal distribution, 4–5, *7*
normetadrenaline, 138
NTBC, for tyrosinaemia type 1, 287
N-terminal-proBNP, 171–172
nuchal translucency, *165*
nucleosides, 253
nucleotides, 253
nutrients, 208–216
 iron, 241
nutrition, 208–223, *see also* malnutrition;
 undernutrition
 assessment of status, 216
 parenteral, 218–220, *221*
nutritional disorders, 208
nutritional support, 216–220
nutrition teams, 220

obesity, 208, 222–223
 causes, **209**, 222
 monogenic, 223
 nonalcoholic fatty liver disease, 194, 196
 polycystic ovarian syndrome, 153
 WHO classification, **221**
obstetric cholestasis, 163–164
occult blood, faecal, 204, 245
occupational hazards, poisoning, 274–275
oedema, 21
 kwashiorkor, 222
 nephrotic syndrome, *57*
oestradiol, 147
 anorexia nervosa, 99
 basal values, **101**
 granulosa-cell tumours, 239
 implants, 156
 menstrual cycle, *148*
 ratio to testosterone, 141
 reference ranges, **148**
oestradiol-17β, 159
oestriol, 159
oestrogens, 147
 pregnancy, 159
 replacement therapy, 103
 on thyroxine-binding globulin, *110*
oestrone, 153, 159
olanzapine, hyperprolactinaemia, 98
oligoclonal bands
 cerebrospinal fluid, 261–262
 serum, 229
oligomenorrhoea, 148, 149, *150*
oliguria, 44, 53, *54*
oncotic pressure, 13, 14
oral contraceptives *see* contraceptives
oral glucose tolerance test, 81, 82
 acromegaly, 95–96
 Cushing's syndrome, 129
 gestational diabetes, 80
 polycystic ovarian syndrome, 152
organic solvents, 275
organophosphates, poisoning, 275
ornithine carbamoyltransferase, X-linked
 deficiency, 286–287
orotic acid, *287*
orthostatic proteinuria, 58
osmolality, 13–14, 23
 fluid deprivation test, 49, 50
 hyperosmolar hyperglycaemia, 86
 methanol poisoning, 273
 urine, 13, 23–24, 48–49
osmole gap, 13
 methanol poisoning, 273, *274*

osmostat, 21
osmotic demyelination syndrome, 18
osmotic diuresis, *88*
    hypernatraemia from, 22, *23*
osmotic gap, faecal, 206
osmotic laxatives, 206
osteoblasts, 63
osteoclasts, 63
osteodystrophy (renal), 55, 71, 73, *75*
osteomalacia, 71–72, 292
osteoporosis, 71, 72
otorrhoea, CSF, 262
ovaries, 147, *see also* polycystic ovarian syndrome
    carcinoma, CA-125, 235–236, 237
    dysfunction, 148–149
    failure, 154–157
overflow proteinuria, 56, **57**
overnight dexamethasone suppression test, 126
oxalate, urine, 59
oximetry, 41, 42
oxygen therapy, *35*, 42
    carbon monoxide poisoning, 251
oxygen transport, 41–42
oxyhaemoglobin, cerebrospinal fluid,
        260, *261*
oxytocin, 104

Paget's disease, **71**, 73, 291–292
pancreas, 199–201
pancreatic polypeptide, **207**
pancreatitis, 200, *201*
panhypopituitarism, 100
paracetamol, 270–272
paraneoplastic conditions, hypoglycaemia, 90
paraproteinaemias, 229–230, 231–232, *233*
parathyroidectomy, 67–68
parathyroid hormone, 63
    assay, 65–68
    magnesium and, 75
    metabolic bone disease, **71**
parenteral nutrition, 218–220, *221*
Patau's syndrome, 164
PCSK9 gene, 178
pegvisomant, 95
pellagra, 215
pentagastrin-stimulated calcitonin test, 240
peptic ulceration, 198–199
perimenopause, 154
    thyroid function, *155*
peripheral thyroid hormone resistance, 118
periportal tracts, liver, 183
pernicious anaemia, 215
pesticides, poisoning, 275

pH, *see also* hydrogen ions
    urine, 50
phaeochromocytoma, 137–138
pharmacogenomics, 268
phenylalanine, 283
phenylketonuria, 283–284
    screening, tyrosinaemia type 1, 287
phenytoin, monitoring, 266
phosphate
    chronic renal disease, 55
    metabolic bone disease, **71**
    metabolism, 73–74
    neonate, 278
    renal osteodystrophy, 73
    serum levels, 64
    TPN, **218**, 219, 220, *221*
    urinary buffer, 31
    vitamin D deficiency, 70
phospholipids, 173
5-phosphoribosyl-1-pyrophosphate, 253
photosensitivity, porphyrias, 249
phylloquinone, 214
physiological jaundice, neonate, 279
phytomenadione *see* vitamin K
PI alleles, AAT deficiency, 227
pigmentation, 93, 132
P-isoamylase, 200
pituitary function tests, Cushing's syndrome, 129
pituitary gland, *see also* anterior pituitary hormones;
        posterior pituitary hormones
    adenomas, *96*, 97–98, 100, 102–103
    psychiatric patients, 98
    tumours, adrenocortical insufficiency, 132
pituitary hypothyroidism *see* central hypothyroidism
pituitary thyroid hormone resistance, 118
placenta, 158–159
plasma, 1, **2**
    ACTH, 128–129
    calcium, 62–63
    cholesterol, 176
    creatinine, 46–47
    drug levels, 264–265
    glucose, 81, 82, **83**
        hypoglycaemia, 87
        metabolic syndrome, 222
    intravenous saline on, 40
    LDL, 177
    metadrenalines, 137
    potassium, 24–25
    proteins, 224–233
        electrophoresis, 224, *225*
        glycated, 84
        pregnancy, *165*

plasma (*cont'd*)
  sodium, 16–17
  volume, 12
    pregnancy, 160
plasma cells, paraproteinaemia, **232**
platelets, HELLP syndrome, 163
plumboporphyria, 246–247, 248
point of care testing (POCT), 3–4
poisoning, 263–275
  acute, 269–274
  carbon monoxide, 251
  iron, 246, 274
  lead, 250, *275*
  liver, 192, 270–272
polyclonal hypergammaglobulinaemia, 229
polycystic ovarian syndrome (PCOS), *150*, 151–154
polysaccharides, 209
polyunsaturated fats, 209
polyuria, 23–24, 48, 50
populations, reference ranges from, 6, *7*
population screening *see* screening
porphobilinogen (PBG), 247, 248
porphyria cutanea tarda, 249–250
porphyrias, acute, 246–249
porphyrins, 246–250
portal hypertension, serum-ascites albumin
    gradient, 197
post-analytical errors, 2
posterior pituitary hormones, 104
post-natal care, diabetes mellitus, 160–161
post-operative patients, hyponatraemia, *20*
post-partum thyroiditis, 162
  vs Graves' disease, 120
post-prandial hypoglycaemia, 89
post-renal proteinuria, 55
posture
  aldosterone, 124
  effect on test results, 5
posture stimulation test, hyperaldosteronism, 136
potassium, *see also* hyperkalaemia; hypokalaemia
  acute kidney injury, 53
  on aldosterone, 124
  balance, 24–28
  coefficient of variation, **6**
  daily requirements, 29
  deficiency, *76*
  diabetic ketoacidosis, 85, 86, *87*
  digoxin and, 266, *267*
  ectopic ACTH production, 129
  excess intake, 27
  gastric outlet obstruction, *37*
  plasma concentrations, 24–25
  renal excretion, 52
  TPN, **218**, 219, *221*

Prader–Willi syndrome, 94, 223
pre-albumin
  cerebrospinal fluid, 259
  pregnancy, 160
  variants, on thyroid function tests, 119
pre-analytical errors, 2
precision, 4, *5*
predictive values, 9–10
pre-eclampsia, 163
pregnancy, 158–166
  on creatinine levels, 46
  ectopic, 160, *200*
  gestational diabetes, 80, 160–161
  molar, hCG, 238
  serum iron, 243
  thyroid function, 116, 161–163
pregnancy-associated plasma protein A (PAPP-A), *165*
pre-hepatic hyperbilirubinaemia, 190
premature ovarian failure, 155
pre-natal diagnosis, foetal abnormalities, 164–166
pre-renal causes, renal failure, 44, 47
prevalence, effect on predictive values, 9–10
primary biliary cirrhosis, *187*
primary hyperaldosteronism, 135–136
primary hyperoxaluria, 59
primary sclerosing cholangitis, CA 19-9, 239
primidone, 266
profiles, 1
progesterone, 147
  infertility, *152*
  menstrual cycle, *148*
  pregnancy, 159
progestogen-only pill, 157
pro-hormones, 104
prolactin, 96–99, *see also* hyperprolactinaemia
  basal values, **101**
  pregnancy, 159
prolactinoma, 97–98, *151*
pro-opiomelanocortin, 93
proprotein convertase subtilisin/kexin type 9
    (PCSK9), 176, 178
prostate-specific antigen (PSA), 146, 237–238
protease inhibitors
  α_1-antitrypsin as, 227
  hypertriglyceridaemia, 180
proteases, 227
protein-bound drugs, 266
protein: creatinine ratio, 163
protein-energy malnutrition (PEM), 222, 288
proteins
  as buffers, 32
  cerebrospinal fluid, 259, 261–262
  on colloid osmotic pressure, 14
  dietary, 210, 218

glycation, 83, 84
liver disease, 186–187
malabsorption, 205
plasma, 224–233
electrophoresis, 224, *225*
glycated, 84
pregnancy, *165*
pseudohyponatraemia, 21
proteinuria, 55–58
pre-eclampsia, 163
tests for, 163
prothrombin, **225**
prothrombin time, 187, **193**, 214
paracetamol poisoning, 272
protoporphyrinogen IX, 247
protoporphyrins, 249, *see also* zinc protoporphyrin
provocation tests, growth hormone, 289–290
proximal convoluted tubules, 43
proximal renal tubular acidosis, 51
pruritus, pregnancy, 163–164
pseudo-Cushing syndrome, 128
pseudogynaecomastia, 147
pseudohyperkalaemia, 27
pseudohyponatraemia, 13, 21–22
pseudohypoparathyroidism, 70
psychiatric patients, hyperprolactinaemia, 98–100
psychogenic diabetes insipidus, 50
PTHrP, hypercalcaemia of malignancy, 68
puberty, gynaecomastia, 146
pulmonary embolism, 172
pulmonary emphysema, 227, *228*
pulse oximetry, 41, 42
purines, 252–258
pyridoxal 5′-phosphate, 216
pyridoxine *see* vitamin B$_6$

Quadruple Test, second trimester screening, 165

race
effect on test results, 6
plasma cholesterol, 176
radioiodine, 111
radiotherapy, to pituitary gland, 103
random venous plasma glucose, 81
rasburicase, 258
reabsorption
bicarbonate, 31–32, 36, 50–51
potassium, 24
sodium, 12, 43
water, 14, 44
reactive hypoglycaemia, 89
reagent strips *see* urine test sticks
receiver operating characteristic curves, 8
recombinant growth hormone, NICE criteria, 95

recombinant TSH test, 239
5α-reductase, 141
re-feeding syndrome, 220
reference ranges, 6, *7*
blood gases, 37
cholesterol and, 176
creatinine, 46
elderly patients, 290
iron status, **243**
sex hormones, **148**
thyroid hormones, 108, *163*
remnant hyperlipoproteinaemia, **178**, 179
renal concentration tests, 49–50
renal disease, 43–59, *see also* chronic renal disease;
nephrotic syndrome; stones
hyponatraemia, 21
microalbuminuria, 84
renal failure, 21, 44, 47, *see also* acute kidney injury;
chronic renal disease
hyperkalaemia, 27
potassium excretion, 52
pre-eclampsia, 163
sodium excretion, 52
tertiary hyperparathyroidism, 68
renal function
elderly patients, 290–291
parathyroid hormone on, 63
renal osteodystrophy, 55, 71, 73, *75*
renal tubular acidosis, 51
metabolic acidosis, 41, 51
potassium loss, 26
renal tubules, 43
in acid–base balance, 31–32
function tests, 48–52
potassium reabsorption, 24
urate excretion, 255
Wilson's disease, 195
renin, 123, 136
renin–angiotensin–aldosterone system, 15, 123–124
requests for tests, 1–2
respiratory acidosis, 34–35, 37
respiratory alkalosis, 35, 38
on calcium levels, 64
hypophosphataemia, *75*
tetany, 69
respiratory insufficiency, 42
retinoic acid, 213
retinol *see* vitamin A
reverse T3, 105–107
rhabdomyolysis, *see also* crush injury
hyperkalaemia, **28**, 54
rhamnose, test for intestinal permeability, 201
rheumatoid factors, 233
rhinorrhoea, CSF, 262

riboflavin, **212**, 214–215
rickets, 71–72
  neonate, 278
  vitamin D-resistant, 70, 71–72
Ringer's lactate, **29**
risk of malignancy index, 236, **237**
Rotor syndrome, 190–191

salbutamol, hypokalaemia, 25
salicylates
  poisoning, 272
  urate excretion, 255
saline (intravenous), **29**
  diabetic ketoacidosis, 86, *87*
  plasma chloride from excess, 40
saline suppression test, *137*
saliva
  drug monitoring, 266
  late night cortisol, 126–128
salvage pathway, purine metabolism, 253, *254*
samples *see* specimens
sandwich assays, parathyroid hormone, 65–67
sarcoidosis, hypercalcaemia, 68
saturated fats, 209
Schilling test, 216
scoline apnoea, 268
screening, 3
  congenital hypothyroidism, 116, 287
  cystic fibrosis, 289
  drug abuse, 274
  elderly patients, 290
  foetal abnormalities, 164–166
  for gestational diabetes, 80
  hyperaldosteronism, 136
  inborn errors of metabolism, 281
  phenylketonuria, tyrosinaemia type 1, 287
  predictive values and, 9–10
  thyroid dysfunction, 109
    elderly patients, 292
    pregnancy, 161
  toxicology, 270
  tumour markers and, **235**, 237, 238
  X-linked ornithine carbamoyltransferase
    deficiency, 286–287
scurvy, 214
secondary hyperaldosteronism, 136
secondary hypogammaglobulinaemia, 229
second trimester screening, 165
secretin, **207**
  test for gastrinomas, 199
secretory IgA, 228
selective venous sampling, ACTH, 129
selenium, 210, 211
^{75}Se homotaurocholate, 202

self-poisoning, 269
semen, *142*
seminomas, hCG, 238
sensitivity, 7–8
serotonin, 206, 207
SERPINA1 gene, 227
Sertoli cells, 140
serum, 1, **2**, *see also* electrophoresis
serum-ascites albumin gradient, 197
serum free light chains, **230 231**
serum transferrin receptor, 244
sex differentiation disorders, 144
sex (gender)
  effect on test results, 6
  plasma cholesterol, 176
  urate levels, 253
sex hormone-binding globulin (SHBG), 120,
    141, 143
  polycystic ovarian syndrome, 153
  pregnancy, 159
sex hormones, reference ranges, **148**
shock, urea levels, 47
short bowel syndrome, 218
short stature, 289–290
short tetracosactrin test, 103, 132–133
sick cell syndrome, 21
sick euthyroid syndrome, 115–116
sirolimus, monitoring, 266
skin, acute porphyrias, 246, 249
skin-fold thickness, 216
SLC39A4 gene, *212*
small intestine, 201–205
smoking
  α_1-antitrypsin deficiency, 227
  carbon monoxide, 251
sodium
  anion gap, 40
  balance, 12–24
  coefficient of variation, **6**
  daily requirements, 29
  diabetic ketoacidosis, 86
  plasma concentrations, 16–17
  population distribution, *7*
  reabsorption, 12, 43
  renal excretion, 52
  retention, 52
  TPN, **218**, 219, *221*
  urine, 24
sodium activity, 22
sodium bicarbonate, diabetic ketoacidosis and, 86
sodium fluoride, plasma glucose tubes, 82
sodium-glucose cotransporter 2 inhibitors, 85
solitary toxic thyroid nodule, **110**
solvents, organic, 275

somatomedin C *see* insulin-like growth factor 1
somatostatin, 94
  on TSH release, 107
specific gravity, urine, 49
specificity, 7–8
specimens
  acid–base balance, 33
  ACTH, 93, 128
  acute porphyrias, 247
  artefactual hyperkalaemia, 27
  cerebrospinal fluid, 260
  collection, 1–2, *see also* 24-hour urine collection
  cryoglobulinaemia, 233
  glucose, 82
  hyperammonaemia, 282
  lipids, 177
  myocardial infarction, timing, 169
  paediatrics, 277
  therapeutic drug monitoring, 264–265
spectrophotometry, cerebrospinal fluid,
      260, *261*
spermatogenesis, 140–141
standard deviation (SD), 4–5
starvation, urea levels, 47
statins, *6*
  creatine kinase, 171
steatohepatitis, nonalcoholic, 196
steatorrhoea, *201, see also* malabsorption
  gastrinomas, 199
steroids, *see also* aldosterone; glucocorticoids;
      mineralocorticoids
  biosynthetic pathways, *125*
  congenital adrenal hyperplasia, 287
  osteoporosis, *72*
  pregnancy, 159
  regulation, 121–124
stomach, 198–199
  outlet obstruction, *37*, 40
stones
  biliary, *200*
  renal, 58–59, *67*, 255–256, 257
stress, on adrenal cortex, 122
stunting, 221
subacute combined degeneration of the spinal
      cord, 216
subarachnoid haemorrhage, 260, *261*
subclinical hyperthyroidism, 111
subclinical primary hypothyroidism, 113, *114*
  perimenopause, *155*
  T4 replacement therapy, 115
subclinical vitamin deficiencies, 213
succinylcholine apnoea, 268
sugar, intake recommendation, 209
sulphaemoglobin, 250

sulphonylurea receptor gene, 277
sulphonylureas, *89*
surgery
  fluid and electrolytes, 28–29
  post-operative hyponatraemia, *20*
suxamethonium apnoea, 268
sweating, potassium loss, 26
sweat test, cystic fibrosis, 289
Synacthen test, 103, 132–133
syndrome of inappropriate ADH secretion (SIADH),
      19–21, 104
  acute porphyrias, *247*
  urine osmolality, 24

T3 hyperthyroidism, 110
tacrolimus, monitoring, 266
Tamm–Horsfall mucoprotein, 55
tandem mass spectrometry, MCAD deficiency, 284
Tangier disease, 181
Tau protein, 260, 262
teicoplanin, monitoring, 266
temperature, on acid–base balance measurement, 33
testicular teratoma, 158
testosterone, 140, 141, 143
  androgen insensitivity syndrome, 144
  basal values, **101**
  deficiency, 144
  factors affecting, 146
  measurement, 145
  pregnancy, 159
  reference ranges, **148**
  replacement therapy, 103, 146
tetany, 69
tetracosactrin test, 103, 132–133
tetrahydrofolic acid, 215
theophylline, monitoring, 267
therapeutic drug monitoring, 263–269
therapeutic ranges, 265
thiamin, **212**
  deficiency, 214, *215*, 220
thiamin diphosphate, 214
thiamin pyrophosphate, 214
thiazides, *291*
  hypercalcaemia, 68
6-thioguanine nucleotides, 268
thionamides, 111
thiopurine methyl transferase, deficiency, 192,
      268, *269*
thirst, 14
thromboembolic disease, 172
thyroglobulin, 106, 239, *240*
thyroid cancer, tumour markers, 239–240
thyroidectomy, 239, *240*
  subtotal, 111–112

thyroid function
  abnormalities, 105–120
    tests affected by, 120
  anorexia nervosa, 99
  drugs affecting, 116–117
  elderly patients, 292–293
  investigations, 107–111
    causes of misleading, 115–119
    hyperthyroidism, **113**
    pregnancy, 159–160
  perimenopause, *155*
  post-partum, 162
  pregnancy, disorders, 116, 161–163
  regulation, 107
thyroid hormone resistance, 118
  TSHoma *vs*, 119
thyroiditis, **110**, *111*, 113
  Hashimoto's, 113, *114*, 119
  post-partum, 162
    Graves' disease *vs*, 120
thyroid-stimulating hormone (TSH), 94, 107
  adenoma secreting, *102*
  basal values, **101**
  causes of abnormal levels, **108**
  drugs affecting, 116–117
  elderly patients, 292
  hyperthyroidism, 109, 111, 112, **113**
  hypothyroidism, 113, 115
  measurement, 107, 108
  perimenopause, *155*
  pregnancy, 161, 162, *163*
  receptor antibodies *see* thyrotrophin receptor
    antibodies
  recovery from illness, 116
  suppression therapy, 239, *240*
  thyroglobulin measurement and, 239
thyroliberin (TRH), 107
thyrotrophin *see* thyroid-stimulating hormone
thyrotrophin receptor antibodies, 110, 119–120
  pregnancy, 161–162
thyrotrophin-releasing hormone, 94
  test, 119
thyroxine, 105–107, *see also* free T4
  drugs affecting absorption, 115
  pregnancy, 159, 161
  replacement therapy, 103, 114–115
  after thyroidectomy, 239, *240*
  total, 108
thyroxine-binding globulin (TBG), 107, 118–119
  oestrogens on, *110*
  pregnancy, 160, *163*
tissue transglutaminase (tTG), antibodies, 203, 204, 290
tobramycin, monitoring, 266
tocopherols *see* vitamin E

tonicity, 13
TORCH, infections, **280**
total body water, 12
total cholesterol, 176–177
total CO_2, 39
  potassium balance, 28
total iron binding capacity, **243**, 244
total parenteral nutrition, 218–220, *221*
total protein
  cerebrospinal fluid, 261
  plasma, 224–225
total T4 and total T3, 108
toxic multinodular goitre, 110
TPMT gene, 192
trace elements, 210–213
  TPN monitoring, 219
transcortin, *122*
transferrin, **225**, 244
  carbohydrate-deficient, 196
  desialylated, 260, 262
  iron bound to, 242
  iron overload, 245
transthyretin, 107
transudates, ascites, 197
trauma
  acute phase response, 225–227
  fluid and electrolytes, 28–29
TRH (thyroliberin), 107
triglycerides, 173, 209
  breath test, 202
  excess, 178–179, *180*
  Friedewald equation, 177
  levels, 177, 178–179
  metabolic syndrome, 222
  metabolism, *175*
  pregnancy, 160
tri-iodothyronine, 105–107, *see also* free T3
trisomies, 164, *165*
trophoblastic disease, hCG, 238
trophoblastic hyperthyroidism, **110**
trophoblastic tumours, hCG secretion, 158
troponins, 167–168, 169–170
trypsin, immunoreactive, 289
tryptophan, carcinoid syndrome, 206, 215
TSHoma, 111, 118
  thyroid hormone resistance *vs*, 119
TSH-receptor antibodies *see* thyrotrophin receptor
    antibodies
tube feeding, 217
tubular proteinuria, 55–56, **57**, 58
tumour lysis syndrome, 258
tumour markers, 234–240
  ectopic ACTH production, 129
  nonmalignant conditions, **236**

24-hour urine collection
  cortisol, 126
  protein, 163
two-hit model, nonalcoholic steatohepatitis, 196
type 1 diabetes, 79, **80**
  coeliac disease and, *204*
  pregnancy, 160
type 2 diabetes, 79–80
  hyperglycaemia, *88*
tyrosinaemia type 1, 287
tyrosine, deficiency, 283

UDP-galactose epimerase, 284
ultraviolet light, vitamin D formation, *63*
unbound calcium *see* ionised calcium
unconjugated hyperbilirubinaemia, neonate,
    279–280
undernutrition, 221–222
  causes, **209**
  children, 221, 288
  hospital patients, 217
unsaturated fats, 209
urea
  acute kidney injury, 53
  coefficient of variation, **6**
  diabetic ketoacidosis, 86
  elderly patients, 290
  liver disease, 188
  plasma concentrations, 47
  pre-eclampsia, 163
  water and sodium depletion, 23
urea breath test, 198
urea cycle defects, 285–287
uric acid, 252–258
  as antioxidant, 258
  excretion, 255
  pre-eclampsia, 163
uricosuric agents, 255, 257
urinary free cortisol, 126
urine, *see also* 24-hour urine collection
  acidification tests, 50–51
  acute porphyrias, 247
  buffers, 31–32
  calcium, 58–59
  carcinoid syndrome, 207
  copper, 195
  creatinine clearance, 46
  drug screening, 274
  electrophoresis, 55–56, 230–231
  factitious diarrhoea, 206
  free cortisol, 126
  glucose, 81
  magnesium, 76
  MCAD deficiency, 284

  metadrenalines, 137, 138
  microalbumin, 84
  osmolality, 13, 23–24, 48–49
  output, acute kidney injury, 52
  potassium, 28
  proteins, 55–58
  sodium, 24
urine test sticks, 4
  ketone bodies, 85
  proteins, 56
urobilinogen, 186, **189**

vancomycin, monitoring, 266
vanillylmandelic acid, 137
variable regions, immunoglobulins, *228*
variance, 6
variation in results, 4–10
  analytical sources, 4–5
  biological causes, 5–6
  from disease, 6–7
variegate porphyria (VP), 246, 247, 248
vasoactive intestinal peptide, 207
vasopressin, 14, 19, 44, 104
vegetable proteins, 210
venous plasma glucose, 81, 82, **83**
  hypoglycaemia, 87
ventilatory failure, 42
Verner–Morrison syndrome, 207
very low density lipoproteins (VLDLs), 173, 175,
    178–179
viral hepatitis, 191–192
  hepatocellular carcinoma, *238*
  neonate, **280**
virilism, 151
vitamin A, **212**
  deficiency, 213
vitamin B_1 *see* thiamin
vitamin B_2, **212**, 214–215
vitamin B_3 *see* niacin
vitamin B_6, **212**
  deficiency, 216
  homocysteine and, 181
vitamin B_{12}, **212**
  deficiency, 215–216
  homocysteine and, 181
vitamin C, **212**, 214
vitamin D, **212**, *see also* cholecalciferol
  deficiency, 69–70, 71, 205, 278, 292
  excess, 68
  renal osteodystrophy, 73, *75*
  ultraviolet light, *63*
vitamin D_2, 63
vitamin D_3 *see* cholecalciferol
vitamin D-resistant rickets, 70, 71–72

vitamin E, **212**, 213–214
vitamin K, 187, **193**, **212**, 214
vitamins, **212**, 213–216
   malabsorption, 205

waist circumference, 222
Waldenström macroglobulinaemia, 230
water
   deprivation test, 49–50
   reabsorption, 14, 44
water balance, 12–24
   daily requirements, 29, 218
   diabetic ketoacidosis, 86
   disorders, 16–24
   elderly patients, 291
   intake and output, **14**
water retention, 19–20

water-soluble vitamins, **212**
   deficiencies, 214–216
weight loss score, MUST, **217**
well-population screening, 3
Wernicke's encephalopathy, 214
Wilson's disease, 194–195

xanthine oxidase inhibitors, 257
xanthinuria, 213, 257
xanthochromia, CSF, 260, 261
X-linked ornithine carbamoyltransferase deficiency,
   286–287
xylose absorption test, 201

zinc, 211, *212*
zinc protoporphyrin, 249, 250, *275*
Zollinger–Ellison syndrome, 199

Printed and bound by CPI Group (UK) Ltd, Croydon, CR0 4YY

27/10/2024

14580370-0001